Psychological Therapy for Paediatric Acquired Brain Injury

Children, young people and families living with an acquired brain injury (ABI), whether through accident, illness, injury or abuse, are rarely offered psychological therapy, and yet the benefits of such interventions can be profound. This important new book, providing a selection of practice examples and insights from frontline practitioners, will be essential reading for any paediatric therapist or clinician.

Beginning with a "life story" of the brain where emphasis is placed on how brain development is fundamentally related to its environment, the book offers key background knowledge before showcasing the core topics of assessment, psychological formulation and intervention. It features a range of therapeutic models, includes direct and indirect work, group work and family therapy, with settings varying from inpatient neurorehabilitation to community work and the transition to education. The long-term needs of those in the criminal justice system are also addressed. The closing chapters focus on the debate around effective outcome measurement and outline a vision for better services.

Elevating the voices of our children, young people and families living with ABI, this pioneering book will provide practitioners with the confidence to work collaboratively across a range of children and young people with disorders of consciousness or communication to those with behaviour that challenges others to manage. It offers new ways to understand both children's pasts and their futures, and will be essential reading for anyone in the field.

Jenny Jim (DClinPsy, MSc, BSc (Hons)) is a Consultant and Principal Clinical Psychologist with a passion for improving the lives of children, young people and families affected by acquired brain injury. Dr. Jim is the Deputy Programme Director (Clinical) of the Professional Doctorate in Clinical Psychology at the University of East London. She is a clinical academic who works with families, develops and researches innovations, lectures and trains clinical psychologists for the NHS. Jenny is the recipient of the British Psychological Society, Division of Neuropsychology's Early Career Award (2020).

Esther Cole (PsychD, MA (Oxon.)) is a Highly Specialist Clinical Psychologist who worked in the NHS for 12 years in different roles and now works in the private sector across the lifespan. Her most recent position is within a community multidisciplinary paediatric therapy centre in South West London. Dr. Cole's therapeutic orientations and research interests are broad and include investigating the effective integration of psychological approaches for adults and children with mental health and neurological conditions.

The Brain Injuries Series

Series Editors: Dr. Giles Yeates and Dr. Fergus Gracey

This series is dedicated to psychological therapies, social interventions and psychosocial issues following acquired brain injury, emphasising both theoretical exploration and the "how-to" of therapeutic work. These titles stand in contrast with previous clinical titles in the brain injury literature that have been assessment focussed and offered little in the way of intervention. Every jobbing clinician and therapist working with survivors of brain injury and their significant others should have this series on their shelves.

Previous titles in the series:

For further information about this series please visit: www.routledge.com/The-Brain-Injuries-Series/book-series/KARNACBI

Psychological Therapy for Paediatric Acquired Brain Injury

Innovations for Children, Young People and Families

Edited by Jenny Jim
and Esther Cole

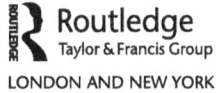 Routledge
Taylor & Francis Group

LONDON AND NEW YORK

First published 2020
by Routledge
2 Park Square, Milton Park, Abingdon, Oxon OX14 4RN

and by Routledge
52 Vanderbilt Avenue, New York, NY 10017

Routledge is an imprint of the Taylor & Francis Group, an informa business

British Library Cataloguing-in-Publication Data
A catalogue record for this book is available from the British Library

Library of Congress Cataloging-in-Publication Data
A catalog record for this book has been requested

ISBN: 978-0-36727-619-5 (hbk)
ISBN: 978-0-36727-620-1 (pbk)
ISBN: 978-0-42929-693-2 (ebk)

Typeset in Times New Roman
by Apex CoVantage, LLC

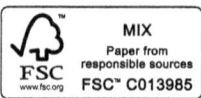

Printed in the United Kingdom
by Henry Ling Limited

"For Leo, my irresistibly captivating son who arrived mid-book manuscript, and, his father, Ed, my partner, who helped deliver them both!"
JJ

"As ever, in all areas of life, I would like to thank my loving husband, Ayo Cole, for his unwavering encouragement, strength, faith and generosity. Thank you to our beautiful children, who continue to fascinate, amaze and teach me as their incredible worlds and minds develop."
EC

Contents

Illustrations

Tables

Editors' acknowledgements

We are indebted to all the wonderful and learned contributors who agreed to join us in this endeavour. To the many people behind the scenes who have given us words of guidance or encouragement, we have not forgotten you. Special thanks to Dr. Heather Liddiard, Consultant Clinical Neuropsychologist, for her steadfast support and to Danielle Pearce, Assistant Psychologist, for helping with proof-reading and formatting challenges!

This book is a reflection of so many of the seminal influences on one's life. For those who inspired and scaffolded, Jenny would like to thank Professor Peter Fonagy, University College London, UK, for his validation throughout her early career as faculty on the Doctorate in Clinical Psychology Programme. To Professor Liam Dorris, University of Glasgow, UK, and Professor Peter Rankin, Institute for Child Health, University College London, UK, for their unwavering support and wise words from the start of her professional training in clinical paediatric neuropsychology. To Professor Piet Hut at the Institute for Advanced Study, Princeton, US, for his invitation to join his Program for Interdisciplinary Studies to exchange ideas with a multitude of great minds. To Professor Barry Beyerstein, Simon Fraser University, Vancouver, Canada, who sparked intrigue and amazement through teaching with endless compassion and excitement, unravelling and explaining mysteries of consciousness with such vim. To Dr. Ann Miller, Marlborough Family Service, UK, who helped support her growth as a systemically informed practitioner personally and professionally. To Professor Alan Parkin, who first inspired her love of neuropsychology during undergraduate studies.

We would also like to thank Ste Weatherhead for being Esther's mentor through the editorial and publication process. He was instrumental in giving her the confidence, as a newly qualified psychologist, to gather a team of editors and contributors together to pitch a proposal to Karnac Books. We would like to thank all the children and families who inspired us. It is your life stories that make the book truly authentic and of value. As your therapists, it is your lives and those of others affected for whom we want to make the difference. We also thank Ethan Murtagh-Kelly, Caroline Murtagh and Gary Kelly, who were the inspiration for this book.

Furthermore, the editors and contributors gratefully acknowledge the permission granted to reproduce the copyrighted material in this book: 'Figure 3.2: A Model for Pediatric Neurocognitive Interventions: Considering the Role of Development and Maturation in Rehabilitation Planning' by J. Limond, A-L.R. Adlam & M. Cormack, *The Clinical Neuropsychologist* Vol. 28: 2 pp. 181–198 (2014). (Permissions from www.tandfonline.com).

About the editors

Jenny Jim is a Consultant and Principal Clinical Psychologist working in paediatric acquired brain injury. Dr. Jim practises at The Children's Trust, the UK's leading charity for children with brain injury, and, is also the Deputy Program Director (Clinical) of the University of East London's Professional Doctorate in Clinical Psychology. She is an Honorary Associate Professor for University College London and regularly lectures for the Clinical Paediatric Neuropsychology MSc at the Institute of Child Health. She has over 15 years of postdoctoral qualified experience working in mental and physical health services with children, young people, adults and families.

Dr. Jim has interests in integrating brain and behaviour relationships within a holistic understanding of a child or young person's context and family. She considers herself a biopsychosocial scientist-practitioner. She has sought postdoctoral qualifications in family therapy and clinical paediatric neuropsychology. Jenny is committed to improving the lives of children and young people with brain injuries, and their families. Jenny recently co-produced a film with the Ridd Family (experts by experience), about the experience of paediatric neurorehabilitation. Titled *From Me to You*, the film was made by families for families to pass on messages of realistic hope. It won the Special Award for User Engagement at the British Medical Association, Patient Information Awards (2018). Jenny is the recipient of the British Psychological Society, Division of Neuropsychology's Early Career Award (2020).

Esther Cole is a Highly Specialist Clinical Psychologist working in private practice across the lifespan. Dr. Cole worked in the NHS for 12 years in different roles. Her most recent position is as an Associate Clinical Psychologist at Therapy4Kids, an independent community multidisciplinary paediatric therapy clinic in South West London. She has a Master's degree in Experimental Psychology from Oxford University, Foundation Level Systemic Training from the University of Surrey and a Diploma in Cognitive Behavioural Therapy from University College London. Her research interests and therapeutic orientations are broad, investigating the integration of psychological approaches to working with people with mental health and neurological conditions, across the lifespan. www.lifespanpsychology.co.uk

Contributors

Rachel Ames is a Clinical Psychologist and a Systemic Psychotherapist. She has worked with children and young people with acquired brain injuries (ABIs) and with a range of neurodevelopmental difficulties. She has worked in the NHS, in a charity and in private practice. She currently works in the NHS in a child and adolescent mental health service (CAMHS) disability team. In her clinical work, she has a particular interest in combining knowledge and practice from paediatric neuropsychology with systemic and narrative models of work.

Katie Byard is a Consultant Clinical Psychologist and co-founder of Recolo UK Ltd, specialising in providing neuropsychological rehabilitation to children, young people, young adults and their families. Dr. Byard has nearly 20 years experience as a clinical psychologist. Prior to moving into the independent sector and specialising in child brain injury rehabilitation, she worked in the NHS in paediatric psychology, child neuropsychology and child mental health and adult neurorehabilitation inpatient services. Dr. Byard's clinical, writing and research interests include the integration of brain and behaviour relationships and systemic thinking and practice in child neuropsychological rehabilitation. She is also committed to contributing to the development of neuropsychological rehabilitation that is evidence based, measurable and meaningful to the young person and his or her family.

Laura Carroll is a Specialist Educational Psychologist. She has an MSc in cognitive neuropsychology and sought post-doctoral qualifications in clinical paediatric neuropsychology. Dr. Carroll works at The Children's Trust within a multidisciplinary team in both a residential rehabilitation setting for children with ABI and a national specialist outreach team who offer assessment and support to children with ABI around the UK. In addition, she has extensive experience working with schools, local authorities and in private practice.

Gemma Costello is Psychology Lead at The Children's Trust. Dr. Costello is a Specialist Educational Psychologist in paediatric neuropsychology working as part of a multidisciplinary team, providing neurorehabilitation to children, young people and their families following ABI. The psychology teamwork across inpatient and national specialist outreach services for young people with

ABI, alongside a non-maintained special school and residential service for children and young people with neurodisability. Gemma is an active member of special interest groups in both paediatric neuropsychology and neurorehabilitation. She is committed to promoting the role of Educational Psychology in paediatric ABI, working with services across the UK and more recently contributing to educational psychology and paediatric neuropsychology training.

Simone Fox is a Consultant Clinical and Forensic Psychologist. Dr. Fox has extensive experience with both adult and adolescent offenders in custody, in secure settings and in the community. She was Deputy Clinical Director on the Royal Holloway University of London Doctorate in Clinical Psychology course until 2016. She is currently employed by South London and Maudsley NHS Foundation Trust as a multisystemic therapy (MST) expert and consults to MST teams across the country and in Scotland.

Anne Fullalove is a Play Therapist, Filial Therapist, Video Interaction Guidance Supervisor and Advisory Teacher, with 30 years of experience working with children with additional needs and their families. She now works in private practice, following her post as Play Therapist within the psychosocial team at the Children's Trust, a residential rehabilitation centre for children with acquired brain injury. She is Associate Tutor in the BSc Hons programme in Child Health and Well Being at Edge Hill University, West Lancashire.

Sophie Gosling is a Consultant Clinical Psychologist. Dr. Gosling joined Recolo UK Ltd in 2011, and since 2015, has been the Clinical Lead for the organisation. Her area of special interest and expertise is paediatric brain injury rehabilitation. She seeks to work with families collaboratively and systemically. Dr. Gosling has over 25 years' experience as a Clinical Psychologist. She has worked in the NHS and university and independent sectors in the UK, and has also worked in Australia and Belgium. She has co-authored over 30 papers, articles and conference presentations in the fields of outcome measurement, rehabilitation, cerebral palsy and health services evaluation.

Fergus Gracey is a Clinical Neuropsychologist and Clinical Senior Lecturer who initially worked at the Oliver Zangwill Centre for Neuropsychological Rehabilitation (OZC) with adults with acquired brain injury presenting with complex, interacting cognitive, social and emotional challenges to participation. Dr. Gracey then took on the role of leading the development of the new Cambridge Centre for Paediatric Neurorehabilitation (CCPNR) service. He currently works in the Department of Clinical Psychology at the University of East Anglia, leading the neuropsychology and research modules and pursuing research interests in qualitative and quantitative approaches to understanding cognitive, emotional and social changes after ABI.

Sarah Helps is a Consultant Clinical Psychologist, Systemic Psychotherapist and Paediatric Neuropsychologist. Dr. Helps works both in the NHS in clinical and training roles and in private practice. She has worked with children with acquired and neurodevelopmental disorders over the past 20 years. Her current writing and research interests include writing collaboratively with service users and the processes of therapeutic work.

Isobel Heyman qualified in medicine at University College London and gained a PhD in developmental neurobiology before training as a child psychiatrist at the Maudsley Hospital and Institute of Psychiatry, London. Dr. Heyman works at Great Ormond Street Hospital for Children in London, UK, where she leads a team specialising in liaison/consultation psychiatry and neuropsychiatry. She is an Honorary Professor at the Institute of Child Health, University College London. Her current research programme focusses on integrating physical and mental health care, particularly in relation to neurological conditions. Common treatable psychiatric disorders are often undetected in this population – she aims to improve early evidence-based intervention in these children. She was awarded UK Psychiatrist of the Year in 2015 by the Royal College of Psychiatrists.

Liz Ireland is a Specialist Clinical Psychologist who works part time at Great Ormond Street Hospital in London. Dr. Ireland specialises in working with children with a diagnosis of cancer, specifically children with brain tumours, and their families. She also works for Recolo UK Ltd, an independent community neurorehabilitation service for children and young people with ABI. Having completed the post-graduate diploma in paediatric and clinical neuropsychology, she combines her knowledge of neuropsychology with systemic ideas in her clinical work.

Heather Liddiard is a Consultant Clinical Neuropsychologist and Head of Neuropsychology at Blackheath Brain Injury Rehabilitation Services (the Huntercombe Group). Dr. Liddiard has spent the majority of her career to date working in the field of intellectual disabilities and ABI in both the NHS and private sectors. She has particular interests in the assessment, formulation and intervention around challenging behaviours. As such, she has an additional qualification in positive behaviour support.

Tara Murphy is a Consultant Paediatric Neuropsychologist and Clinical Psychologist. Dr. Murphy worked at Great Ormond Street Hospital between 2003 and 2017 in neuropsychology and intervention services. She has expertise in providing and supervising neuropsychological assessment of children with a range of ABI and neurodevelopmental conditions. She has also been involved in leading research on quality of life, educational interventions, neuropsychological assessment and psychological treatment. Dr. Murphy believes in the importance of supporting families, teachers and other important people in the system on how to understand a child's cognitive strengths and weaknesses and mental health. She volunteered in Uganda during 2018, providing training, teaching and being involved in child mental health and neuropsychological services. She currently works and is leading research in Saint Helena in the South Atlantic.

Alison Perkins is a Clinical Psychologist working in paediatric ABI. Dr. Perkins practises as part of a multidisciplinary team at The Children's Trust, which provides neurorehabilitation for children with an ABI and their families. Over many years of working within the field of paediatric ABI, she has developed a particular interest on the impact of an ABI on the young person's developing identity. She believes that promoting the development of a resilient self-construct is an essential part of holistic paediatric neurorehabilitation.

Sara Portnoy is a Consultant Clinical Psychologist who works at University College Hospital in London working with children who have a chronic illness, where she developed and runs the "Beads of Life" programme. She also works for Life Force, a community multidisciplinary paediatric palliative care and bereavement team, which works in the London boroughs of Camden, Haringey and Islington. She also volunteers for the Refugee Resilience Collective, which is a group of systemic and narrative therapists who work with refugees and long-term volunteers in Northern France. She has over 25 years of experience working with children with physical illnesses.

Suresh Pujar is working as a Locum Consultant in Paediatric Neurology at Great Ormond Street Hospital for Children, and his research interest is in understanding the long-term effects of neuronal injury in the developing brain. For his doctoral thesis at Great Ormond Street UCL Institute of Child Health, Dr. Pujar conducted a prospective population-based study to investigate the long-term outcomes following prolonged seizures (convulsive status epilepticus) in childhood.

Elizabeth Roberts is a Specialist Educational Psychologist in Paediatric Neuropsychology. Dr. Roberts has undertaken post-doctoral qualifications in Clinical Paediatric Neuropsychology. She works within a multidisciplinary team at the Children's Trust, a residential rehabilitation setting for children with ABI. She also has several years of experience working as a local authority Educational Psychologist, providing psychology support to nurseries, schools and colleges.

Jackie Solaiman is an Occupational Therapist and mother to four children, the youngest of which is Rafi who experienced a severe acquired brain injury, due to a bleed in 2012, at the age of 12. Jackie has written from the perspective of an Expert by Experience for this book. Jackie is passionate about enabling Rafi to have an interesting and fulfilling life, and is motivated by his positivity to have a go at anything! Rafi has been selected to represent Team GB in Race-Running at the 2019 World Para Athletics in Dubai.

Daniel Stark is a Paediatric Neuropsychologist and Clinical Psychologist who works at Great Ormond Street Hospital. Dr. Stark has extensive experience in neuropsychology as well as child and adolescent mental health. This includes providing and supervising neuropsychological assessments of children with neurodevelopmental conditions and ABIs, as well as specialist mental health assessment and treatment. He has expertise in providing evidence-based treatments and interventions for these children and families. His research to date has incorporated interests in neuropsychology as well as the provision of mental health interventions.

James Tonks has a PhD in paediatric neuropsychology and a doctorate in clinical psychology from the University of Exeter. Dr. Tonks is a Consultant Paediatric Clinical Neuropsychologist with Haven Clinical Psychology Practice, Cornwall, UK. He specialises in youth offending and assessment of capacity to participate in criminal proceedings after brain injury. He is an Honorary Lecturer at the University of Exeter Medical School, UK, and is Visiting Fellow in Paediatric Neuropsychology and Neuroscience at the University of Lincoln, UK.

Suzanna Watson is a Clinical Psychologist who worked with children, young people and their families in community neurodevelopmental services before specialising in acute rehabilitation for children with ABIs at the Royal London Hospital. This post was funded by the Helicopter Emergency Services and the East London Mental Health Trust at the time that the major trauma networks were established. Having worked with Recolo UK Ltd in community paediatric rehabilitation, Dr. Watson moved to the CCPNR to have the opportunity to work in community paediatric neurorehabilitation in the NHS with Fergus Gracey. She now has a role in developing acute and community paediatric neuropsychology services for Cambridgeshire and Peterborough NHS Foundation Trust.

Huw Williams is an Associate Professor of Clinical Neuropsychology at Exeter University and a registered Clinical Neuropsychologist. Professor Williams has a PhD in in the area of intellectual disability and a doctorate in clinical psychology. He is the past Chair of the Division of Clinical Neuropsychology of the British Psychological Society. He has contributed to development of cognitive behavioural approaches for people with intellectual disability and neurodisability.

Preface

I think it is fair to say that this is a vitally important book. It joins less than a handful of books worldwide that outline psychological therapy for children and families affected by paediatric acquired brain injury (ABI). It has a market in this expanding client population, which is growing with improvements in emergency medicine, surgery and intensive treatments. Clinicians are facing dilemmas of addressing such an overwhelming level of need that cuts across all domains of functioning. We hope this book can provide a resource to help clinicians make sense of, prioritise and intervene appropriately and realistically within the service contexts they find themselves.

We use storytelling in a therapeutic capacity within this book. I would like to open it by telling the story of how the book came to life. It was initiated in an entirely unconventional way. I first saw Dr. Jenny Jim speak at an event in London for widening access to the profession of clinical psychology in 2006. During my final placement as a trainee clinical psychologist in Autumn 2012, I was later fortunate enough to meet a young man with an ABI who made me realise the gap in psychological therapy provision for children and young people affected by brain injury, and their families.

After giving a well-received talk on "James" (Chapter 9) to the Paediatric Neuropsychology Special Interest Group in 2015, I contacted Ste Weatherhead. He was the only author of a book on narrative approaches for brain injury, and I asked him why there was no similar book for children: *Narrative Approaches for Childhood Brain Injury*. It was he who suggested I initiate and edit this book, and he gave me the confidence, as a newly qualified clinical psychologist, to approach specialists in the area to write the book proposal with me – serendipitously, one of whom was Jenny Jim.

So, this is a unique book for many reasons: one of which is that it is edited by a specialist clinical psychologist who works in paediatric ABI and me, a clinical psychologist who has worked predominantly in mainstream mental health and dementia services. However, our hope is that this book will appeal to a much wider audience of therapists; therapists who, unexpectedly, come across a history of paediatric brain injury in mainstream child and adult mental health settings, as I do. I represent the majority of clinicians who will come across adults and children with ABI histories in other contexts. They are, poignantly, more likely to meet a psychologist, therapist or counsellor than a paediatric neuropsychologist, throughout their lifespans.

With a child sustaining a brain injury through illness, accident, injury or abuse every 30 minutes in the UK alone (CBIT, 2018), it has been suggested that up to five children in any given classroom may have sustained a brain injury (HC Deb, 2018). We, therefore, hope that childhood brain injury features on everybody's agenda.

It has been a privilege for me to write with a team of experts breaking new ground in paediatric psychological therapy and neurorehabilitation. As mentioned, brain injury can affect all domains of functioning, so the breadth of needs of the children and young people affected cut across many different services: the health, social, education and justice sectors, to name a few. I, therefore, also hope this book will appeal to commissioning bodies, researchers and the government: the ministries of health, education and justice in the UK and internationally.

There are a range of professionals, stances and theoretical orientations in the book: clinical and educational psychologists, a psychiatrist, neurologist and a play therapist. I want to thank everyone who collaborated on this project and had faith in the process. This enabled me to contribute to the project management, co-ordination, development and editing of this book from the position of an outsider looking in on real excellence, expertise and innovation.

Esther Cole

References

Child Brain Injury Trust (CBIT). (2018). Take on the Peak District Challenge for the Child Brain Injury Trust! Retrieved June 11, 2019, from https://childbraininjurytrust.org.uk/2018/02/take-on-the-peak-district-challenge-for-the-child-brain-injury-trust/

HC Deb. (2018, June 18). Acquired Brain Injury. Vol. 643, col. 132. Retrieved July 24, 2018, from https://hansard.parliament.uk/commons/2018-06-18/debates/6619D69D-616C-4EEC-A2A5-5F3A5C082FA1/AcquiredBrainInjury

Series editors' foreword

Our brain injury series takes a bold new step forward in this publication edited by Drs. Jenny Jim and Esther Cole into therapeutic work with children and young people who have survived acquired brain injury (ABI) and their families. It is a privilege to host this innovative work within our book series for several reasons. Firstly, I (GY) remember looking to the paediatric ABI literature nearly 20 years ago for inspiration when we were developing our initial perspectives on family work in adults with ABI. The paediatric ABI outcome studies led by Keith Yeates and Stephanie Taylor operationalised non-linear complex path modelling to explore the interrelationship between injury-related, individual survivor-related and family/social context–related factors in the evolution of outcomes over time. This was conceptually leaps ahead of thinking in the adult ABI field at the time. What has struck me then and since is that this sophistication of thinking in the outcome literature was not visibly matched by an applied therapeutic engagement with such ideas in the published paediatric literature. When asking UK colleagues about this, I was assured that such work was going on, but the innovative clinicians concerned were too busy to write up and disseminate their work. There were disparate moments when the potential of this community's work did become visible to the reader, notably Sarah Helps's (2013) edited special issue of *Context* (a systemic and family therapy journal) on family work with paediatric ABI. Alongside this, other psychotherapeutic approaches to child ABI and explicit presentations of neurorehabilitation models that engage with both injury, child and contextual factors have become more numerous in the last ten years (referenced throughout this book).

We have been awaiting with interest a more substantial presentation of systemic, family therapy and narrative ideas in this field that engage with neurology, context and everything in between to fully realise the applied potential of the conceptual advancements mentioned earlier. Well, here it is, and we proudly believe that this book meets such expectations and takes the field on significantly further – once again inspiring related clinician communities such as adult neurorehabilitation and paediatric work with other long-term conditions. To our knowledge, this is the most developed exposition of systemic and social context-oriented therapeutic ideas in the field, but retaining a core innovation in paediatric applied clinical neuropsychology too. The inclusion of academics and rehabilitation clinicians using other models or with wider remits serves to broaden the scope of the book, resulting in an integrated and coherent set of ideas across the contributors (all leaders and innovators in their fields). Both established clinical concerns and new frontiers in practice are approached within this corpus of vibrant and challenging ideas and practices. The productivity and innovation within this community of clinicians and academics in paediatric neurorehabilitation is now visible to all.

We hope the reader will agree with our excitement and enjoy this stimulating read, and more importantly will feel equipped with both new therapeutic tools that are practically accessible and a new lens through which to view complex challenges inherent in this clinical field.

Dr. Giles Yeates
Series Editor
Dr. Fergus Gracey
Series Co-editor

Reference

Helps, S. L. (2013). Special issue editorial: Effects of acquired brain injury on the child, the family and the wider system. *Context, 125,* 1–2.

Experts by Experience Reflections – Jackie Solaiman

We invited Jackie Solaiman, mother to Rafi, a young man affected by a severe acquired brain injury (ABI) in childhood to write about her experience. We hope this will situate our book in the context of what is important to our families. Jackie has the unique perspective of being an occupational therapist as well as a mother trying to navigate a path through this life-changing experience.

"At age 12, my son was struck down by a severe intracranial brain haemorrhage. Rafi was ill for a very long time. Family life as we knew it was over. For a long time, life for myself, my husband and my three daughters revolved around Rafi: initially at his bedside wondering if he would survive and then separated as I went with him to spend time in a specialist rehab centre. Rafi is now 18; he is different than what he may have been but is usually happy and amazes everyone with his energy and determination.

I remember the complete shock and speed with which Rafi deteriorated and our lives changed. When he was being given CPR at the local A&E, I thought he was going to die, but my emotions seemed to be paused as I waited to see what would happen. Before his brain surgery, we were told it was highly likely he wouldn't make it. We waited for him to come round, but he didn't for a very long time; we were told he was "locked in". We did what we could to let him know we were there.

When Rafi was medically stable, he was transferred to the Children's Trust. For us as a family, it was an exciting place where Rafi would get specialist rehab, but Rafi could not engage with the therapies. This period of his recovery was the hardest to deal with due to his lack of insight. He was often violent and abusive. We made the decision for Rafi to leave early as he was too emotionally disturbed, continuing to battle post-traumatic amnesia. Once in his familiar home environment, Rafi began to thrive; he settled emotionally and was able to cooperate with therapists. He had good multi-agency meetings prior to his return to school, and his phased return went well.

Rafi needed his family around him to feel secure and safe. Services that helped us stay strong as a family were invaluable. We didn't know what recovery Rafi would make but having knowledge of neuroplasticity and knowledge of other people who had been "locked in" and made good recovery gave us hope and encouraged us to keep positive. I found my sessions with the clinical psychologist at the Children's Trust helped me to cope with a very demanding time and with the strain on the family, and to understand what Rafi was going through and make the difficult decision to leave prematurely.

With hindsight, I feel that Rafi may have benefitted from being discharged straight home from hospital if there were services that could have supported us (which there weren't). Access to psychology services in the community were very limited. It has been difficult to get any support with issues that have arisen since we have been home (cognitive and emotional). He has developed anxieties and borderline obsessive behaviours, which the GP did not take seriously; we have to muddle along on our own. Since leaving children's services, he has no reviews apart from for physical issues. Access to specialist brain injury services throughout Rafi's life would be very reassuring but are not available."

Introduction

Jenny Jim and Heather Liddiard

> As the old adage goes, once you have seen one child with a brain injury, you have seen one child with a brain injury.
>
> (Wilde, 2016)

Hearing these words was a Eureka moment for me, (Jenny Jim), as I sat in the audience of Professor Elisabeth Wilde's keynote speech at the 2016 Recolo conference. It encapsulated the importance for respecting the centrality of heterogeneity when working with our children and young people with brain injuries when as a clinician, you really do not see the same presentation twice (the same diagnosis often but, not presentation). Therein lies the uniqueness, but also the continual challenges, for all those committed to helping our children and young people living with the aftermath of a brain injury.

Terminology to describe the causes of brain injury such as "RTA", for road traffic accident, can give us a false sense of uniformity but in reality, it does little to explain what life is really like for our children and families affected. More of our children are surviving with serious injuries due to advances in intensive medicine, and the therapeutic field is challenged to come up to speed to meet the myriad sequelae. No two injuries are the same, and thus our approach to be of help needs to dovetail differently to each family we see. Embracing the heterogeneity rather than disguising it with labels is vitally important for our work as clinicians.

Paediatric neurorehabilitation is a burgeoning field, growing exponentially in the past few decades. Robust empirical studies from Professor Vicki Anderson's team at the Murdoch Research Institute (Melbourne) have been central in demonstrating the devastating effects of early and severe childhood brain injury, challenging common myths around children having a greater ability to "bounce back". Theoretical ideas from Professor Faraneh Vargha-Khadem's team at the Institute of Child Health (UCL, UK) also contribute greatly to understanding why greater childhood brain plasticity may not necessarily equal positive brain recovery not only due to the fundamental negative impact the primary injury may have but also due to its ability to hinder and derail normative ongoing childhood development.

Concurrent with this dose of "bad news" punctuating our knowledge is the counterweight of an increasing recognition of how the relationships and support around a child or young person positively affect organic brain recovery and psychological resilience (which interact with each other). Dr. Rima Shore's seminal book *Re-thinking the Brain* (1997) eloquently presents the "new news" of seeing the brain as ever changing, especially in response to nurturing relationships – that it is simply impossible that our fundamental neural architecture cannot change in relation to the love and care it receives. The work of Dr. Allan Schore at UCLA makes vital connections between psychology, attachment and neuroscience – further breaking through from the myth of mind-body dualism that seems to implicitly pervade clinical work and organisation of our clinical services to this day.

Systematic reviews of risk and resiliency factors in paediatric TBI provide yet more evidence for the interplay of social and environmental context on recovery (Gerring & Wade, 2012; see also Wade, Carey, & Wolfe, 2006; Wade, Michaud, & Brown, 2006; Wade, Walz, Carey, & Williams, 2008). This is not only behavioural or emotional recovery but also neuropsychological recovery. For instance, parental mental health and distress affect emotional outcomes for the child but also affect cognitive and behavioural outcomes such as verbal IQ, fine motor control, social competence, adaptive behaviour and levels of behaviour problems (Taylor et al., 1999). Likewise, positive parenting is predictive of IQ and practical judgement (Gerrard-Morris et al., 2009). Strengthening the capabilities of the family system around our children is paramount (see the work of Gan, Gargaro, Kreutzer, Boschen, & Wright, 2010; Gan & Ballantyne, 2016). It is also now widely recognised that severity of injury does not show a linear relationship to quality of life and disability (Hurst, 2009). These findings further propel our practice with children with brain injuries to evolve, embracing both traditional clinical and neuropsychological practices. Remits of current services can be based on outdated ideas about the nature of brain development and recovery, and so can limit chances for innovation.

Why has it taken so long to recognise that rehabilitation through therapy is vital for childhood brain injury? If we look to the field of adult neuropsychology, such brain and behaviour relationships have been widely recognised, certainly since the world wars and prior to that through the infamous 19th-century "case study" of Phineas Gage. Perhaps the starkness of the changes in personality and functioning made it easier for an observable cause-and-effect relationship to be determined. For children, as they only have a subset of the skills that they will eventually acquire when they meet with say an accident or neurological illness, it is much harder to discern that their functioning is compromised. Think about a 3-month-old baby sustaining a brain injury – his or her realm of self-expression is limited arguably to subtle motor abilities – measuring an impact on those is extremely hard. It is only later when baby grows up and miss his or her milestones that one is likely to see the actual effects of injury months earlier.

Such "sleeper effects" are likely to have added to the hiddenness and invisibility of childhood brain injury and thus why we as a society have not provided nearly enough rehabilitation for our children and young people. Consequently, there is a potentially very large and desperately underserved population that must manage growing up into adulthood without ever accessing appropriate rehabilitation. Many of these people may have been labelled with various misdiagnoses, such as having anger problems, intellectual disability or deemed socially odd without ever realising the difference that could have been made if their brain injuries were recognised earlier, their own understandings facilitated of what that would mean to them and how to self-manage with the help of support systems around them.

If we take seriously the statistic that a child sustains a brain injury every 30 minutes (Childhood Brain Injury Trust, 2017), we must know that any clinician working in children's services is very likely to encounter one of our children or young people with a brain injury. Whilst dedicated services have increased and specialist services do exist, such as charitable organisations like the Children's Trust in the UK, they are by no means adequate in number (often with long waiting lists). Furthermore, these are services for only the very seriously injured, which are a small (but very important) portion of the population. Expertise needs to be spread across all types of services and provisions (NHS, health, education and criminal justice – government-funded, charitable and private). Even in the more established world of adult neurorehabilitation, services are oversubscribed and geographically very varied. Thresholds to entry can make access very difficult and have unintended consequences, unwittingly sustaining a system that refuses those without their exact criteria, but nonetheless have stark needs that will not be met in mainstream or other services.

On a more positive note, therapeutic input for our children and young people with brain injury is at a very exciting stage, embracing complexities and seeing interdisciplinary integration across psychology, neuropsychology and neuroscience (e.g. Ashton, 2015; Byard, 2015; Gracey, Olsen, Austin, Watson, & Malley, 2015; O'Doherty & O'Connor, 2015; Perkins, 2015). Clinicians are rising to the challenge of developing therapeutic rehabilitation that pushes the boundaries of their own traditional professions (be it clinical psychology, educational psychology, family therapy or play therapy) to truly encompass and dovetail to the wholistic world of our children or young people with brain injuries and their families. We hope this book is a helpful addition to innovations that are happening across the globe.

Who is this book for?

The audience for this book is all clinicians in specialised and mainstream services who work with our children and young people. If you are a clinician working in children's services, it is likely that you would have come in contact with children and young people who have had a brain injury. However, you may not have been aware at the time, as often these injuries are invisible unless accompanied by stark physical disabilities. We can't "see" cognitive and emotional problems as easily, and often behaviour is interpreted without the crucial lens of an injured brain.

This book is designed to help clinicians with the process of "dovetailing", of bringing together a family's needs and expertise with our own as professionals. We, alongside pioneering contributors of this book, seek to do this by setting out some background knowledge followed by examples of innovations in current practice. We shine a light on therapeutic practice for psychosocial needs versus cognitive remediation, as very little is written on the former (this book assumes both to be necessary and equally important for comprehensive care).

It is clear that many jobbing clinicians are innovating practice, as using traditional approaches without adaptation is simply not possible. Much of this innovation involves weaving in narrative, systems and systemic ideas with more established cognitive and behavioural models.

Aims of the book

Our aim is to share ideas that help to put together a comprehensive clinical picture to guide innovative practice regardless of setting. There are only a limited number of specialist services with a specific remit to support our children and young people who face living with a brain injury. Specialist services are strictly time limited, with high thresholds for entry. Children and young people unable to access these services face a battle to get their needs assessed and met between learning disability and mental health provisions. Consequently, their uniqueness and struggles are often not understood within a framework that respects the impact of the injury on their psychological well-being.

Ethos of the book

This book has a pluralistic ethos that reflects the contributors' orientations and methods of working. The book began life predominantly focussed on narrative approaches (White & Epston, 1990) because this appeared to reflect a trend in current innovative practice. Ste Weatherhead and David Todd's (2014) *Narrative Approaches to Brain Injury* encouraged us to add to the literature with more of an emphasis on children and families. Over time, it became apparent that a wider focus would be a more authentic representation of the breadth of the work being undertaken. Many of the practice examples are influenced by narrative or systemic theories, though these are built upon a foundation of core clinical skills that typify wholistic clinical neuropsychology, such as multimodal assessment, formulation and working in partnership across multiple systems.

A main concept underpinning this book is that all children and young people with brain injuries are placed within a biopsychosocial context and thus cannot be seen in isolation – always existing in relationships within multiple systems. Change is an additional key concept relevant to respecting the child and young person's development and recovery. It is also echoed in how the systems and agencies that support the child into adulthood change over time. These systems often relate to each other with varying degrees of success. The major challenge is how to achieve a good enough fit between the dynamic needs of the child (and his or her family) with what services can provide at a specific point in time. This attunement is essential to maximising quality of life. Producing a practical book which others can use as a springboard for their own practice was also a major motivating factor.

We feel privileged to work with these children, as we recognise how we can have an important impact on their recovery at a time when their brains are exquisitely sensitive to external influences on their fundamental sense of self and their life goals. Within this framework, it is not surprising to us that narrative principles have been used alongside more traditional therapies, such as behavioural or cognitive behavioural interventions. Narrative therapy sees problems as separate from the person and promotes a stance of curiosity. It assumes that the stories that we construct about ourselves, others and the future serve to constrain or liberate our lived experiences. This happens through the meanings that are attached to these stories. Thus, new conversations we have with others are powerful ways to "re-story" who we are and what is possible within our lives.

For our children and young people with brain injuries, having a means to understand themselves as more than just their brain injuries and to develop new valuing stories of themselves is particularly important. Narrative approaches give opportunities for them to author multiple stories of resilience rather than allowing a dominant story of "deficits" to engulf their identities. Having a cohesive narrative has also been shown to be a key ingredient in allowing a person to recovery from traumatic experiences (Brewin, 2001), thus this innovative approach could be beneficial by addressing the psychological issues on multiple related levels. The way in which narrative principles can be used alongside wholistic clinical neuropsychology is demonstrated in chapters described next.

What's in the book?

The first part of this book focusses on the useful things to know before embarking on therapeutic work, setting out an introduction to brain development plus facts about types of brain injuries, their outcomes and their medical management. An innovative approach is used to present the development of the brain in the form of imagining a "Brain" telling you its "life story". With a more medical lens, essential knowledge regarding incidence and outcomes of acquired brain injuries (ABIs) and their treatment is presented.

Part I then moves onto how clinicians work together with our children and families in order to understand their priorities and thus our focus. It outlines an example of an assessment process and user-friendly formulation models to guide intervention. The assessment method presented encompasses a comprehensive and inclusive approach with attention paid to the importance of feedback from families and professionals. This is further reflected when presenting formulation models that help clinicians make sense of an array of complex information to guide options for intervention.

Part II of the book describes a range of current innovations in therapy. Using the perspective of another imaginary "Brain", this time seeking help following an injury, it demonstrates narrative processes through deconstruction of dominant stories and identities alongside the reconstruction of alternative preferred stories and identities.

Examples of practice are presented using narrative-influenced play therapy and autobiographical work approaches for when talking therapy with a child or young person is not an option due to age or severe communication challenges.

When a child is more profoundly injured and direct therapeutic work is not possible, clinicians can feel deskilled and disempowered. Systemic and narrative ideas for supporting families are offered.

Behaviour challenges are frequent after a brain injury, thus a collaborative approach with a young person that builds upon positive behaviour support using narrative ideas is presented. Following on from this the "Beads of Life" approach is described in helping children and young people within a group intervention to develop stories of self besides the brain injury.

Next follows a description of how clinicians can help families to open up space for stories lived and untold to find ways to look to their future. Looking at the bigger picture, we know that our children with brain injuries (who may have faced behavioural challenges) are much more likely to come into contact with the criminal justice system. It is true to say that it is only through the pioneering work of a few leading researchers that the frequency of brain injury in prison populations is being recognised. The impact of the injury is now beginning to be considered in relation to traditional interventions. Important considerations for psychotherapy, including multisystemic therapy, for our children and young people with brain injuries in conflict with the law is described.

A major factor for ensuring high-quality care of our children and young people is doing as much as we can so that systems work together for positive transition across educational settings. A model of practice to support this is outlined.

Part III of the book speaks to the question of "What differences do we make?" and takes a considered approach to using measures of clinical outcome in our work. The book concludes with a chapter offering views that speak to the heart of the chief medical officer's report in 2012 (Davies, 2013), which argued that "our children (*especially with neurological disorders*) deserve better" and what that "better" might look like.

We hope clinicians use this book as a springboard for further innovation and gain the same sense of validation through reading it as was felt from Professor Wilde's words.

References

Ashton, R. (2015). Educational neuropsychology. In J. Reed, R. Byard, & H. Fine (Eds.), *Neuropsychological rehabilitation of childhood brain injury, a practical guide* (pp. 237–253). London: Palgrave Macmillan.

Brewin, C. (2001). A cognitive neuroscience account of posttraumatic stress disorder and its treatment. *Behaviour Research and Therapy, 39*, 373–393.

Byard, K. (2015). A contextual, systemic perspective in child neuropsychological rehabilitation. In J. Reed, R. Byard, & H. Fine (Eds.), *Neuropsychological rehabilitation of childhood brain injury, a practical guide* (pp. 173–190). London: Palgrave Macmillan.

Childhood Brain Injury Trust (CBIT). (2017). Retrieved July 14, 2018, from https://child braininjurytrust.org.uk

Davies, S. C. (2013). *Annual report of the chief medical officer 2012, our children deserve better: Prevention pays.* London: Department of Health.

Gan, C., & Ballantyne, M. (2016). Brain injury family intervention for adolescents: A solution-focused approach. *NeuroRehabilitation, 38*(3), 231–241. doi:10.3233/NRE-161315

Gan, C., Gargaro, J., Kreutzer, J., Boschen, K., & Wright, F. (2010). Development and preliminary evaluation of a structured family system intervention for adolescents with brain injury and their families. *Brain Injury, 24,* 651–663.

Gerrard-Morris, A., Taylor, H. G., Yeates, K. O., Walz, N. C., Stancin, T., Minich, N., & Wade, S. L. (2009). Cognitive development after traumatic brain injury in children. *Journal of International Neuropsychological Society, 16,* 1–12.

Gerring, J. P., & Wade, S. (2012). The essential role of psychosocial risk and protective factors in pediatric traumatic brain injury research. *Journal of Neurotrauma, 29*(4), 621–628.

Gracey, F., Olsen, G., Austin, L., Watson, S., & Malley, D. (2015). Integrating psychological therapy into interdisciplinary child neuropsychological rehabilitation. In J. Reed, R. Byard, & H. Fine (Eds.), *Neuropsychological rehabilitation of childhood brain injury, a practical guide* (pp. 191–214). London: Palgrave Macmillan.

Hurst, R. (2009). The international disbilty rights movement and the ICF. *Disability and Rehabilitation, 25*(11–12), 572–576.

O'Doherty, S., & O'Connor, R. (2015). Music therapy and neurospsychology: An innovative and integrated approach. In J. Reed, R. Byard, & H. Fine (Eds.), *Neuropsychological rehabilitation of childhood brain injury, a practical guide* (pp. 254–270). London: Palgrave Macmillan.

Perkins, A. (2015). Psychological support using narrative psychotherapy for children with brain injury. In J. Reed, R. Byard, & H. Fine (Eds.), *Neuropsychological rehabilitation of childhood brain injury, a practical guide* (pp. 215–236). London: Palgrave Macmillan.

Shore, R. (1997). *Rethinking the brain.* New York: Families and Work Institute.

Taylor, H. G., Yeates, K. O., Wade, S. L., Drotar, D., Kline, S., & Stancin, T. (1999). Influences on first-year recovery from traumatic brain injury in children. *Neuropsychology, 13,* 76–89.

Wade, S., Carey, J., & Wolfe, C. (2006). The efficacy of an online cognitive-behavioral, family intervention in improving child behavior and social competence following pediatric brain injury. *Rehabilitation Psychological, 51*(3), 179–189.

Wade, S., Michaud, L., & Brown, T. (2006). Putting the pieces together: Preliminary efficacy of a family problem-solving intervention for children with traumatic brain injury. *Journal of Head Trauma Rehabilitation, 21*(1), 57–67.

Wade, S., Walz, N., Carey, J., & Williams, K. (2008). Preliminary efficacy of a web-based family problem solving treatment programme for adolescents with traumatic brain injury. *Journal of Head Trauma Rehabilitation, 23,* 269–277.

Weatherhead, S. & Todd, D. (2014). *Narrative Approaches to Brain Injury.* Karnac.

Wilde, E. (2016). Neuropsychological consequences of childhood brain injury. Keynote speech. Neuropsychological consequences of childhood brain injury: Improving child brain injury outcomes: From science to innovation in practice conference, 11 February, London: Recolo.

White, M., & Epston, D. (1990). *Narrative means to therapeutic ends.* New York: W.W. Norton & Company.

Part I

Getting started

Chapter 1

"My life story" by the brain

Jenny Jim

Making concepts simple: using language and metaphor

I have written two chapters from the perspective of the brain speaking, "'*My life story*' by the brain" (Part I) and "Narrative-inspired interview with the brain" (Part II). The aim was to help introduce complex concepts around brain development and brain injury to readers using simple, accessible language. I believe in making complex concepts user-friendly; otherwise, knowledge can be lost to language. Stories seem to me to be a natural forum open to children and adults alike, allowing us to connect to our innately creative and fantastic imaginations.

Story lines and characters can be used to form a bridge between semantic knowledge and our natural ways of weaving meaning in conversation and stories. "Mini-worlds" can capture enormous detail, as long as meaning connects the details together. I wanted both chapters to demonstrate this idea. I hope they will be a springboard to others to use fun and creative means to connect crystallised knowledge to our natural ways of making meaning in our lives together.

For instance, another project I am currently developing with Jon Ettey, a doctorate student, uses narrative principles to personify and externalise the different lobes of the brain so that children and adults can better hold on to their functions, their vulnerabilities and what they need from themselves and others to recovery from injury. "The Lobe Family" will be one of the first (if not the first) theoretically and therapeutically grounded psychoeducational packages co-constructed directly with children with an acquired brain injury (ABI). Each character will have a personality demonstrating the main functions of the lobe and will "talk" to the user. The way they interact will demonstrate what we know about the development of the brain and principles of connectivity, plasticity, environmental-dependency/expectancy and effects of rehabilitation.

All of these resources can be used with children and adults to increase their mastery of knowledge that forms a solid basis for understanding and reclaiming their own agency in a situation where they may often feel stripped of their role and expertise. In Part II, "The Narrative-inspired interview with the brain" purposefully does not include academic references but follows the work of Michael White

(2007) as a basis for the questions the fictitious narrative therapist uses. I felt that making this more explicit, in the actual interview, deflated its emotional impact. "'*My life story*' by the brain", as a more complex endeavour, required endnotes throughout, as I felt this would enhance the reading and rigour of the chapter. The Brain will now talk you through its "life story" from birth to old age.

Conception to birth: the worm in the womb

I was born just three weeks after conception. Funny to think that I began life as a plate and then a tube![1] When I look at my electron microscopic baby pictures, I cringe, as I resemble a fat earthworm. Thank goodness they didn't have social media back then. I develop at the "head" of the worm, and the "tail" then becomes the spinal cord. Together, we are the central nervous system, the figurative and literal "backbone"; of our minds and bodies.

The spinal cord gets off the blocks fast and begins to develop its first synapses[2] by week five. This allows the first movements of my embryonic body just a week later and at ten weeks even more refined actions, such as hiccupping and sucking my thumb. I am more of a slow burner when it comes to ripening, playing the "long game" as they say. In this game of "heads or tails", this flip is always rigged to "Tails".

Whilst I may mature at a slower rate, I am still rapidly generating my brain cells[3] and by week five, I have formed three bulgy areas of my wormy and tube-like self, towards my front, middle and back. Two weeks later, the front and back areas have both divided into two.[4] These each become more intricate with time. It's rather like building a house and making sure the floorplan and basic wiring is down so that all rooms are connected. Of course, the house needs a water supply, so I make four interconnected internal chambers that produce my favourite *eau de vie*,[5] the supply of which extends into the space between me, my skull and the canal in the spinal cord.

Incidentally, within the walls of my two biggest chambers is also where I manufacture my brain cells. I make two varieties of brain cells: the vocal communicating neurones and their support act, the glia. To say I run a busy production line would be a *slight* understatement given that I usually make up to 80–100 billion *of each variety* of brain cell in the womb![6] I issue each neurone with its own passport and travel itinerary so it can immediately migrate from its place of birth to a specific destination.[7] By week 24, I have almost all my neurones made.

Returning to my house-building metaphor, my front rooms are by far the largest because I need a lot of cells to make my most complex areas. Also known as my "cerebrum", it is the prime location that I invest in to become my cerebral hemispheres. I guess you could see them as my HQ offices.

I put most of the grey cell bodies of my neurones on the outer layer of the hemispheres – i.e. grey matter. Scientists named this the "cortex" – the Latin word for tree bark because of the grooves they saw. Underneath my grey matter are the tails of my neurones that will eventually look white when they are covered in fat – i.e. white matter.[8] I have to mention that I am careful to shrink wrap myself[9] and, of course, ensure an oxygen supply to all my rooms.[10]

You could say I am a natural architect rather than *avant-garde*, I follow a similar genetic building plan to other brains, so I put things where they seem to make sense and rarely get maverick with my blueprint.[11] However, this doesn't stop me from adding my individual sparkle by customising my rooms and how well they are connected to one another. A big influence on my overall interior structure and design are the experiences I am exposed to. I'll talk more about this later.[12]

Once I have my cells in place, I can get my vital jobs done. Firstly, I decorate the back rooms, which are the seat of control of all my critical reflexes (this area is known as the brainstem). The moment I finish furnishing this room and do the lights-on "big reveal" is like flicking the switch for "autopilot mode" – it means I no longer have to worry about controlling things such as breathing, how fast my heart beats and the pressure that blood is pumped through my body. By the end of the second trimester (week 28), my brainstem is almost completely mature, which means my foetal body stands a chance of surviving outside of the womb.

Once I am sure my autopilot mode is in place, I get to work on the "thinking" part of my brain so I can learn about the world I am in. Scientists discovered that if they crept up and startled me with loud noises, I would eventually learn to ignore their silly games.[13] Honestly, sometimes I think they assume I am just resting on my laurels as if in some kind of suspended animation, but I am busy studying – learning all about my mother: her smell, her heartbeat and her voice.[14,15]

Of course, I can't say that I am consciously doing this – conscious thinking comes later when my cerebral cortex comes online. You might have noticed that I have been decorating my house from back to front, a bit topsy-turvy, but when you think about it, the tail also came before the head, so I guess when it comes to my story, it is one that doesn't follow expectations.

Throughout my time in the womb, I must make sure I get enough folic acid; otherwise, the "head" of my tube never closes, and this would be the end of me (technically before I am even born!).[16] If the "tail" does not seal, then the spinal cord will grow without the protection of the spine.[17] Also, infections, malnutrition or drug/chemical exposure can wreak havoc on my newly born neurones that are hitch-hiking[18] across to their forever homes and so are particularly vulnerable to attack.

Another thing I must mention before I tell you about my next big life event is that I haven't quite told you my story from the *very* beginning. Scientists are now reliably informing me that long before I start emerging as a plate, the "instruction manual and programme of works" for my development have already been influenced, not only by the genes of my parents, but the life experiences of my mother[19,20] in particular.

Birth: eviction to exuberance

I was evicted from my lovely womb-home when I was ready enough to live without it.[21] What a shock to be "outside" and having lots of new sounds, smells and things I could see! I had to get used to my body not being supported by the comfort of my bathing liquid, and it was very scary at first. Luckily, I had learnt the smell, voice and heartbeat of my mother, so I knew I wasn't really alone. But I do have to admit that it took a while to really learn I was safe – because I was so dependent on my parents, I made sure they were close, by crying (*a lot*) so that I was gradually convinced that they hadn't forgotten about me. Flashing a few winning smiles[22] seemed to make them forget the pain of those early days.

I weigh around 1 pound now, and my neurones are so excited by the world around them that they can't stop talking to one another. I am using up energy like nobody's business, and by the time I am 1-year-old, I am at young adult levels of power; this increases exponentially so that by the time I am 3, I am sapping 2.5 times adult levels![23] This is perhaps not surprising because in these years, I am producing 700 new neural connections every second![24] Scientists call this time my "exuberant period". At an almost unimaginable rate, my cerebral cortex bursts into life – like the crescendo of a thousand New Year's Eve fireworks displays, my neurones make up to two million new synapses every second.[25] Anything that happens to me makes a big impression. Scientists describe this as "plasticity"[26] – repeated experiences can easily become part of my "go-to" templates about the world[27]

Because I don't yet know what things are going to be important to me, I employ a "wide-net" strategy and try to lay down the building blocks for as many memories as possible. I am glad I spent a lot of time making my neurones (approximately 86 billion of them!) before I was evicted, as now they bolt into action like a spread of runners in a relay team, each having migrated in strategic locations forming highways across my landscape of interiors.

Networks are laid down between my neuronal cell bodies in parallel with me insulating the tails of the neurones. Just like cabling a wire, the fat[28] I put down means the messages relay faster and more efficiently.[29] These networks are like the first imprints of my experiences,[30] and the more the routes are run the more distinct they become. I put on a lot of weight after I am out of the womb because of this. In fact, I lay down so many networks, as a baby I have twice as many connections than an average adult.[31]

The early years equations

Brains + love = development

Bowlby[32] was right when he said the first 18 months of life are inordinately important to a person's sense of belonging in this world. At this time, I am constructing my templates of how I expect to be treated, by whom and how I can get my needs met. This is my neural blueprint for relationships for the rest of my life.

If my parents spend time getting to know me and my foibles,[33] a remarkable thing happens – my gelatinous being becomes synchronised with theirs.[34] Our brains communicate, and their affection shapes the fundamental development of the rest of my nervous system. Brain role models help me understand my emotions and bring peace to my networks. One particularly important "room" I develop only after I am out of the womb is just for understanding people and emotions.[35] Given that this is the basis of empathy, it makes sense that I can't develop this on my own.[36] I sometimes think about what it would be like if I was born without toys, days out, people talking to me, enough milk and love – what would I have become?[37]

Brains + love + new experiences = development

In the early months, I am driven to obsession with my parents.[38] I naturally find their faces, voices, touch and smell simply irresistible. I also think humans in general are just great. I would much rather listen to them speak or sing than just general sounds. It is good that my parents feel the same way about me. They love giving me cuddles, comfort and even speak to me in a funny baby-speak.[39] This makes me grow and develop even more, and my neurones become more densely connected.

It may surprise you to know that my body had fully developed vocal chords by week 12,[40] and I already began to put the earliest building blocks down for speaking through silent crying and sucking. Adding the baby-speak when I am born is critical to consolidating the wiring of the neurones that are responsible for me to learn language when I am older. If this time passes by without anyone talking to me, then I will never be able to learn language to my full potential. This is an example of what scientists call a "critical period".[41, 42] The way I see it is more basic than that. Simply put, I know that love means that I get what I need to be the best I can be.[43]

Underpinning my new emerging skills[44] there are mini-fireworks displays going off at different times at different locations inside of me. As you know, this is my cerebral cortex's chance to get on the map. Without this, I wouldn't be able to have conscious thoughts, feelings, memories or actions. The displays start at the back (visual cortex), in an Alice band that runs ear to ear (somatosensory cortex) and its neighbouring area (motor cortex). This happens later in the side (temporal cortex) and front (frontal cortex) areas. This allows me to get up and running several "processing centres": visual, sensory and motor, and then language and emotions. Last, but not least, I develop my HQ centre for reasoning.

It's amazing to think that when I left the womb, each single neurone had about 2,500 synapses, but by the time I am 2 or 3, each one has about 15,000![45] At the mere age of 2 years, my cerebral cortex contains over a hundred trillion synapses.[46]

Brains + cells = development

You may be wondering how on earth I can keep accommodating these new cells and synapses, especially as I have limited space to expand within my skull. I mentioned earlier that scientists named the outer layer of grey matter the cortex because of the grooves they saw, and so you have a clue that I have transformed from my early days as a smooth tubelike earthworm. I now bear more resemblance to a walnut! It's like I have undergone a form of in-skull aging – I develop wrinkles pretty fast and no amount of beauty treatment can stop that!

In fact, these grooves and crevices[47] start forming as early as 14 weeks[48] and thank goodness it happens, as it gives me more surface area, which equals more processing power. Groovy is definitely cool when it comes to brainpower. Imagine if you will, a heady pairing of an image-conscious brain and an unscrupulous backstreet cosmetic brain surgeon – a dose of Botox would remove all its wrinkles but with that a wiping out of the poor brain's ability to learn and survive.[49]

Brains – cells = development!

Not all the cells I make survive . . . now don't be sad about this because I actually programme them to die[50] – I did say that my story might not follow expectations! Before you think I am some kind of self-sadomasochistic psychopath, let me explain. Think of these cells as willing lemmings, happy with a short cameo role in this complex story of development. Effectively, they sign short-term contracts to perform and accept when they are no longer needed . . . I can see that you are still not with me on this, so let me give you an example, and I'll try not to shock you further. We all had webbed fingers and toes when we were in the womb. OK still with me? Well, you would still have them if I wasn't allowed to programme the webbing to die off. See, now you understand!

Scientists can actually be quite poetic at times, and they named this process "apoptosis", which is from the Greek for "falling off" as leaves of a tree.[51] This is one way I keep myself as streamlined and efficient as possible. Staying with the arboreal analogy, I also start engaging in a new hobby of "pruning"[52] from around the age of 6. This is where I remove the weaker synaptic connections – think of it as a sort of neurological topiary.

Growing up: From the apprentice to the specialist

Topiary is my favourite hobby from the start of puberty, and this makes everything run more efficiently, like a sort of neural spring clean. I keep this up all the way through adolescence and even into adulthood.[53] The experiences I have determine how strong the connections are between the neurones and, therefore, which ones are spared the neurological pruning shears. Once I have reached adolescence, I have happily pruned about 50% of my synapses, leaving around 500 trillion as my core synapse family.[54]

This process means that parts of my brain become better at doing their jobs, graduating to higher levels with more experience. Different areas become specialised for certain vocations. They do say geniuses are not born but made – put in 10,000 hours into a skill and anyone can reach boss level.[55]

It is *generally* a case of "use it or lose it" when it comes to sculpting which cells stay and which ones go. An interesting aberration of this could explain a condition known as synaesthesia, when brains do not distinguish each sensory modality as separate but can, for instance, experience colours as painful or single letters of the alphabet as invoking colours. Some scientists believe that perhaps all brains started as "cross-wired", but for a rare number of brains, they did not prune away these connections.[56]

Like an unruly hedge, I have to always keep an eye on what is happening as the network never just "logs off" or goes offline. In this way, my topiary always has to change with it. Neurones are born chatterboxes and love communicating with each other; it's like they are afraid of letting go of any new experience they have. However, I need to draw the line at just keeping a whisper here and there. I will only allow the conversations that either happen repeatedly or with great impact to survive. For instance, imagine if I was auditioning to see if a trace memory could become a consolidated one, I may give the direction of *"and once more with feeling"*.

Plastic fantastic?!

I guess you will be getting the picture that I am somewhat of a chameleon in my earlier years – changing and adapting to the experiences I have. In this way, my neural architecture is fundamentally shaped by what happens to me and what I expect to happen in the future. I make sure I am always prepared by forming pathways that are required to respond to experiences.

It is as if all memories are sketched out in pencil and certain ones then get written over with permanent marker until they are etched as neural signatures of my life experiences.

My neural topiary can shape-shift a lot more when I am younger, imbuing the experiences I have then with a very special significance. That is why some scientists refer to plasticity as a "double-edged sword".[57]

The reason for this is that my core job is adaptation; I do what I need to do to survive at the time. What's the problem with this you may say? Well, the issue is that when I am busily pruning and shaping my pathways, I am doing this without the benefit of my HQ. As you know, this matures last and with it comes my ability to reason and sense-make; I am particularly vulnerable in not being able to use HQ to reassure the rest of myself (self-regulate) and problem solve.

Brains − love + trauma = aberrant development

The flipside of plasticity is that I am forever imprinted by all experiences, good and bad. I am fundamentally altered by severely stressful interactions, especially so if I can't predict them (which is very hard without an HQ) and if they go on for a long time. My anxiety and fear networks become activated often and thus overly developed. They are more reactive − it's like my house burglar alarm is always on intermittent and can be triggered to full alarm by a feather dropping on a trip wire. Even when my HQ comes online, it finds the task of managing a constant alarm exhausting. Battling with a legacy of emotional tinnitus disrupts it from getting on with its job of reasoning and thinking.

I haven't yet told you that I make many chemicals that are really important in controlling my body's behaviour and emotions.[58] When I get stressed, a part of me releases a hormone which then triggers a whole chain of events affecting my mind and body.[59] This is really unpleasant − if I am put in lots of stressful and unpredictable situations when I am really young (such as being physically or emotionally abused by someone I should trust), then I am forever changed by them, and unless I get help or learn ways to deal to with what has happened, they can dictate my life in terrible ways. For instance, abused brains can sometimes paradoxically seek out abusive relationships/interactions so that they at least feel in control of them (always believing they will be abused in the end anyway, so what do they have to lose?).[60]

In this circumstance, developing full capacity to regulate my own emotions is hard, and I don't really have space on my "to-do list" to be concerned with the emotions of others. Early childhood abuse means young plastic brains adapt in ways that may be highly disadvantageous to them when they are adults.[61]

To prevent negative neural signatures influencing my life uncontrollably and maladaptively, I need to return to my brain role models. As you know by now, brains develop through interaction with other brains. If I find even just one brain that understands me, tunes in to my wavelength (rather than forces me to listen at its frequency) and we have *reciprocal* interactions, I become better at reducing the intensity of my intermittent burglar alarm. Eventually, I might be able to time when it is not activated at all.[62]

The *Oxford English Dictionary* defines "reciprocal" as an adjective of the English language meaning "given, felt or done in return", but I feel mathematicians hit the nail on the head even better "(of a quality or function) related to another so that their product is unity".

Other brain strains

Most brains grow up pretty well, but I thought it would be helpful for you to know about some other risks that young brains face. Now that you know all the things that are happening, even before birth, I guess it's not too much of a stretch to realise it can be a delicate time laying down all my foundations. Sometimes my movement pathways do not develop as usual, and this can result in the most common childhood physical disorder, cerebral palsy.[63] There are also a range of other difficulties that can arise before, during or after birth.[64]

Ageing: boom and bust?

Of course, all brains get older, and throughout my teenage years to young adulthood, my social brain[65] is the main part to take off. Society sculpts me more and more – my front rooms become more intricate and closely wired to other parts of the house. This means I develop distinctly more uniquely human traits of being able to regulate my behaviour in relation to others, to think about myself as having an identity of my own, to have ambitions and hopes for the future. Crucially, I develop brain areas that will actually help achieve my dreams, which underpin skills such as planning, organisation and strategy formation.

If all goes to plan, I learn to "roll with the punches" of adulthood and enjoy the highs too. It's an ever-changing playing field, but as I said, my main job is about adapting to the "slings and arrows" of life. In fact, this probably is fundamentally what keeps me healthy throughout my life.

Some brains are worried about getting older, but I think they might be just overfocussing on the bad and not the good. Yes, it's true that brains do change,[66] and we do need perhaps a little longer to process stuff, but we also have accumulated more knowledge, and our library of words is so much more extensive and eloquent.[67] I do also make some new brain cells in certain areas.[68]

It is by no means a "boom and bust" picture – spiralling into decline is not an inevitable part of getting older. I myself am looking forward to the days when I age gracefully, full of complexity, like a great Saint-Émilion Bordeaux.

My parting words

Isn't it a curiosity that brains are the only organs that can actually study themselves, perhaps an exercise in narcissism?![69]

I hope you agree that *all* brains (including yours) are amazing – to think that a piece of brain the size of a grain of rice actually contains 10,000 nerve cells and can make between 1–10,000 connections,[70] I can't imagine how artificial intelligence could ever match our potential. No wonder no brain could be the same as another. "You" and your unique snowflake personality will only grace this world once.

It's been such a pleasure to have your attention, and I hope, above all, that your brain in now different than when we first met.

Notes

1 The neural plate is formed from the neuroectoderm, which is derived from the ectoderm – the outermost of the three germ layers of the embryo. The other layers being the mesoderm and endoderm. The neural tube is formed when the neural groove fuses. The neural groove results from folding of the neural plate. The neural tube is complete by 4.5 weeks of embryonic development (Crossman & Neary, 2010).

2 A synapse is a gap (or cleft) between two neurones that allows a nerve impulse/action potential travelling from the dendrites and toward the axon of one neurone to trigger an onwards impulse in the dendrites of the receiving neurone/s. Whilst the action potential is an electrical signal the communication across the synapse is chemical and relies on the release of neurotransmitters to trigger the electrical impulse in the next neurone/s. (Crossman & Neary, 2010).

3 This is the process of neurogenesis of brain nerve cells known as neurones and glia (Crossman & Neary, 2010).

4 The front of the brain is also known as the forebrain/prosencephalon, middle of the brain as the midbrain/mesencephalon and the back of the brain as the hindbrain/rhombencephalon. The front areas further divide into the telencephalon and diencephalon, and the back areas into the metencephalon and myelencephalon (Crossman & Neary, 2010).

5 This liquid is the cerebral-spinal fluid (CSF) and is produced by the choroid plexus in the chambers – i.e. ventricles. CSF functions to protect the CNS, as a shock absorber and giver of nutrients. There is a barrier that protects the brain from absorbing harmful substances present in the blood via CSF circulation. CSF is circulated from inside the brain to the space below the middle meningeal lining called the arachnoid mater. This space is thus termed the "sub-arachnoid" space. CSF is constantly produced and requires reabsorption at the same rate by the body via the venous sinuses (Crossman & Neary, 2010).

6 This figure relates to neurones and glia, totalling an awesome 160–200 billion brain cells in total (the Wellcome Trust, 2017).

7 This relates to the process of neuronal migration.

8 Within this layer, there are also some selected cell bodies – i.e. the basal nuclei. The process by which axons are covered with fat is called myelination (Crossman & Neary, 2010).

9 This refers to the brain's out coverings collectively known as the meninges, comprising of the dura matter, arachnoid layer and pia matter (Crossman & Neary, 2010).

10 The brain has an extensive vasculature of brain vessels that ensure it is fed by oxygen and glucose.

11 For instance, the majority of brains will have four lobes and connecting white matter tracts. White matter tracts are now visible in live brains thanks to diffusion tensor imaging (DTI). Other methods of imaging the brain are computed tomography (CT scan, or computerised axial tomography, CAT scan), electroencephalograph (EEG), positron emission tomography (PET), magnetic resonance imaging (MRI), functional magnetic resonance imaging (fMRI) and magnetoencephalography (MEG) (see PBS, 2001a for a user-friendly resource explaining these major scanning methods).

12 See the theory of ontogenetic specialisation (Vargha-Khadem et al., 2000).

13 Using in utero monitoring, foetus' can demonstrate habituation to stimuli and learning according to brain maturation (Morokuma et al. 2004).

14 Likewise, Graven and Browne (2008) have shown a selective learning of the mother's voice from in utero exposure.

15 There is a movement known as "foetal origins" based on findings of foetal abilities to learn a range of information whilst in utero spanning from maternal accent to more controversially perhaps, how safe or dangerous the world (Murphy Paul, 2011).

16 This refers to anencephaly, whereby the brain and skull bones are unable to develop normally (Crossman & Neary, 2010).

17 This refers to spina bifida, whereby the spinal cord and spine do not close, resulting in a gap. There are various types of spina bifida with differential impacts (NHS Choices, 2017).

18 Newborn neurones use existing radial glial cell fibres to travel to their destinations (Crossman & Neary, 2010).

19 Maternal enrichment has been shown to produce favourable effects on offspring who have brain damage, increasing their likelihood of recovery (Gibb et al., 2014).

20 See Murphy Paul (2011).

21 Some brains are born too early. Prematurity carries particular risks for future brain development, which then relate to cognitive difficulties (see Peterson et al., 2000). Similarly, extremely low birth weight babies also show risks to brain development and cognition (see Vohr et al. 2000).

22 Smiling and positive looks are thought to stimulate endogenous neurobiological processes underlying pleasure and reward (endorphin and dopamine release) that stimulates neuronal growth in the pre-frontal cortex and orbitofrontal cortex. Respectively, these areas can function to predict/anticipate future pleasurable interactions/contingencies and develop empathic interactions (Schore, 1994).

23 See the work of Chugani (1997) who uses PET scanning to monitor glucose utilisation in the developing baby's brain. For some, this is evidence that babies and infants are biologically primed for learning.

24 Zero to Three (2017).

25 Zero to Three (2017).

26 See Kolb and Gibb (2011) for a review of plasticity and eight key factors which deconstruct types of experience that are important, as well as genetic factors that influence brain development.

27 See the work of Bliss and Collingridge (1983) on long-term potentiation; Hebb's (1949) principle of "neurones that fire together, wire together" and Kandel (2009) on the neurobiological underpinnings of learning and memory.

28 Known as myelin.

29 Messages along the tail/axon are known as action potentials are electrical in nature, hence myelin acting as a conductant. Continuation of the "message" at the end of the tail/axon at the synapse is chemical.

30 This is thought to be the neural basis of learning

31 PBS (2001b).

32 John Bowlby (1907–1990), pioneer of Attachment Theory.

33 It is generally agreed that babies are born with individual temperaments vs. being tabula rasa. Furthermore, difficult temperaments do not predict worse outcomes, what matters is the way in which parents are able to adapt and co-regulate baby's brains (see Belsky et al. 1998)

34 Human infant brains have been shown to mirror their caregivers with relationships between emotional availability and fundamental development of the sympathetic and parasympathetic nervous systems (see Davidson & Fox, 1992).

35 See Gerhardt (2004) for a discussion about the importance of the orbitofrontal cortex and experience dependence development.

36 Shared neural activity is also seen in the mirror neurone system, which is thought to allow mimetic development in humans.

37 See the seminal work of Michael Rutter (1981) and the development of children kept in Romanian orphanages and Music (2016) who looks at the relationship between attachment, maltreatment, brain impacts and socio-emotional development.

38 Newborns prefer their mothers' voices (see DeCasper & Fifer, 1980).

39 This refers to "motherese", "baby talk" or "child-directed speech", which shows repetition, exaggerated prosody, elongated phonemes, higher pitch, simplification of speech, etc., different than that of adult speech (see Kaplan et al. 2001). This is thought to accelerate language acquisition. Babies have been shown to prefer this type of speech over adult-directed speech (Cooper & Aslin, 1990).

40 NHS Scotland (2011).

41 Lenneberg (1967).

42 Critical periods can be seen within a "chicken or egg" type of debate. Some believe these correspond to times of synaptic excess enhancing readiness to grasp certain skills, others believe exposure to conditions to learning of skills itself brings forth critical periods.

43 See Gerhardt's (2004) book *Why Love Matters. How Affection Shapes a Baby's Brain* for deeper discussion of the interface between affection, psychological development and neuroscience.

44 See the work of Mary Sheridan in Sharma & Cockerill (2014).

45 Gopnick, Meltzoff & Kuhl (1999).

46 Zero to Three (2017).

47 The grooves are known as gyri and the crevices as sulci.

48 Monteagudo and Timor-Tritsch (1997).

49 This is analogous to "lissencephaly" which means "smooth brain" (see NINDS, 2017).

50 This refers to the process of apoptosis, programmed cell death that starts to happen in the womb. This is distinguished from cell death resulting from a process of necrosis which is unexpected (due to external forces/injury, poisons, infection, metabolic issues or lack of blood supply due to stroke).

51 Alberts et al. (2002).

52 See Huttenlocher (1990).

53 Petanjek et al. (2011).

54 The brain is a dynamic system, incapable of *not* changing (see Shore, 1997)

55 Gladwell (2009).

56 An alternative hypothesis for this is that there may be a failure in inhibitory feedback processes akin to phantom limb pain (Ramachandran & Hubbard, 2001).

57 Shonkoff & Phillips (2000, p. 94)

58 This refers to the endocrine system.

59 This refers to the relationship between developmental trauma cortisol levels and the sensitisation of the hypothalamic-pituitary-adrenal axis (Schore, 1994). See also Polyvagal Theory (Porges, 2003) for discussion of a "face-heart" connection that purports that phylogenetic development of the vagal system allowed humans to use social interaction to regulate the visceral system.

60 This refers to what is known as a cycle of abuse.

61 Some structural and functional brain changes that have been reported are smaller left hemisphere, sensitised limbic system, reduced hippocampal volume and reduced hemispheric connectivity (Child Welfare Gateway: protecting children, 2017).

62 Sensitivity of caregiver's responses, their attunement, co-regulation leading to a child's brain to self-regulate has been studied by several leading clinical psychologists: see mentalisation (Fonagy, Gergely, Jurist, Target, 2002); intersubjectivity (Trevarthen & Aitken, 2001), brain-based parenting (Hughes & Baylin, 2012), parenting with the brain in mind (Siegel, 2004). Though this was not explicitly within Vygotsky's (1896–1934) zone of proximal development, I would argue that this is also an example of attunement and co-regulation leading to learning.

63 Cerebral palsy can have many causes, such as bleeding in the brain, disrupted oxygen supply or infection in pregnancy but often exact causes are not clear (NHS England, 2017). Cerebral palsy may also have cognitive effects.

64 Premature baby brains are at higher risk of seizure disorders. Risks of the perinatal period are of stroke, epilepsies, hydrocephalus, meningitis, encephalitis and neurodevelopmental disorders (First Signs, 2014) such as ADHD. In the postnatal period, risks are of acquired brain injury, tumours, dementias and other neurological disorders such as Parkinson's (Mayo Clinic,1998–2017; Child Neurology Foundation, 2017)

65 See the work of Blakemore (2006).

66 Reported changes include shrinkage of the pre-frontal cortex and hippocampus, less efficient neurotransmission due to reduced myelin and aging vasculature that may affect blood and oxygen transportation; further, there are more plaques and tangles, and greater risk of inflammation (NIA, 2017)

67 Whilst processing speed may decline, the evidence shows that older people get there in the end and that blanket cognitive decline is not an inevitable consequence of aging. Additionally, older people show improved recognition (vs. recall) memory, though word-finding and visuo-spatial skills can show decline (Howieson, 2011).

68 Neurogenesis is a controversial concept with some believing that there is evidence of this for neurones that migrate to the olfactory bulb in dentate gyrus of the hippocampus and striatum (see Gould, 2017). Further, there is also evidence, that the neurone's support act, the glia also regenerate (Gould, 2017). However, others believe these claims are not substantiated enough by hard evidence (see Costandi, 2012, for a journalist's synopsis of this debate).

69 This point also speaks to the idea of consciousness and identity, perhaps the biggest enigma of neuroscience and neuropsychology, which even defies adequate definition. How does the activity of some 86 billion neurones give rise to a sense of a singularity? Returning to the mathematical definition of reciprocal, "(of a quality or function) related to another so that their product is unity", it is almost this on a mass production scale. Rhythmic convergence of neural activity is thought to describe the neurobiological process that aligns with our own sense of "being conscious" but this is only part of the puzzle. How does consciousness "emerge" and why does it arise at all (see Crick & Koch, 1998)? For a radical stance equating identity to the human connectome, see Seung (2010).

70 PBS (2001b).

References

Alberts, B., Johnson, A., Lewis, J., Morgan, D., & Raff, M. (2002). *Molecular biology of the Cell* (4th ed.). New York: Garland Science.

Belsky, J., Hsieh, K., & Crnic, K. (1998). Mothering, fathering and infant negativity as antecedents of boys' externalising problems and inhibition at age 3 years: Differential susceptibility to rearing experience? *Development and Psychopathology, 10*, 301–319.

Blakemore, S. J., & Choudhury, S. (2006). Development of the adolsecent brain: Implications for executive functions and social cognition. *Journal of Child Psychology and Psychiatry, 47*(3–4), 296–312.

Bliss, T. V. P., & Collingridge, G. L. (1983). A synaptic model of memory: Long-term potentiation in the hippocampus. *Nature, 361*, 31–39.

Bowlby, J. (1965). *Maternal care and mental health. The master work series*, 2nd ed. London: Jason Aronson.

Chugani, H. T. (1997). Neuroimaging of developmental non-linearity and developmental pathologies. In R. W. Thatcher, G. R. Lyon, J. Rumsey, & N. Krasnegor (Eds), *Developmental neuroimaging: Mapping the development of brain and behavior* (pp. 187–195). San Diego: Academic Press.

Cooper, R. P., & Aslin, R. N. (1990). Preference for infant-directed speech in the first month after birth. *Child Development, 61*, 1584–1595.

Crick, F., & Koch, C. (1998). Consciousness and neuroscience. *Cerebral Cortex, 8*, 97–107.

Crossman, A. R., & Neary, D. (2010). *Neuroanatomy: An illustrated colour text*. China: Churchill Livingstone Elsevier.

Davidson, R., & Fox, N. (1992). Asymmetrical brain activity discriminates between positive v. negative affective stimuli in human infants. *Science, 218*, 1235–1237.

DeCasper, A. J., & Fifer, W. P. (1980). Of human bonding: Newborns prefer their mothers' voices. *Science, 208*, 1174–1176.

Fonagy, P., Gergely, G., Jurist, E., & Target, M. (2002). *Affect regulation, mentalization, and the development of the self*. New York: Other Press.

Gerhardt, S. (2004). *Why love matters. How affection shapes a baby's brain*. East Sussex: Routledge.

Gibb, R. L., Gonzalez, C. L., & Kolb, B. (2014). Prenatal enrichment and recovery from perinatal cortical damage: Effects of maternal complex housing. *Frontiers in Behavioral Neuroscience, 8*, 223.

Gladwell, M. (2009). *Outliers: The story of success*. London: Penguin.

Gopnick, A., Meltzoff, A., & Kuhl, P. (1999). *How babies think: The science of childhood*. London: Phoenix.

Graven, S. N., & Browne, J. V. (2008). Auditory development in the fetus and infant. *Newborn and Infant Nursing Reviews, 8*(4), 187–193.

Hebb, D. O. (1949). *The organisation of behavior*. New York: Wiley & Sons.

Hughes, D. A. & Baylin, J. (2012). *Brain-based parenting: The neuroscience of caregiving for healthy attachment*. New York, NY: W.W. Norton.

Huttenlocher, P. R. (1990). Morphometric study of human cerebral cortex development. *Neuropsychologia, 28*(6), 517–527.

Kandel, E. R. (2009). The biology of memory: A forty-year perspective. *Journal of Neuroscience, 29*(41), 12748–12756.

Kaplan, P. S., Bachorowski, J., Smoski, M. J., & Zinser, M. (2001). Role of clinical diagnosis and medication use in effects of maternal depression on infant-directed speech. *Infancy, 2*, 537–548.

Kolb, B., & Gibb, R. (2011). Brain plasticity and behaviour in the developing brain. *Journal of the Canadian Academy of Child and Adolescent Psychiatry, 20*(4), 265–276.

Lenneberg, E. H. (1967). *Biological foundations of language*. New York: Wiley.

Monteagudo, A., & Timor-Tritsch, I. E. (1997). Development of fetal gyri, sulci and fissures: A transvaginal sonographic study. *Ultrasound Obstetrics Gynecology, 9*(4), 222–228.

Morokuma, S., Fukushima, K., Kawai, N., Tomonaga, M., Satoh, S., & Nakano, H. (2004). Fetal habituation correlates with functional brain development. *Behavioural Brain Research, 153*(2), 459–463.

Music, G. (2016). *Nurturing natures: Attachment and children's emotional, social and brain development*. Abingdon: Routledge.

Petanjek, Z., Judas, M., Simic, G., Rasin, M. R., Uylings, H. B. M., Rakic, P., & Kostovic, I. (2011). Extraordinary neoteny of synaptic spines in the human prefrontal cortex. *Proceedings of the National Academy of Sciences of the United States of America, 108*(32), 13281–13286.

Peterson, B. S., Vohr, B., Staib, L. H., Cannistraci, C. J., Dolberg, A., Schneider, K. C., . . . Ment, L. R. (2000). Regional brain volume abnormalities and long-term cognitive outcome in pre-term infants. *Journal of the American Medical Academy, 284*(15), 1939–1947.

Porges, S. W. (2003). The polyvagal theory: Phylogenetic contributions to social behaviour. *Physiology and Behavior, 79*, 503–513.

Ramachandran, V. S., & Hubbard, E. M. (2001). Synaesthesia – a window into perception, thought and language. *Journal of Consciousness Studies, 8*(12), 3–34.

Rutter, M. (1981). *Maternal deprivation reassessed* (2nd ed.). Harmondsworth: Penguin.

Schore, A. (1994). *Affect regulation and the repair of the self.* Hillsdale, NJ: Lawrence Erlbaum Associates Inc.

Siegel, D.J. (2004). Attachment and self-understanding: Parenting with the brain in mind. *Journal of Prenatal and Perinatal Psychology and Health, 18*(4), 273–286.

Sharma, A., & Cockerill, H. (2014). *Mary Sheridan's from birth to five years: Children's developmental progress* (4th ed.). London: Routledge.

Shonkoff, J. P., & Phillips, D. A. (Eds.). (2000). *From neurons to neighbourhoods: The science of early childhood development.* Washington, DC: The National Academies Press.

Shore, R. (1997). *Rethinking the brain.* New York: Families and Work Institute.

Trevarthen, C., & Aitken, K. J. (2001). Infant intersubjectivity: Research, theory and clinical applications. *Journal of Child Psychology and Psychiatry, 52*, 3–48.

Vargha-Khadem, F., Isaacs, E., Watkins, K., & Mishkin, M. (2000). Ontogenetic specialisation of hemispheric function. In J. M. Oxbury, C. E. Polkey, & M. Duchowney (Eds.), *Intractable focal epilepsy: Medical and surgical treatment* (pp. 405–418). London: Harcourt Publishers.

Vohr, B., Wright, L. L., Dusick, A. M., Mele, L., Verter, J., Steichen, J. J., . . . Kaplan, M. D. (2000). Neurodevelopmental and functional outcomes of extremely low birth weight infants in the national institute of child health and human development neonatal research network, 1993 – 1994. *Pediatrics, 105*, 1216.

White, M. (2007). *Maps of narrative practice.* New York, NY: W. W. Norton.

Website resources

Child Neurology Foundation. (2017). Retrieved August 2017, from www.childneurol ogyfoundation.org/patients-or-caregivers/living-neurological-condition/what-is-a-neurologic-disorder/

Child Welfare Information Gateway: Protecting Children. (2001). *Understanding the effects of maltreatment on early brain development.* U. S. D. o. H. a. H. Services. Washington, DC: Child Welfare 21, Information Gateway. Retrieved January 2017, from www.childwelfare.gov/pubs/focus/earlybrain/index.cfm

Costandi, M. (2012). Does your brain produce new cells? A sceptical view on adult human neurogenesis. *The Guardian.* Retrieved August 2017, from www.theguardian.com/science/neurophilosophy/2012/feb/23/brain-new-cells-adult-neurogenesis

First Signs. (2014). *Other developmental and behavioral disorders.* Retrieved August 2017, from www.firstsigns.org/delays_disorders/other_disorders.htm

Gould, E. (2017). Are you born with all your brain cells or do you grow new ones? *Brainfacts. org.* Retrieved August 2017, from www.brainfacts.org/About-Neuroscience/Ask-an-Expert/Articles/2012/Are-you-born-with-all-your-brain-cells-or-do-you-grow-new-ones

Howieson, D. B. (2011). *Cognitive skills and the aging brain: What to expect.* The Dana Foundation. Retrieved August 2017, from www.dana.org/Cerebrum/2015/Cognitive_Skills_and_the_Aging_Brain__What_to_Expect/

Mayo Clinic. (1998–2017). *Division of child and adolescent neurology.* Retrieved August 2017, from www.mayo.edu/research/departments-divisions/department-neurology/programs/division-child-adolescent-neurology

Murphy Paul, A. (2011). What we learn before we're born. *TEDGlobal.* Retrieved August 2017, from www.ted.com/talks/annie_murphy_paul_what_we_learn_before_we_re_born

National Institute of Neurological Disorders and Stroke, NINDS. (2017). *Lissencephaly information page.* Retrieved August 2017, from www.ninds.nih.gov/disorders/lissencephaly/lissencephaly.htm

National Institute on Aging, NIA. (2017). *How the aging brain affects thinking.* Retrieved August 2017, from www.nia.nih.gov/health/how-aging-brain-affects-thinking

NHS Choices. (2017). *Spina bifida.* Retrieved August 2017, from www.nhs.uk/conditions/Spina-bifida/Pages/Introduction.aspx

NHS England. (2017). *Cerebral palsy.* Retrieved July 2017, from www.nhs.uk/Conditions/Cerebralpalsy/Pages/introduction.aspx)

NHS Scotland. (2011). *Healthier Scotland maternal and early years for early years workers.* Retrieved August 2017, from www.maternal-and-early-years.org.uk/speech-in-unborn-babies

PBS. (2001a). *The secret life of the brain: Scanning the brain.* Retrieved August 2017, from www.pbs.org/wnet/brain/scanning/meg.html

PBS. (2001b). *The secret life of the brain.* Retrieved August 2017, from www.pbs.org/wnet/brain/

Seung, S. (2010). I am my connectome. *TEDGlobal.* Retrieved August 2017, from www.ted.com/talks/sebastian_seung

The Wellcome Trust. (2017). *Big picture: Bringing cutting edge science to the classroom and beyond.* Retrieved August 2017, from https://bigpictureeducation.com/are-we-born-all-brain-cells-we%e2%80%99ll-ever-have

Zero to Three. (2017). Retrieved August 2017, from www.zerotothree.org

Chapter 2

An introduction to paediatric acquired brain injury

Daniel Stark, Suresh Pujar, Isobel Heyman and Tara Murphy

The high prevalence of childhood acquired brain injury (ABI) is a major public health concern worldwide (Gerrard-Morris et al., 2010). In addition to trauma, the incidence of ABI is increasing in the context of advances in medical technology and treatment, with greater numbers of children surviving the acute stages of the ABI, but often with increased rates of morbidity. Adverse effects are seen across a range of domains, including impacts on physical, cognitive, social, emotional and behavioural functioning.

Correspondingly, the research focus has shifted from the acute and post-acute stages of ABI to children's longer-term cognitive, emotional, behavioural, social and academic outcomes. Hence ABI is a topic of interest across many fields – for example, neurology, rehabilitation medicine, psychiatry, psychology, social care – for both practitioners and researchers. The following chapter presents an overview of the literature on factors affecting the incidence and outcomes of ABI, including a summary of the medical aspects affecting children's care.

Definition

The term "acquired brain injury" is expansive, referring to any traumatic or non-traumatic brain insult sustained in the post-neonatal period (Chevignard, Toure, Brugel, Poirier, & Laurent-Vannier, 2009) and is a leading cause of death and disability in childhood (Forsyth & Kirkham, 2012). Traumatic injury is caused by an external force such as a collision, fall, assault or blast injury. Non-traumatic injury may be due to brain tumours, central nervous system (CNS) infection, hypoxia or a cerebrovascular event.

The definition of ABI excludes hereditary, congenital and degenerative conditions, or injuries caused by birth trauma, although, clearly, these are also a form of injury or atypical change which can occur to a child's brain. Cerebral palsy is an example of an umbrella term – describing children traditionally thought to have predominantly motor difficulties, whose brain injuries occur before, during or immediately after birth. Although this group will not be further discussed here, the cerebral palsy literature is informative for ABI, as these children are now known to additionally have extensive rates of cognitive, emotional and behavioural difficulties – similar to many cases of ABI (see for example Parkes et al. 2008).

Further, ABI is distinct from neurodevelopmental conditions such as hyperkinetic disorder/attention deficit hyperactivity disorder (ADHD), autism spectrum disorder, chromosomal disorder or specific learning disorder, which are associated with an innate atypical course of development, although many children with ABI acquire atypical development after the injury (Ball & Karmiloff-Smith, 2014).

Epidemiology

It is estimated that non-traumatic acquired brain injuries (including infection and hypoxia – ischemia, stroke and brain tumours) resulting in major neurological morbidity affect about 1,300 children in the UK (population about 60 million) each year. This is equivalent to the all-severity incidence of cerebral palsy (Forsyth & Kirkham, 2012). In a UK study by Hayes and colleagues (2017), 4,508 children aged 1–18 years in England had an ABI severe enough to warrant substantial rehabilitation over a nine-year period.

Traumatic brain injury (TBI) is one of the most common causes of death or disability in children worldwide. In more economically developed countries, childhood mortality from TBI is second only to death from congenital disease (Feickert, Drommer, & Heyer, 1999). The prevalence of paediatric TBI is difficult to determine, and in 2004, the World Health Organisation (WHO) reported that more high-quality research was required (Cassidy et al., 2004). Current estimates vary: a study from New Zealand estimated the prevalence in individuals under the age of 25 years to be 110–236 per 100 000 (McKinlay et al., 2008).

Factors affecting incidence of ABI

Identifying factors affecting the incidence of ABI is difficult due to its heterogeneous nature. For example, there are clearly established risk factors for the development of brain tumours (e.g. environmental and infectious agents; Baldwin & Preston-Martin, 2004). ABI as a result of injury or accident varies according to a number of factors, which can result in differing insults to the developing brain.

Population-based studies have indicated that age has a strong relationship with TBI, with a bimodal peak incidence – first in early childhood and then in late-adolescence/early adulthood (Bruns & Hauser, 2003), reflecting greater independence of activities with age. Non-accidental injury due to child abuse is an important cause of ABI in infants. Parslow et al. (2005) described the most common causes of TBI in children admitted to ten paediatric intensive care units in the UK and Ireland, with results presented in Figure 2.1.

Previous research has highlighted that male children from more vulnerable socioeconomic backgrounds (Amram et al., 2015) with pre-existing cognitive or behavioural problems are at greatest risk for sustaining a TBI (McKinlay et al., 2010). For example, children who sustain repeated head injuries are more likely

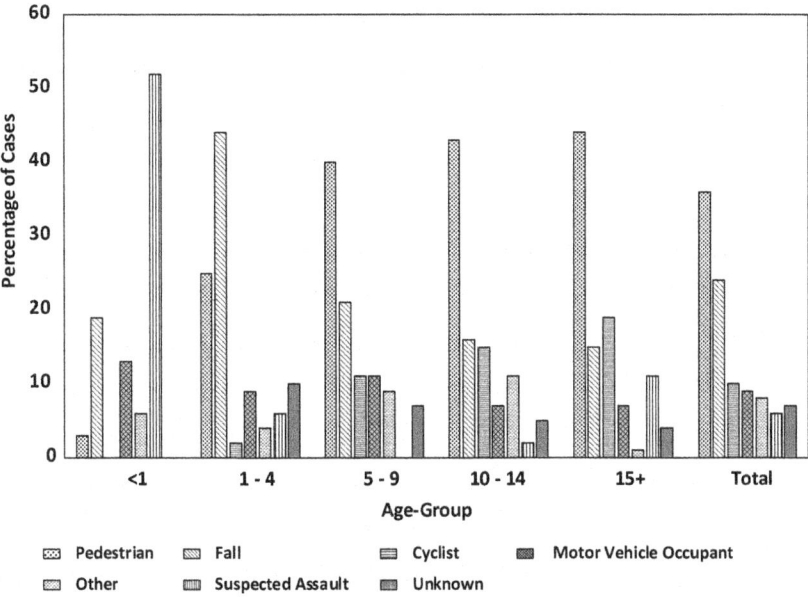

Figure 2.1 Data extracted from Parslow et al. (2005) highlighting the relationship between age and cause of TBI

to be described pre-injury as disobedient, destructive, hyperactive and prone to fighting with other children (Murgio, 2003). Similarly, using a virtual reality paradigm, children with ADHD performed significantly poorer on a road-cross safety task (Clancy, Rucklidge, & Owen, 2006). This risky, premorbid behaviour is thought to increase the risk of sustaining a TBI.

However, data from real-world studies have produced conflicting findings on the relationship between ADHD and TBI (Adeyemo et al., 2014). The rate of TBI has also been found to vary with socioeconomic status (SES). Many studies have found that a significantly higher proportion of children from poor social backgrounds sustain TBIs (Hippisley-Cox et al., 2002; Parslow et al., 2005; Taylor et al., 1999). This has been attributed to decreased supervision; lower levels of information about the use of preventative strategies, such as helmets; and exposure to more hazardous environments and exposure to a higher volume of fast-moving traffic (Murgio, 2003).

A further substantial factor affecting the prevalence of ABI are the advances in diagnostics and improvements in acute management of conditions involving the central nervous system. This has led to increases in survival rates across a range of conditions. As a result, there are significantly more children surviving following moderate to severe ABI, but with considerable morbidity (Anderson, Fenwick, Manly, & Robertson, 1998).

Mechanism of injury and recovery following ABI

There are a diverse range of aetiologies for ABIs, including multiple forms of traumatic injury as well as a range of medical conditions influenced by genetic, epigenetic and environmental factors (e.g. infection and tumours). In recent decades, additional iatrogenic causes of ABI are emerging, such as assertive cancer treatments involving surgical treatment and cranial irradiation (for example, Tonning Olsonn et al. 2014). Despite this, the pathophysiological processes underlying the neuronal injury are common to all.

In addition to the direct injury caused by trauma/ischaemia, the mechanisms of inflammation, oxidative injury and excitotoxicity may all be triggered and work synergistically to precipitate necrotic and apoptotic neuronal loss (Morrison, Fraser, & Cepinskas, 2013). In addition, in the immediate aftermath, individuals with ABI are at risk of secondary brain injury due to preventable factors such as cerebral hypoperfusion, hypoxia, acidosis, hypo/hyperglycemia and hyperthermia. Further, many of the drugs routinely utilised after ABI in intensive care setting, such as some sedatives, analgesics and anti-epileptics, have been shown to up-regulate pathological apoptosis and increase neuronal loss in experimental studies (Morrison et al., 2013).

Plasticity is a core property of the CNS, reflecting its ability to change and re-organise over the course of development as well as in the face of changing environmental stimuli (Kolb & Gibb, 2011). Modern research has highlighted the bidirectional role of genetics, neurobiology, cognition/behaviour and environmental factors in the development of the CNS, which are core features of Interactive Specialisation Theory (IST; Johnson, 2011). Under typical developmental processes, IST indicates how cortical regions develop greater specialisation and localisation of function, resulting in more efficient processing of information and more adult-like levels of performance. However, ABI is associated with differing cascades of ionic response, neurotransmitter release, cellular changes, synaptic remodelling and, potentially, altered network connectivity (Giza et al., 2009), with corresponding impact on behavioural and cognitive outcome.

In certain instances, plasticity allows the transfer of important functions from damaged to undamaged areas of the brain, leading to recovery of function, whilst at other times, specific developmental processes can be impeded, with poorer functional outcome recorded (e.g. Anderson, Catroppa, Morse, Haritou, & Rosenfeld, 2005). The individual course of recovery and, ultimately, the developmental outcome of the child, are shaped by a range of factors. These include pre-injury factors, factors related to the injury itself in addition to individual and environmental variables.

A range of approaches and treatments are available following injury. Medications such as amantadine, apomorphine and zolpidem can be used to treat disorders of consciousness following severe brain injuries (Gosseries et al., 2014). There is also promising experimental and clinical data showing the efficacy of the 5-HT1A receptor agonist therapy in conferring histological protection and facilitating neurobehavioural and cognitive recovery after adult or paediatric brain trauma (Cheng et al., 2016). Encouraged by the beneficial effect in newborns with hypoxic-ischaemic encephalopathy (Jacobs et al., 2013), therapeutic hypothermia was tried in children with TBI, but this was associated with increased mortality and adverse outcomes and, therefore, not recommended (Crompton et al., 2017).

Whilst there is emerging evidence for neuroprotective therapies, morbidity remains commonplace. Multidisciplinary rehabilitation remains the predominant form of clinical response. In the UK, the NHS aims to refer children with severe ABIs to regional paediatric neuroscience centres and emphasises the importance of early access to specialist neurorehabilitation following the acute management. There is no data available on the implementation of this, and marked geographic variability of access to services has been noted in the UK (Hayes et al., 2017). The need for longer-term psychosocial rehabilitation in which a multidisciplinary approach is primary has been recognised but is covered within other chapters in this volume.

Within the broader scope of rehabilitation, cognitive training is an area ripe for further research and implementation. To date, research is growing in cognitive rehabilitation, although limited by generalisation of transfer to real-world experience, small sample sizes, assessment of long-term outcome and over focus on specific cognitive domains (Slomine & Locascio, 2009; Cox et al., 2015; Eve at al., 2016; Fuentes & Kerr, 2017; Gorman, Barnes, Swank, & Ewing-Cobbs, 2017). Overall, there is a paucity of research on the long-term effectiveness of rehabilitation on the child's cognitive, behavioural, social, educational and emotional outcomes following ABI.

Outcomes after ABI and predictors of outcomes

Prognostic factors

There is a clear need to identify factors affecting outcome in ABI so that the child's current and future needs can be identified and managed. The cause of the ABI is a major determinant of outcome; consequently, most of the literature concerning outcome prediction is aetiology specific. Factors related to outcome have been most extensively studied in the TBI literature, and the need for further research in the non-TBI literature is well recognised (Schagen et al., 2014). However, even amongst children with TBI, there is a paucity of research, and extant studies are characterised by small samples, which often preclude the analysis of factors contributing to outcome, such as age, socioeconomic effects and characteristics of the ABI.

Injury variables

Given the diverse range of aetiology in ABI, there are multiple factors related to the ABI that impact on outcome. Amongst the best-established predictor of outcome is injury severity (usually defined on the basis of the Glasgow Coma Scale (GCS) score combined with clinical findings), with the strongest evidence coming from the TBI literature (Babikian & Asarnow, 2009). Whilst the impact of mild TBI remains a controversial area, moderate and severe TBIs are associated with negative outcomes across a range of cognitive domains, including attention, information processing, memory and executive function. There are also persisting deficits in social functioning, behavioural difficulties in addition to increased rates of mental health difficulties, such as anxiety and depression (Di Battista, Godfrey, Soo, Catroppa, & Anderson, 2014).

Whilst some clinical severity indices such as the motor component of the GCS, post-traumatic amnesia and pupil reactivity have been shown to be of predictive value, there is much individual variability and, therefore, recovery following ABI is difficult to predict. The cause of TBI has also been associated with outcome. For example, inflicted TBI is associated with particularly poor outcomes, with high rates of mortality and significant morbidity amongst survivors (Lind et al., 2016).

Other forms of ABI are associated with different outcomes, with a diverse range of variables thought to impact on outcome. For instance, long-term follow-up studies of children with brain tumours have resulted in mixed findings. Maddrey et al. (2005) reported ten-year, follow-up data on children with medulloblastomas who had been treated with resection and radiotherapy, with additional chemotherapy in a sub-sample. Mean FSIQ scores were low (FSIQ = 75), indicating substantial combined impact on children's broader intellectual functioning. In contrast, Aarsen et al. (2009) reported that three years post-diagnosis, the intellectual abilities of children with pilocytic astrocytomas were in the average range. However, difficulties with sustained attention, visual-spatial memory and executive functioning, as well as poorer verbal IQ scores, were found. Greater difficulties in cognitive functioning were associated with different tumour locations (e.g. supratentorial vs. infratentorial tumours) as well as additional factors such as the presence of hydrocephalus, radiotherapy, residual tumour size after treatment and age.

Hypoxic and hypoxic-ischaemic injuries represent a further distinct form of ABI, with brain injury mediated by a combination of the degree of metabolic demand of the affected tissue and the degree of innervation/proximity to blood-supply (Caine & Watson, 2000). Specific outcomes are again dependent on aetiology of injury. Cardiac arrest in children is associated with particularly poor outcome (6.4% survival rate when occurring out of hospital; Atkins et al., 2009). In contrast, near drowning is associated with higher survival rates. A meta-analysis (Quan et al., 2016) demonstrated that duration of submersion was the most significant predictor of neurological outcome. Other factors that have been proposed as protective (e.g. low water temperature) were not found to significantly impact on outcome.

Other authors have emphasised the role of the temporal pattern of the ABI. For example, better outcomes have been reported amongst children with slow-growing tumours compared to acute lesions, such as stroke (Desmurget, Bonnetblanc, & Duffau, 2007). Such data suggest greater compensatory plasticity in the face of gradually developing ABIs compared to acute injuries such as stroke and TBI.

Cognitive reserve

In assessing outcome, the concept of a "cognitive reserve" has been researched in the adult brain injury literature. It is seen as a complex moderating variable, which often poses clinicians with the puzzling question of why individuals with the same level of brain pathology show different levels of impairment. Cognitive reserve can be conceptualised as the ability of the brain to cope with damage or insult by using pre-existing cognitive processes or compensatory mechanisms (Stern, 2009). This process allows certain individuals to sustain damage and maintain cognitive function compared to others.

The concept is assessed by socioeconomic status, family function and education status in addition to measures of language (Dennis et al., 2006). Adults with higher levels of education pre-injury (alongside estimates of larger pre-injury brain size) show more intact cognitive outcome post-injury (Kesler, Adams, Blasey, & Bigler, 2003). However, the results are more equivocal in paediatric populations post-ABI. In one study, performance on literacy and language tasks, which are thought to be the best predictors of premorbid intellectual ability in adult populations, did not predict cognitive outcome (Fuentes, McKay, & Hay, 2010). Other studies showed that pre-injury academic ability and learning disorder, alongside maternal education and severity of brain injury, were predictive of outcome following ABI (Fay et al., 2010; Farmer et al., 2002; Kesler, Tanaka, & Koovakkattu, 2010).

Age at injury

Whilst injury severity has a long-established relationship with outcome, the timing of brain insult has also emerged as a significant prognostic factor in the last 15–20 years. In direct contrast to long-held views of greater plasticity and recovery of function the younger the child (i.e. "the Kennard principle"), recent research has highlighted strong interactional effects between the severity of injury and the age at which it is sustained. Such data indicates a "double-hazard", with poorest outcomes for young children sustaining severe injuries (Anderson et al., 2005).

Subsequent studies have indicated that TBI before the age of three years is associated with particularly poor outcomes across a range of intellectual, cognitive and functional outcome domains (Anderson et al., 2014). These findings would suggest that brain insult before the age of three has a substantial impact on the development and specialisation of multiple cortical networks which adversely affects the development of cognitive skills. Earlier age at injury diminishes cognitive reserve by preventing the child from acquiring efficient cognitive strategies that may have otherwise been recruited to maintain function after brain insult

(Dennis et al., 2006). Amongst survivors of drowning, age has not been found to significantly contribute to outcome (Quan et al., 2016).

Biomarkers of outcomes after ABI

Brain imaging may aid in predicting outcomes as damage to particular brain regions can result in specific cognitive and behavioural difficulties. For example, frontal and temporal lesions have been associated with impaired executive functioning and poorer memory and learning outcomes (A. R. Johnson, DeMatt, & Salorio, 2009). Likewise, left hemisphere injury is associated with poorer language and communication abilities (Fyrberg, Horneman, Asberg Johnels, Thunberg, & Ahlsen, 2017).

In addition to conventional structural neuroimaging, diffusion tensor imaging (DTI), functional neuroimaging techniques such as functional MRI (fMRI), positron emission tomography (PET), single-photon emission computed tomography (SPECT) and transcranial magnetic stimulation (TMS), using resting state, passive and active paradigms, have been employed in the assessment and prognosis of disorders of consciousness often associated with ABI (Gosseries et al., 2016).

A meta-analysis of resting state functional neuroimaging studies in disorders of consciousness showed markedly reduced activity within the midline cortical and subcortical structures, anatomical structures linked to the default-mode network (Hannawi, Lindquist, Caffo, Sair, & Stevens, 2015). Similarly, white matter integrity measured using DTI has been shown to predict recovery following ABI. Whilst fractional anisotropy (FA) increase, particularly in corticospinal tracts, is associated with a favourable outcome, FA remained depressed in those with poor recovery following TBI (Sidaros et al., 2008; Kraus et al., 2007; Galanaud et al., 2012). In a recent study, Ryan and colleagues demonstrated association between increased cognitive fatigue and volumetric reductions in the cortico-striatal network (CSN) circuitry and its putative hub regions, 24 months post-TBI in children (Ryan et al., 2016). Whilst these advanced neuroimaging techniques could provide useful prognostic information, further validation is required before such research techniques are integrated into clinical practice (Gosseries et al., 2016).

Neurophysiological studies such as electroencephalogram (EEG) and evoked potentials may have predictive value following ABI (Forsyth & Kirkham, 2012). Certain findings in conventional EEG, such as burst suppression and α coma, are recognised as indicators of major disruption of brain function, but they may also be induced by anaesthetic drugs. Persistent absence of somatosensory evoked potentials (in the absence of subdural haemorrhage or severe selective brain stem injury) is specific for a poor outcome after ABI in adults but has not been specifically validated in children.

In addition to brain imaging and neurophysiology, several authors have investigated injury biomarkers in cerebrospinal fluid (CSF) and blood, thought to be largely expressed in brain parenchyma, for their ability to predict outcomes mostly after severe TBI. In a systematic review, correlations were found between elevated

CSF biomarkers and either poor outcomes (interleukin-8, interleukin-1β, neuron-specific enolase, endothelin-1, High-Mobility Group Box 3.1, and cytochrome C) or good outcomes (nerve growth factor, doublecortin and interleukin-6; Daoud et al., 2014). Blood biomarkers correlated with outcomes were glial fibrillary acidic protein, hyperphosphorylated neurofilament, Ubiquitin C-Terminal Hydrolase-L1, αII-Spectrin breakdown product 145 kDa, and leptin. In this review, outcomes were defined as either in-hospital mortality or functional outcomes such as Glasgow Outcomes Scale or Pediatric Cerebral Performance Category. The review suggests that no single biomarker has the sensitivity or specificity in predicting outcomes and highlights the need for identifying and validating novel brain injury biomarkers and/or biomarker panels with greater sensitivity and specificity.

Pre-injury variables

When considering TBI, in addition to injury variables, pre-injury factors have been found to be strong predictors of long-term behavioural outcomes. A number of studies have demonstrated that pre-injury levels of anxiety, anger, aggression and behavioural difficulties are strong predictors of behavioural problems post-TBI (e.g. Cole et al., 2008; Catroppa, Anderson, Morse, Haritou, & Rosenfeld, 2008), with the latter study accounting for comparable levels of variance as injury severity. Pre-injury ADHD may be a risk factor for sustaining a TBI, and it is also associated with poorer recovery and increased rates of disability (Bonfield, Lam, Lin, & Greene, 2013). Similar trends have also been found for adaptive outcomes (Catroppa et al., 2008), with pre-injury levels remaining strong predictors ten-years post-injury (Anderson, Godfrey, Rosenfeld, & Catroppa, 2012).

Environmental variables

Enriching environments have a long-standing relationship with optimal developmental outcomes, which have also been proposed to be a substantial factor in recovery from ABI. Animal models have demonstrated greater cortical thickness and increased numbers of dendrites and synapses amongst animals housed in enriched environments after injury (Giza, Kolb, Harris, Asarnow, & Prins, 2009). Involvement of the family and broader system around the child within the rehabilitation network suggests more positive outcome for function (McKinlay et al, 2016).

A number of environmental factors have been found to be predictive of outcome amongst children sustaining TBI. Amongst the most robust factors are socioeconomic effects, with lower SES most significantly associated with adverse behavioural outcomes (Li & Liu, 2013). Other studies have also linked SES with cognitive and intellectual outcomes, accounting for approximately 20% of the variance in Full Scale IQ at three years post-injury (Crowe et al., 2012). However, with conflicting data presented from other samples (e.g. Anderson et al., 2014), SES may be best conceptualised as a proxy variable, and without studies examining the specific constituent variables, it's use in clinical interventions is questionable.

The family environment has been identified as an important predictor of the child's functioning after brain injury. For example, higher ratings of family function (e.g. family communication and supportiveness) have been associated with better behavioural adjustment and improved adaptive outcomes 18-months post-injury. Furthermore, authoritative parenting has been found to be predictive of better social competence, whereas permissive parenting styles were associated with poorer social outcomes (Yeates, Taylor, Walz, Stancin, & Wade, 2010). A number of studies have demonstrated high rates of parental mental health difficulties following ABI in their children, with demonstrable relationships between parental psychological functioning and rates of both internalising (e.g. Peterson et al., 2013) and externalising difficulties (e.g. Raj et al., 2013) in children. However, there are clearly a range of complex, inter-related reciprocal relationships between family and environmental factors and outcomes following ABI. This has been investigated longitudinally; using statistical controls in their methodology, child behavioural difficulties 6-months post-TBI predicted higher parental distress at 12-months, and, conversely, parental distress at 6-months predicted more behavioural difficulties at 12-months (Taylor et al., 2001).

Emotional and behavioural function

Children with ABI have a substantial risk (10%–50%) for a new psychiatric disorder emerging after the injury (Li & Liu, 2013). As mentioned, some pre-existing conditions such as ADHD may be a risk factor for acquiring a brain injury (impulsive or reckless behaviour making a child more accident-prone), but many more children have a psychiatric disorder for the first time post-injury (Brown, Chadwick, Shaffer, Rutter, & Traub, 1981). All of the common childhood psychiatric conditions are over-represented in children with ABI.

From studies that have compared the impact of a severe orthopaedic injury (non-head/brain) with a brain injury, it is apparent that the major component of the increased risk is mediated by direct brain effects on behaviour and emotional function, as children suffering the painful, disabling and often chronic impact of non-brain injury do not have markedly elevated rates of psychiatric disorder seen in brain injured children (see Heyman et al., 2015). Changes in cognitive functioning, especially abnormalities in executive functioning and social abilities may in turn have a negative impact on emotions and behaviour, especially as the child matures and becomes more aware of the differences between themselves and other children their age.

Detection and evaluation of any new emotional and behavioural problems in children with ABI is important, as the impact of these on day-to-day life for the child and family may be significant. When considering intervention for mental health difficulties following ABI, there is a well-recognised paucity of research. As such, it should be assumed that the same mechanisms of change that underpin evidence-based interventions in typically developing populations will also be effective in ABI populations. Interventions are likely to include parent training for challenging behaviour and psychological treatments and medication for anxiety and depression.

However, evidence-based interventions may require adaptation so that they can be accessed effectively by children and families. These may well include accounting for the child's developmental stage and premorbid functioning, the impact of the ABI on their developmental trajectory across various domains and the broader family's functioning and resources. Services need to prioritise interventions for mental health problems in these children, as their successful treatment can markedly improve the quality of life for the child and family (e.g. Brown, Whittingham, Boyd, McKinlay, & Sofronoff, 2014).

Conclusions

ABI is a leading cause of neurological disability in children and is associated with a range of long-term, negative, cognitive, social, psychiatric, psychological and academic outcomes (Treble-Barna et al., 2017). Research is beginning to reveal high-risk groups and to identify factors which may be predictive of outcome. These associations are complex, often bidirectional and involve biological and environmental factors. However, much of the research is based on TBI, which leaves questions about how these findings apply to children with ABI with its range of differing aetiologies. With ongoing research, our understanding of the biological, psychological and social mechanisms underlying the impairment in ABI are improving and there is, therefore, an expectation that rehabilitation can be more effectively tailored to the child and family's individual needs. This is an area ripe for further research and an opportunity for scientists and clinicians to work collaboratively with the aim of improving outcomes for children and families affected by ABI.

References

Aarsen, F. K., Paquier, P. F., Arts, W. F., Van Veelen, M. L., Michiels, E., Lequin, M., & Catsman-Berrevoets, C. E. (2009). Cognitive deficits and predictors 3 years after diagnosis of a pilocytic astrocytoma in childhood. *Journal of Clinical Oncology*, *27*(21), 3526–3532. doi:10.1200/JCO.2008.19.6303

Adeyemo, B. O., Biederman, J., Zafonte, R., Kagan, E., Spencer, T. J., Uchida, M., . . . Faraone, S. V. (2014). Mild traumatic brain injury and adhd: A systematic review of the literature and meta-analysis. *Journal of Attention Disorders*, *18*(7), 576–584. doi:10.1177/1087054714543371

Amram, O., Schuurman, N., Pike, I., Yanchar, N. L., Friger, M., McBeth, P. B., & Griesdale, D. (2015). Socio economic status and traumatic brain injury amongst pediatric populations: A spatial analysis in greater vancouver. *International Journal of Environmental Research and Public Health*, *12*(12), 15594–15604. doi:10.3390/ijerph121215009

Anderson, V., Catroppa, C., Morse, S., Haritou, F., & Rosenfeld, J. (2005). Functional plasticity or vulnerability after early brain injury? *Pediatrics*, *116*(6), 1374–1382. doi:10.1542/peds.2004-1728

Anderson, V., Fenwick, T., Manly, T., & Robertson, I. (1998). Attentional skills following traumatic brain injury in childhood: A componential analysis. *Brain Injury*, *12*(11), 937–949.

Anderson, V., Godfrey, C., Rosenfeld, J. V., & Catroppa, C. (2012). Predictors of cognitive function and recovery 10 years after traumatic brain injury in young children. *Pediatrics*, *129*(2), e254–e261. doi:10.1542/peds.2011-0311

Anderson, V., Spencer-Smith, M. M., Coleman, L., Anderson, P. J., Greenham, M., Jacobs, R., . . . Leventer, R. J. (2014). Predicting neurocognitive and behavioural outcome after early brain insult. *Developmental Medicine & Child Neurology*, *56*(4), 329–336. doi:10.1111/dmcn.12387

Atkins, D. L., Everson-Stewart, S., Sears, G. K., Daya, M., Osmond, M. H., Warden, C. R., . . . Resuscitation Outcomes Consortium, I. (2009). Epidemiology and outcomes from out-of-hospital cardiac arrest in children: The resuscitation outcomes consortium epistry-cardiac arrest. *Circulation*, *119*(11), 1484–1491. doi:10.1161/CIRCULATIONAHA.108.802678

Babikian, T., & Asarnow, R. (2009). Neurocognitive outcomes and recovery after pediatric TBI: Meta-analytic review of the literature. *Neuropsychology*, *23*(3), 283–296. doi:10.1037/a0015268

Baldwin, R. T., & Preston-Martin, S. (2004). Epidemiology of brain tumors in childhood – a review. *Toxicology and Applied Pharmacology*, *199*(2), 118–131. doi:10.1016/j.taap.2003.12.029

Ball, G., & Karmiloff-Smith, A. (2014). Why development matters in neurodevelopmental disorders. *Neurodevelopmental Disorders: Research Challenges and Solutions*, 19.

Bonfield, C. M., Lam, S., Lin, Y., & Greene, S. (2013). The impact of attention deficit hyperactivity disorder on recovery from mild traumatic brain injury. *Journal of Neurosurgery: Pediatrics*, *12*(2), 97–102. doi:10.3171/2013.5.PEDS12424

Brown, F. L., Whittingham, K., Boyd, R. N., McKinlay, L., & Sofronoff, K. (2014). Improving child and parenting outcomes following paediatric acquired brain injury: A randomised controlled trial of stepping stones triple p plus acceptance and commitment therapy. *Journal of Child Psychology and Psychiatry*, *55*(10), 1172–1183. doi:10.1111/jcpp.12227

Brown, G., Chadwick, O., Shaffer, D., Rutter, M., & Traub, M. (1981). A prospective study of children with head injuries: Iii. Psychiatric sequelae. *Psychological Medicine*, *11*(1), 63–78.

Bruns, J., Jr., & Hauser, W. A. (2003). The epidemiology of traumatic brain injury: A review. *Epilepsia*, *44* (Suppl 10), 2–10.

Caine, D., & Watson, J. D. (2000). Neuropsychological and neuropathological sequelae of cerebral anoxia: A critical review. *Journal of the International Neuropsychological Society*, *6*(1), 86–99.

Cassidy, J. D., Carroll, L. J., Peloso, P. M., Borg, J., von Holst, H., Holm, L., . . . WHO Collaborating Centre Task Force on Mild Traumatic Brain Injury. (2004). Incidence, risk factors and prevention of mild traumatic brain injury: Results of the WHO Collaborating Centre Task Force on Mild Traumatic Brain Injury. *Journal of Rehabilitation Medicine*, (43 Suppl), 28–60.

Catroppa, C., Anderson, V. A., Morse, S. A., Haritou, F., & Rosenfeld, J. V. (2008). Outcome and predictors of functional recovery 5 years following pediatric traumatic brain injury (tbi). *Journal of Pediatric Psychology*, *33*(7), 707–718. doi:10.1093/jpepsy/jsn006

Chevignard, M., Toure, H., Brugel, D. G., Poirier, J., & Laurent-Vannier, A. (2010). A comprehensive model of care for rehabilitation of children with acquired brain injuries. *Child: Care, Health and Development, 36*(1), 31–43. doi:10.1111/j.1365-2214.2009.00949.x

Cheng, J. P., Leary, J. B., Sembhi, A., Edwards, C. M., Bondi, C. O., & Kline, A. E. (2016). 5-hydroxytryptamine 1a (5-ht 1a) receptor agonists: A decade of empirical evidence supports their use as an efficacious therapeutic strategy for brain trauma. *Brain Research, 1640*, 5–14.

Clancy, T. A., Rucklidge, J. J., & Owen, D. (2006). Road-crossing safety in virtual reality: A comparison of adolescents with and without ADHD. *Journal of Clinical Child & Adolescent Psychology, 35*(2), 203–215. doi:10.1207/s15374424jccp3502_4

Cole, W. R., Gerring, J. P., Gray, R. M., Vasa, R. A., Salorio, C. F., Grados, M., . . . Slomine, B. S. (2008). Prevalence of aggressive behaviour after severe paediatric traumatic brain injury. *Brain Injury, 22*(12), 932–939.

Cox, L. E., Ashford, J. M., Clark, K. N., Martin-Elbahesh, K., Hardy, K. K., Merchant, T. E., . . . Conklin, H. M. (2015). Feasibility and acceptability of a remotely administered computerized intervention to address cognitive late effects among childhood cancer survivors. *Neurooncology Practice, 2*(2), 78–87. doi:10.1093/nop/npu036

Crompton, E. M., Lubomirova, I., Cotlarciuc, I., Han, T. S., Sharma, S. D., & Sharma, P. (2017). Meta-analysis of therapeutic hypothermia for traumatic brain injury in adult and pediatric patients. *Critical Care Medicine, 45*(4), 575–583. doi:10.1097/CCM.0000000000002205

Crowe, L. M., Catroppa, C., Babl, F. E., & Anderson, V. (2012). Intellectual, behavioral, and social outcomes of accidental traumatic brain injury in early childhood. *Pediatrics, 129*(2), e262–e268. doi:10.1542/peds.2011-0438

Daoud, H., Alharfi, I., Alhelali, I., Stewart, T. C., Qasem, H., & Fraser, D. D. (2014). Brain injury biomarkers as outcome predictors in pediatric severe traumatic brain injury. *Neurocritical Care, 20*(3), 427–435.

Dennis, M., Yeates, K. O., Taylor, H. G., & Fletcher, J. M. (2006). Brain reserve capacity, cognitive reserve capacity, and age-based functional plasticity after congenital and acquired brain injury in children. *Cognitive Reserve: Theory and Applications*, 53–83.

Desmurget, M., Bonnetblanc, F., & Duffau, H. (2007). Contrasting acute and slow-growing lesions: A new door to brain plasticity. *Brain, 130*(Pt 4), 898–914. doi:10.1093/brain/awl300

Di Battista, A., Godfrey, C., Soo, C., Catroppa, C., & Anderson, V. (2014). Depression and health related quality of life in adolescent survivors of a traumatic brain injury: A pilot study. *PloS One, 9*(7), e101842.

Eve, M., O'Keeffe, F., Jhuty, S., Ganesan, V., Brown, G., & Murphy, T. (2016). Computerized working-memory training for children following arterial ischemic stroke: A pilot study with long-term follow-up. *Applied Neuropsychology Child, 5*(4), 273–282. doi: 10.1080/21622965.2015.1055563

Farmer, J. E., Kanne, S. M., Haut, J. S., Williams, J., Johnstone, B., & Kirk, K. (2002). Memory functioning following traumatic brain injury in children with premorbid learning problems. *Developmental Neuropsychology, 22*(2), 455–469. doi:10.1207/S15326942DN2202_2

Feickert, H. J., Drommer, S., & Heyer, R. (1999). Severe head injury in children: impact of risk factors on outcome. *Journal of Trauma, 47*(1), 33–38.

Fay, T. B., Yeates, K. O., Taylor, H. G., Bangert, B., Dietrich, A., Nuss, K. E., . . . Wright, M. (2010). Cognitive reserve as a moderator of postconcussive symptoms in children with complicated and uncomplicated mild traumatic brain injury. *Journal of the International Neuropsychological Society*, *16*(1), 94–105.

Forsyth, R., & Kirkham, F. (2012). Predicting outcome after childhood brain injury. *CMAJ*, *184*(11), 1257–1264. doi:10.1503/cmaj.111045

Fuentes, A., & Kerr, E. N. (2017). Maintenance effects of working memory intervention (cogmed) in children with symptomatic epilepsy. *Epilepsy & Behavior*, *67*, 51–59. doi:10.1016/j.yebeh.2016.12.016

Fuentes, A., McKay, C., & Hay, C. (2010). Cognitive reserve in paediatric traumatic brain injury: Relationship with neuropsychological outcome. *Brain Injury*, *24*(7–8), 995–1002. doi:10.3109/02699052.2010.489791

Fyrberg, A., Horneman, G., Asberg Johnels, J., Thunberg, G., & Ahlsen, E. (2017). Communication in children and adolescents after acquired brain injury: An exploratory study. *Journal of Rehabilitation Medicine*, *49*(7), 572–578. doi:10.2340/16501977-2243

Galanaud, D., Perlbarg, V., Gupta, R., Stevens, R. D., Sanchez, P., Tollard, E., . . . Recovery, C. (2012). Assessment of white matter injury and outcome in severe brain trauma: A prospective multicenter cohort. *Anesthesiology*, *117*(6), 1300–1310. doi:10.1097/ALN.0b013e3182755558

Gerrard-Morris, A., Taylor, H. G., Yeates, K. O., Walz, N. C., Stancin, T., Minich, N., & Wade, S. L. (2010). Cognitive development after traumatic brain injury in young children. *Journal of the International Neuropsychological Society*, *16*(1), 157–168. doi:10.1017/S1355617709991135

Giza, C. C., Kolb, B., Harris, N. G., Asarnow, R. F., & Prins, M. L. (2009). Hitting a moving target: Basic mechanisms of recovery from acquired developmental brain injury. *Developmental Neurorehabilitation*, *12*(5), 255–268. doi:10.3109/17518420903087558

Gorman, S., Barnes, M. A., Swank, P. R., & Ewing-Cobbs, L. (2017). Recovery of working memory following pediatric traumatic brain injury: A longitudinal analysis. *Developmental Neuropsychology*, *42*(3), 127–145. doi:10.1080/87565641.2017.1315581

Gosseries, O., Charland-Verville, V., Thonnard, M., Bodart, O., Laureys, S., & Demertzi, A. (2014). Amantadine, apomorphine and zolpidem in the treatment of disorders of consciousness. *Current Pharmaceutical Design*, *20*(26), 4167–4184.

Gosseries, O., Pistoia, F., Charland-Verville, V., Carolei, A., Sacco, S., & Laureys, S. (2016). The role of neuroimaging techniques in establishing diagnosis, prognosis and therapy in disorders of consciousness. *The Open Neuroimaging Journal*, *10*, 52–68. doi:10.2174/1874440001610010052

Hannawi, Y., Lindquist, M. A., Caffo, B. S., Sair, H. I., & Stevens, R. D. (2015). Resting brain activity in disorders of consciousness: A systematic review and meta-analysis. *Neurology*, *84*(12), 1272–1280. doi:10.1212/WNL.0000000000001404

Hayes, L., Shaw, S., Pearce, M. S., & Forsyth, R. J. (2017). Requirements for and current provision of rehabilitation services for children after severe acquired brain injury in the uk: A population-based study. *Archives of Disease in Childhood*. doi:10.1136/archdischild-2016-312166

Heyman, I., Skuse, D., Goodman, R., Thapar, A., Pine, D. S., Leckman, J. F., . . . Taylor, E. (2015). Brain disorders and psychopathology. *Rutter's Child Adolesc Psychiatry*, *4*, 389–402.

Hippisley-Cox, J., Groom, L., Kendrick, D., Coupland, C., Webber, E., & Savelyich, B. (2002). Cross sectional survey of socioeconomic variations in severity and mechanism of childhood injuries in Trent 1992-7. *British Medical Journal*, *324*(7346), 1132.

Jacobs, S. E., Berg, M., Hunt, R., Tarnow-Mordi, W. O., Inder, T. E., & Davis, P. G. (2013). Cooling for newborns with hypoxic ischaemic encephalopathy. *Cochrane Database of Systematic Reviews* (1), CD003311. doi:10.1002/14651858.CD003311.pub3

Johnson, A. R., DeMatt, E., & Salorio, C. F. (2009). Predictors of outcome following acquired brain injury in children. *Developmental Disabilities Research Reviews, 15*(2), 124–132. doi:10.1002/ddrr.63

Johnson, M. H. (2011). Interactive specialization: A domain-general framework for human functional brain development? *Developmental Cognitive Neuroscience, 1*(1), 7–21. doi:10.1016/j.dcn.2010.07.003

Kesler, S. R., Adams, H. F., Blasey, C. M., & Bigler, E. D. (2003). Premorbid intellectual functioning, education, and brain size in traumatic brain injury: An investigation of the cognitive reserve hypothesis. *Applied Neuropsychology, 10*(3), 153–162. doi:10.1207/S15324826AN1003_04

Kesler, S. R., Tanaka, H., & Koovakkattu, D. (2010). Cognitive reserve and brain volumes in pediatric acute lymphoblastic leukemia. *Brain Imaging and Behavior, 4*(3–4), 256–269. doi:10.1007/s11682-010-9104-1

Kolb, B., & Gibb, R. (2011). Brain plasticity and behaviour in the developing brain. *Journal of the Canadian Academy of Child and Adolescent Psychiatry, 20*(4), 265–276.

Kraus, M. F., Susmaras, T., Caughlin, B. P., Walker, C. J., Sweeney, J. A., & Little, D. M. (2007). White matter integrity and cognition in chronic traumatic brain injury: A diffusion tensor imaging study. *Brain, 130*(Pt 10), 2508–2519. doi:10.1093/brain/awm216

Li, L., & Liu, J. (2013). The effect of pediatric traumatic brain injury on behavioral outcomes: A systematic review. *Developmental Medicine & Child Neurology, 55*(1), 37–45. doi:10.1111/j.1469-8749.2012.04414.x

Lind, K., Toure, H., Brugel, D., Meyer, P., Laurent-Vannier, A., & Chevignard, M. (2016). Extended follow-up of neurological, cognitive, behavioral and academic outcomes after severe abusive head trauma. *Child Abuse & Neglect, 51*, 358–367. doi:10.1016/j.chiabu.2015.08.001

Maddrey, A. M., Bergeron, J. A., Lombardo, E. R., McDonald, N. K., Mulne, A. F., Barenberg, P. D., & Bowers, D. C. (2005). Neuropsychological performance and quality of life of 10 year survivors of childhood medulloblastoma. *Journal of Neurooncology, 72*(3), 245–253. doi:10.1007/s11060-004-3009-z

McKinlay, A., Grace, R. C., Horwood, L. J., Fergusson, D. M., Ridder, E. M., & MacFarlane, M. R. (2008). Prevalence of traumatic brain injury among children, adolescents and young adults: Prospective evidence from a birth cohort. *Brain Injury, 22*(2), 175–181.

McKinlay, A., Kyonka, E., Grace, R., Horwood, L., Fergusson, D., & MacFarlane, M. (2010). An investigation of the pre-injury risk factors associated with children who experience traumatic brain injury. *Injury Prevention, 16*(1), 31–35.

McKinlay, A., Linden, M., DePompei, R., Aaro Jonsson, C., Anderson, V., Braga, L., . . . Wicks, B. (2016). Service provision for children and young people with acquired brain injury: Practice recommendations. *Brain Injury, 30*(13–14), 1656–1664. doi:10.1080/02699052.2016.1201592

Morrison, G., Fraser, D. D., & Cepinskas, G. (2013). Mechanisms and consequences of acquired brain injury during development. *Pathophysiology, 20*(1), 49–57. doi:10.1016/j.pathophys.2012.02.006

Murgio, A. (2003). Epidemiology of traumatic brain injury in children. *Revista Española de Neuropsicología, 5*(2), 137–161.

Olsson, I. T., Perrin, S., Lundgren, J., Hjorth, L., & Johanson, A. (2014). Long-term cognitive sequelae after pediatric brain tumor related to medical risk factors, age, and sex. *Pediatric Neurology, 51*(4), 515–521. doi:10.1016/j.pediatrneurol.2014.06.011

Parkes, J., White-Koning, M., Dickinson, H. O., Thyen, U., Arnaud, C., Beckung, E., . . . Colver, A. (2008). Psychological problems in children with cerebral palsy: A cross-sectional European study. *Journal of Child Psychology and Psychiatry, 49*(4), 405–413. doi:10.1111/j.1469-7610.2007.01845.x

Parslow, R. C., Morris, K. P., Tasker, R. C., Forsyth, R. J., Hawley, C. A., Group, U. K. P. T. B. I. S. S., & Paediatric Intensive Care Society Study, G. (2005). Epidemiology of traumatic brain injury in children receiving intensive care in the UK. *Archives of Disease in Childhood, 90*(11), 1182–1187. doi:10.1136/adc.2005.072405

Peterson, R. L., Kirkwood, M. W., Taylor, H. G., Stancin, T., Brown, T. M., & Wade, S. L. (2013). Adolescents' internalizing problems following traumatic brain injury are related to parents' psychiatric symptoms. *The Journal of Head Trauma Rehabilitation, 28*(5), E1–E12. doi:10.1097/HTR.0b013e318263f5ba

Quan, L., Bierens, J. J., Lis, R., Rowhani-Rahbar, A., Morley, P., & Perkins, G. D. (2016). Predicting outcome of drowning at the scene: A systematic review and meta-analyses. *Resuscitation, 104*, 63–75. doi:10.1016/j.resuscitation.2016.04.006

Raj, S. P., Wade, S. L., Cassedy, A., Taylor, H. G., Stancin, T., Brown, T. M., & Kirkwood, M. W. (2013). Parent psychological functioning and communication predict externalizing behavior problems after pediatric traumatic brain injury. *Journal of Pediatric Psychology, 39*(1), 84–95.

Ryan, N. P., Beauchamp, M. H., Beare, R., Coleman, L., Ditchfield, M., Kean, M., . . . Anderson, V. A. (2016). Uncovering cortico-striatal correlates of cognitive fatigue in pediatric acquired brain disorder: Evidence from traumatic brain injury. *Cortex, 83*, 222–230. doi:10.1016/j.cortex.2016.07.020

Schagen, S., Klein, M., Reijneveld, J., Brain, E., Deprez, S., Joly, F., . . . Wefel, J. (2014). Monitoring and optimising cognitive function in cancer patients: Present knowledge and future directions. *European Journal of Cancer Supplements, 12*(1), 29–40.

Sidaros, A., Engberg, A. W., Sidaros, K., Liptrot, M. G., Herning, M., Petersen, P., . . . Rostrup, E. (2008). Diffusion tensor imaging during recovery from severe traumatic brain injury and relation to clinical outcome: A longitudinal study. *Brain, 131*(Pt 2), 559–572. doi:10.1093/brain/awm294

Slomine, B., & Locascio, G. (2009). Cognitive rehabilitation for children with acquired brain injury. *Developmental Disabilities Research Reviews, 15*(2), 133–143. doi:10.1002/ddrr.56

Stern, Y. (2009). Cognitive reserve. *Neuropsychologia, 47*(10), 2015–2028. doi:10.1016/j.neuropsychologia.2009.03.004

Taylor, H. G., Yeates, K. O., Wade, S. L., Drotar, D., Klein, S. K., & Stancin, T. (1999). Influences on first-year recovery from traumatic brain injury in children. *Neuropsychology, 13*(1), 76–89.

Taylor, H. G., Yeates, K. O., Wade, S. L., Drotar, D., Stancin, T., & Burant, C. (2001). Bidirectional child-family influences on outcomes of traumatic brain injury in children. *Journal of the International Neuropsychological Society, 7*(6), 755–767.

Treble-Barna, A., Schultz, H., Minich, N., Taylor, H. G., Yeates, K. O., Stancin, T., & Wade, S. L. (2017). Long-term classroom functioning and its association with neuropsychological and academic performance following traumatic brain injury during early childhood. *Neuropsychology, 31*(5), 486.

Yeates, K. O., Taylor, H. G., Walz, N. C., Stancin, T., & Wade, S. L. (2010). The family environment as a moderator of psychosocial outcomes following traumatic brain injury in young children. *Neuropsychology, 24*, 345–356.

Chapter 3

Assessment in paediatric acquired brain injury

Suzanna Watson and Fergus Gracey

We are always going to be indebted to you for all the work you have done and the progress Jordan has made. He wasn't able to understand before. He is making a good job of that now. Emotionally he is a very loving and thoughtful lad with a big heart. We are thankful that you helped him to rediscover that part of himself. Your work restored some calm and brought clarity to a very stormy period for all of us.

(Joanne Dowen, Parent)

Introduction

In this chapter, we describe an interdisciplinary neuropsychological assessment process for children and young people (CYP) with acquired brain injuries (ABI). We have divided this chapter into two parts. In Part 1, we describe the context of our approach to assessment of children with ABIs and our understanding of ideas from the literature that shape this process. Part 2 is dedicated to the practice and process of assessment that we have developed in collaboration with children, families, services and commissioners. It is a work in progress.

Part 1 – the background and context to our approach

Who are we?

We write from the perspective of having both held the role of clinical lead for the Cambridge Centre for Paediatric Neuropsychological Rehabilitation (CCPNR). This is a specialist, community, interdisciplinary, public (National Health Service) rehabilitation service for children with ABIs in the East of England. The team is made up of paediatric neuropsychologists, clinical psychologists, occupational therapists, a speech and language therapist, educational psychologist, neurologist and psychiatrist. It is the first of its kind in the UK.

Fergus is a clinical neuropsychologist who initially worked at the Oliver Zangwill Centre for Neuropsychological Rehabilitation (OZC). This was with adults with ABI who presented with complex, interacting, cognitive, social and emotional challenges to participation. Whilst much of the direct intervention at the OZC fits within a traditional, compensatory and skills-based approach to rehabilitation, the specific holistic model of the programme strongly emphasises group and social context in facilitating change. Having extended his interest in the relationship between context, meaning, identity and cognitive change/potential, Fergus then took on the role of leading the development of the new CCPNR service. Whilst continuing to support the CCPNR as an honorary consultant, Fergus now works as a senior clinical lecturer in the Department of Clinical Psychology at the University of East Anglia. There he leads the neuropsychology and research modules and continues to pursue research interests in qualitative and quantitative approaches to understanding cognitive, emotional and social changes after ABI.

Suzanna is a clinical psychologist who worked with CYP and families in community neurodevelopmental services before specialising to work in neurorehabilitation for children with ABIs. She started in acute rehabilitation for children with ABIs at the Royal London Hospital. This post was funded by the Helicopter Emergency Services and the East London Mental Health Trust at the time that the major trauma networks were established. Here she developed an interest in the individual and contextual influences on the trajectory of recovery for children with ABI. She moved to the CCPNR to have the opportunity to work in community paediatric neurorehabilitation and now has a role in developing acute and community paediatric neuropsychology services for Cambridgeshire and Peterborough NHS Foundation Trust.

Together, we share a curiosity for understanding the impact of ABI on CYP and their families. We seek to deliver interventions that maximise their developmental trajectory post-injury. We see assessment as part of this intervention. We recognise the importance of drawing on multiple perspectives and forms of knowledge in developing both interventions and the services that are able to provide them.

What is the service context?

The interdisciplinary team (IDT) at the CCPNR was established in 2009 and serves as a regional specialist community service for CYP in the east of England. With the help of parents of CYP who have had an ABI, and with established acute and community services, the CCPNR has sought to develop the paediatric neurorehabilitation pathway for CYP who are treated for their ABI in Addenbrookes Hospital in Cambridge, UK. CYP are now typically referred to the CCPNR from acute services as part of their transition from acute to community services. However, CYP with ABI continue to be referred from community services when they require the specialist interdisciplinary expertise to be able to meet their needs. The CCPNR is able to see children up to the age of 19 if they are still engaged in education.

The service is commissioned by Clinical Commissioning Groups and case managers to work with acute and community services to meet the specialist needs of children with ABI. This means that, in addition to assessing children's strengths and needs, the service seeks to understand the strengths and needs of those supporting them within their family, their school, their community and their local services.

What are the theoretical inspirations for our service model?

Rehabilitation psychology is organised around the goal of optimising well-being and meaningful participation for individuals with disabilities in daily living (Dunn, Ehde, & Wegener, 2016). CYP with ABI are a moving target both in terms of recovery of function and in the attainment of new developmental skills (Kaufman, Lahey, & Slomine, 2017). We bring inspiration from the fields of development, neuropsychology, holistic approaches to rehabilitation, systemic theory and social-emotional process research, and as "critical realists", we recognise the importance of flexibility with different epistemological positions when engaging with diverse clinical realities.

Key historical influences are probably best captured in the work of Vygotsky, whose theories of culture, development and cognition provide a map for thinking about the interplay between context, cognition and language. For us, Vygotsky highlights how an overly individualistic neuropsychology risks failure to provide an account of the involvement of neuropsychological processes in the fundamental activities of being human – connection and productivity with others.

The second significant influence is that of Kurt Goldstein. In parallel with others such as Oliver Zangwill and A. R. Luria, Goldstein's ideas (developed through supporting injured soldiers) have had a significant influence on the development of neuropsychological assessment and rehabilitation practice. His "organismic theory" highlights the tendency for people to strive towards a "holism" or completeness of sense of identity, an idea which is a precursor to self-actualisation models such as those of Maslow and Rogers. Goldstein proposed the consequences of ABI to arise from any one or combination of three processes:

- The loss of abilities due to acquired deficits;
- The "catastrophic" emotional reaction to the loss of abilities; and
- The loss of abilities due to avoidance of situations that might trigger a catastrophic reaction.

These three concepts underpin the "holistic" model of rehabilitation developed initially by Yehuda Ben-Yishay (1985) and then George Prigatano (1999) and more recently articulated by Wilson, Gracey, Evans, and Bateman (2009). The holistic principles have also been applied in adult community rehabilitation where the importance of a long-term, psychotherapeutic, flexible approach to addressing lifelong fluctuating needs is emphasised (Coetzer, 2008).

A model for assessment of childhood ABI

We previously presented a cognitive-systemic model (Gracey, Olsen, Austin, Watson, & Malley, 2015) to account for the development of problems following childhood brain injury. This model emphasises the interplay between underlying brain development, the consequences of damage and the impact of the social-cognitive-affective context in terms of the development of higher cognitive functioning in both "cold" cognitive and "hot" social-emotional domains. We described the responses of others (parents, siblings, teachers, friends, peers, etc.) in terms of the "appraisals" they make for the injured child's changed behaviour, in the context of their understanding and their expectations of the child. For example, appraisals of "threat" and of limited ability to cope with such stresses in any one of the systems around the child could compromise the child's social and cognitive development. Thomas-Unsworth and Tucker (2012) have explored the perceptions of parents in a qualitative study that illustrates the extent to which this can have an impact on adolescents' development of independence and autonomy.

However, we recognise that our previous cognitive-systemic model is to an extent deconstructive and does not easily allow prioritisation of the "felt sense" or experiential aspects of these processes. Nevertheless, the model highlights a need for an understanding of the outcome of a child's injury in terms of individual neuropsychological sequelae, the sense-making and responses of others in the child's context, as well as the reciprocal action of these responses on the child's cognitive, emotional and social development. We have attempted to summarise the reciprocal interaction between the individual and contextual impact of ABI on children's developmental trajectories in Figure 3.1.

As an interdisciplinary service drawing on these ideas, we take a social, neurodevelopmental and systemic approach to the assessment of children and families that have suffered from ABI. We see the primary role of our assessment as facilitating a shared understanding of the multiple perspectives of the injury with the child, his or her family and those supporting him or her. Consistent with the Y-shaped model (Gracey, Malley, & Evans, 2009), the perspective of one might be a "threat" to another, or an individual him or herself might hold contradicting or conflicting perspectives. Such processes might reduce the capacity for a system to reflect or mentalise. We aim to provide the space for this to be possible.

Both/and: from the individual to the contextual factors

From the child or young person's individual neuropsychological functioning to the functioning of his or her context, our assessment aims to develop a shared understanding. We begin with the fundamentals of what the literature can tell us about the nature of the type of injury and brain-behaviour relationships in children and as a community neurorehabilitation service, we take a context-sensitive

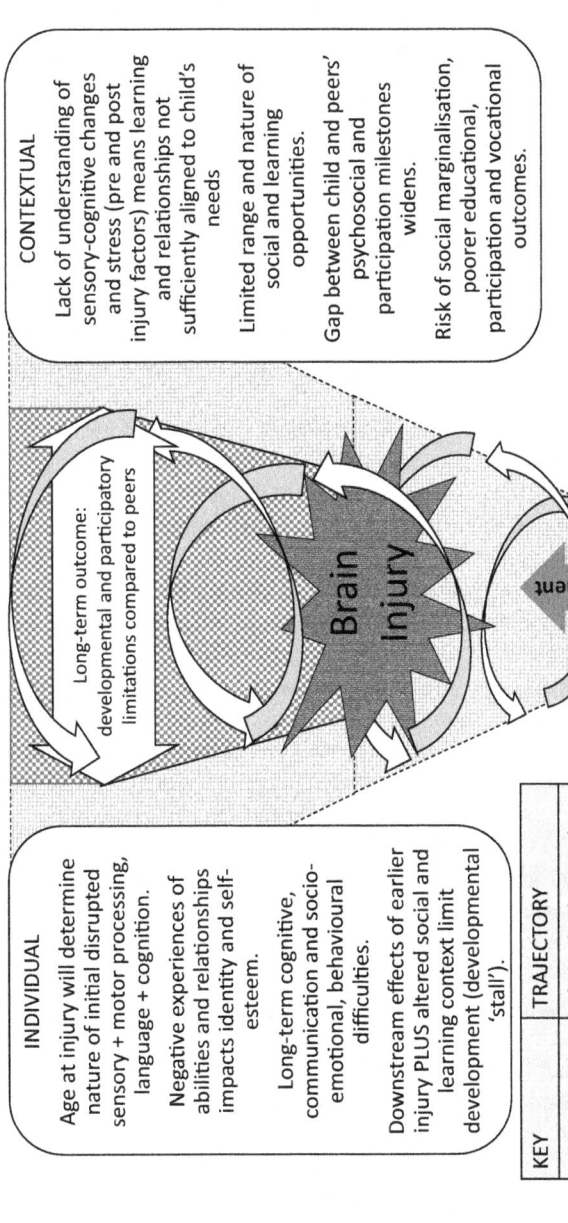

Figure 3.1 Diagram showing the reciprocal interaction between individual and contextual aspects of development, the disruption of this interplay arising following ABI, aligned with key principles for consideration in assessment, formulation and rehabilitation

approach to the assessment process (e.g. Ylvisaker, 2003; Byard, Fine, & Reed, 2011). The team aims to hold the story of what literature there is for CYP with ABI and explores what this means for the child and family following the injury at that time in the child's developmental trajectory. This requires an assessment process that includes hypothesis-driven standardised assessments as well as exploration as to how this does and doesn't have an impact on them in their participation in different environments.

The CYP's individual neuropsychological functioning

The assessment and understanding of a child's injury are ongoing processes that require constant reformulation as the young person recovers from his or her injury, his or her brain continues to develop and he or she develop his or her skills and identity. Our understanding of what literature there is helps to shape this sense-making process and the information we gather. This also enables us to normalise the child and family's experience.

We aim to understand the young person's developmental trajectory before he or she had the injury so that we can consider how this may have changed. We are aware that any standardised assessment is only a snapshot in this new trajectory post-injury, and timing of the assessment post-injury is important. Often, the level of impact of the injury does not become fully apparent until years after the injury. Functional magnetic resonance imaging (fMRI) studies have illustrated that different areas of the brain are recruited for tasks at different stages of brain development (e.g. Schlaggar et al., 2000). The extent to which these areas can be recruited to support cognitive and social functioning is dependent on the injury, stage of development and the context in which it occurs (family, school, etc.). A child may have an IQ score in the average range in comparison to his or her same aged peers three months after the injury but his or her score could be in the extremely low range five years later due to the acquired cognitive difficulties that impede new learning. The extent of a child's executive functioning difficulties is often not fully apparent until he or she is much older. Please see the graph in Figure 3.2 (Limond, Cormack, & Adlam, 2014), which illustrates the importance of assessment at regular intervals to monitor developmental trajectories. Repeat assessment allows us to evaluate whether new interventions need to be applied or previous interventions need to be reinstated.

It is through an understanding of the young person's premorbid trajectory and the monitoring of his or her recovery that can we get a shared sense of the impact of the injury. We often find children to have previously unidentified pre-injury developmental or mental health difficulties (e.g. specific learning difficulties, ASC, ADHD, anxiety and depression) that have an impact on their recovery post-injury. Twenty-six percent of the children we see at the CCPNR have premorbid behavioural diagnoses (Shravat, Wagner, & Gracey, 2017). It is helpful to disentangle the developmental and acquired needs where possible.

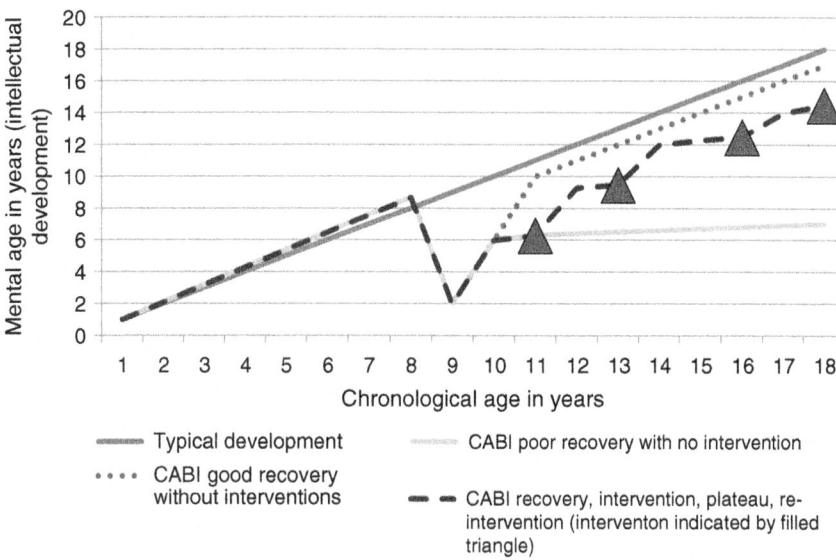

Figure 3.2 Developmental trajectories post-childhood ABI

Source: (Limond et al., 2014)

The contextual factors: family, community and school (or college)

ABI disrupts family interactions, higher cognition and the capacity to engage freely in exploratory behaviour – processes that help provide an autobiographical or episodic account for selfhood. Therefore, we focus on what this means for the CYP and family participation in specific contexts. We are eager to learn about the different narratives, and the metaphoric compaction of these to help engage with families to safely shift towards intervention (Ylvisaker & Feeney, 2000). For example, if a family narrative is about a young person who is "like a train that doesn't stop", we can think about what the train needs and how it can be supported. We see play/creativity/exploration as necessary ingredients for assessment and rehabilitation, including amelioration of the impact of cognitive issues (as elaborated by Limond et al., 2014 in their Paediatric Neuropsychological Intervention model). This requires attention to information and hypotheses regarding neuropsychological functioning alongside subjective experiences and sense-making of the child, family and others.

The whole family unit itself may benefit from engagement in work that facilitates its own re-storying of the child and of family life. Indeed, analysis of goal setting data from our service indicated that the most common type of goal for families related to improving understanding in order to be able to help their children (Watson, 2016). In line with the evidence from Braga, Da Paz Junior, and Ylvisaker (2005), we aim to support the family to be able to understand the young person's needs so that the family members can support the delivery of intervention into the child's everyday life. Thus, the understanding of, and support for, family functioning is at the heart of the assessment process.

We have come to learn that some families have already begun to develop narratives of family life post-injury that provide a ready basis for engaging in rehabilitation and can therefore embark fairly quickly in a focussed plan of rehabilitation based on a detailed formal IDT assessment. However, we are aware that for some, a combination of contextual, service-related, psychosocial, pre-injury and injury factors can present challenges to finding a common rehabilitative narrative. This diversity of family needs at a given time is described in our model of complexity and engagement in rehabilitation (CORe; Gracey et al., 2015). Guided by this model, we include a variety of assessment activities in different contexts. This allows for collecting information *with* the family, greater understanding of the family system and enables joint exploration of problems, issues and strengths.

We would not be able to assess the impact of an injury on the young person without considering the different environments in which he or she participates. As with families, each return to education post-ABI is unique in terms of peers, access to the curriculum and development of independence. As with families, each education system is different in terms of its own strengths and needs in their ability and resources to meet a CYP with ABI's needs.

A shared understanding

The primary aim is to create a safe and reflective environment in which we can bring together what the scans, medical reports and scores on standardised measures tell us with what the child, family, community therapists, social worker and class teacher can tell us. Through this, we aim to develop a shared narrative across the system, the services and agencies supporting the child, recognising that as we enter the family's world, we also become part of the system. We aim to take an executive, metacognitive and regulatory role in this collaborative sense-making process. Therefore, if we see that there are multiple different stories which might not easily come together in a single shared understanding, we take the meta-position of holding and reflecting upon these different stories. We seek to test different hypotheses rather than attempt to "push" for a single dominant understanding. This also requires attention to, and respect for, the multiple perspectives that can arise within the team itself. Routine opportunities for shared discussion of assessment and clinical work are fundamental to this way of working.

The interdisciplinary team process

The rehabilitative process of collaborative narrative construction starts with the assessment process. It requires team members to have the capacity to both hold on to and highlight key factual information whilst enabling meaningful CYP and family narratives. Team members facilitate the process of linking information with the CYP, their siblings and family experience to allow those narratives to be discovered and developed. This means team members need to be open to being compelled by emotive narratives, whilst also retaining a critical faculty and ability to be flexible and attend to what lies outside of that narrative.

If assessment is to align with this developmental self-regulatory and systemic framework, then the clinician is challenged to collect specific, detailed information from a wide range of sources and types, and to co-construct meaningful sense-making with the family at the same time. This requires collaborative hypothesis making and testing, and the integration of key objective information with the experience of the CYP, family and IDT. In our teamwork, we have recognised that more can be gained therapeutically from the shared experiential process of coming to an understanding or realisation together (as a team, with the family, with other professionals). It is important to hold back from making quick conclusions, to maintain curiosity and to seek exploration of perspectives in interactions with other team members. From our experience and reading of the literature, Box 3.1. summarises some of the ideas that shape our practice.

Box 3.1   Ten ideas that influence practice of assessment of paediatric ABI in the community

1   **Assessment is an iterative, collaborative, reflective, person-centred endeavour** involving the CYP, his or her family, professionals and others in the child's specific context.

2   **Childhood brain injury happens to a developing brain:**

   2a)   **The age the child is at injury** is important for understanding the impact of the injury on a young person's developmental trajectory due to the impact of the injury on the ongoing development of the brain (Tonks, Yates, Williams, Frampton, & Slater, 2010; Gracey et al., 2014).

   2b)   **There is a need to understand the change in a child's developmental trajectory by monitoring over time.** Problems don't always show themselves immediately.

3   **Severity of injury and period of post-traumatic amnesia (PTA)** (for children with TBI) are helpful predictors as to the level of impact for CYP (Ponsford, Spitz, & McKenzie, 2016).

4   **CYP with brain injuries have similar mental health needs to those in child and adolescent mental health services** (Tonks et al., 2010; Gracey et al., 2014): It's normal for CYP with ABI to have mental health difficulties.

5   **Community rehabilitation is best delivered in the child's own developmental and participatory context**. Any assessment needs to include an understanding of these to be useful to the child and family.

6   **Premorbid family functioning is a significant predictor of outcome** (Butler et al., 2008). Understanding family functioning is important for outcome (Yeates, Taylor, Walz, Stancin, & Wade, 2010; Gerring & Wade, 2012).

7   **Time and experience post-injury** are important for understanding the trajectory and interplay between the CYP's injury, skill development, context and future support needs.

8   **Paediatric rehabilitation has better outcomes when delivered by trained parents** and those supporting children in schools in their everyday participation than by clinicians alone (Braga, De Paz, & Ylvisaker, 2010).

9   **It is important to understand the consequences and meaning of the injury to family members** and how the family organises itself to maintain a sense of continuity of identity and/or reduces threat to that identity (Roscigno & Swanson, 2011; Roscigno, Swanson, Vavilala, & Solchany, 2011; Gracey, Evans, & Malley, 2009).

10   **The sustainability of intervention is dependent on the psychosocial foundations**. Intervention is best delivered in line with a stepped model in which working relationships and shared understanding are developed (CORe model, Gracey et al., 2015) before developmentally appropriate neurocognitive interventions can be identified to optimise the child and family's outcomes (e.g. Paediatric Neurocognitive Interventions model, Limond et al., 2014).

Part 2 – practical application to assessment in childhood ABI

Part 2 is primarily focussed on the assessment process we have developed at the CCPNR in the community. However, to contextualise this, we begin with a brief description of the early assessments that can be helpful in the acute management of ABI in terms of understanding its neuropsychological sequelae and maximising the trajectory of recovery.

Acute inpatient assessment

Assessment begins as soon as the CYP is brought to hospital. Regardless of the type of injury, it is important to assess for and normalise an acute stress reaction for families when a CYP is in intensive care. Early contact with the child and family can foster a sense of safety, promote calming, a sense of self-efficacy, connectedness and hope (e.g. Hobfoll et al., 2007). If the family members are provided with this reassurance when the young person becomes fully conscious, they are much better able to provide it for their child. At Addenbrooke's Hospital, we are fortunate to have dedicated counsellors for parents of children with ABI who are integrated into the neurology MDT.

Post-traumatic amnesia and head injury symptoms

Once a young person who has had a traumatic brain injury is fully conscious, a PTA assessment helps those supporting the CYP (family and professionals) understand the CYP's level of orientation and ability to lay down continuous memories. Assessments like the Westmead Post Amnesia Scale for Children (Rocca, Wallen, & Batchelor, 2008) help guide modifications to the pharmacological treatments (e.g. sedatives, antiepileptic drugs or antipsychotic medication) and adaptations to the environment to maximise their recovery if the young person is disoriented and unable to make continuous memories (e.g. with the use of photographic visual timetables for what is happening when and who is who). It helps identify the support needed to reduce the distress of this disorientation and to pace early rehabilitation. We have found psychoeducation for families about what to expect with the Rancho Los Amigos Scale a useful concrete guide to normalise PTA as part or recovery and to orientate the family as to where their child is in their recovery post-TBI.

Once clear of PTA, we have found it helpful to assess head injury symptoms (e.g. Rivermead Post-Concussion Symptoms questionnaire, Eyres, Carey, Gilworth, Neumann, & Tennant, 2005) in order to provide a structure for monitoring recovery and the psychoeducation that can be provided by slowly grading up activity post-discharge (e.g. Master, Gioia, Leddy, & Grady, 2012). When a young person is experiencing difficulties with memory, headaches, fatigue and irritability, we can normalise and monitor these symptoms to support a level of participation that maximises the trajectory of their recovery.

The importance of this early support, psychoeducation and positive management of symptoms post-injury can be easily overlooked in terms of the sequalae post-injury. At the CCPNR, we find that the children with ABI who have developed symptoms of post-traumatic stress rarely remember their injury. The trauma stems from perceptions of threat to their life during their hospital stay while they are disoriented and unable to make continuous memories in PTA. In the community, we see many young people who are out of school who present with symptoms of chronic fatigue, anxiety and low mood due to lack of understanding of what is normal post-ABI. This is only exacerbated if the parents are low in resources because they are struggling with their own symptoms of post-traumatic stress.

Informal and formal assessment

Once oriented, informal assessments can be sought with games that are fun, promote engagement and are dependent on higher cognitive skills (e.g. Guess Who?

and Connect Four). Where possible, games from home can give a sense of how the CYP can cope with the sensory, physical, communication, cognitive, emotional and behavioural demands of developmentally appropriate tasks. This understanding (e.g. the damage to the left temporal lobe is making it difficult for them to understand words but we can use pictures) can help to shape the interdisciplinary rehabilitation as well as upskill and support the everyday care from parents and the nursing staff on the ward. We find this early sense-making with parents enables them to become part of their child's rehabilitation from the beginning. We find the collaborative process of putting together a one-page "Top Tips" for those visiting the CYP and family a helpful exercise (e.g. "I'm still in PTA/ I don't always know where I am/ This can be scary/ Please tell me who you are and what you are doing/ I need extra time to understand what you've said to me/ Ask me to tell you what you've said so that you can see if I have understood/ Write information down/ Please keep the curtains closed because I'm very sensitive to light").

In addition to the assessments from individual disciplines (e.g. OT, SLT, neuropsychology and physio), there are interdisciplinary measures that can help shape an holistic approach to acute rehabilitation to enable the re-acquisition of previously attained skills and the discharge planning process (e.g. the Functional Independence Measure + Functional Assessment Measure (FIMFAM, Turner-Stokes, Nyein, Turner-Stokes, & Gatehouse, 1999), the Paediatric Extended Glasgow Outcome Scale (Beers et al., 2012) or the Kings Outcome Scale for Childhood Head Injury (Couchman, Rossiter, Colaco, & Forsyth, 2001). The FIMFAM produces a helpful visual representation of a child's needs that is very accessible for families.

When to assess?

We know that an assessment is going to provide a snapshot in a young person's trajectory. However, when do we want to formally assess the impact of the injury and the possible downstream implications for future developmental and psychosocial milestones? There is often such rapid change once a young person is conscious that it is more helpful to wait to do individual batteries of standardised neuropsychological assessments. We have to recognise that future assessment will be required to understand the child's trajectory post-injury. Depending on the rate of recovery and fatigue, neuropsychological assessment may not be helpful until discharge or even months after discharge. It is a clinical judgement as to when it is going to be most helpful for the CYP and what other services are going to be able to be involved. Early assessment can provide a baseline, facilitate referrals to further rehabilitation providers and help to consider appropriate educational placements and access to community services. However, often, families are so grateful that their children are alive and able to be discharged (from what has been a distressing and traumatic setting) that they cannot begin to think about any cognitive difficulties that might be problematic now, let alone those that might not become apparent until later.

Discharge planning

The CORe model (Gracey et al., 2015) enables us to attend to where a child/young person and the system around them is in relation to engaging with other services, and pritoritise the focus accordingly. From enabling a coming together and ensuring statutory services are in place (for example, where there is a high level of risk/vulnerability or where alternative statutory education provision is required) to where residential rehabilitation is needed, the CORe model can help the transition into the community or watchful waiting and review.

At the CCPNR, we have collaborated with neurology colleagues at Addenbrookes to establish a follow-up brain injury clinic for this very reason: to be able to monitor outcome, triage into community services where necessary and establish sufficient relationship with the family that might facilitate future contact should it be required.

Community neurorehabilitation assessment

As an IDT at the CCPNR, we have found it helpful to have a framework for assessment. We have developed the use of the Children and Youth Version of the International Classification of Functioning (World Health Organisation, 2007; McDougall, Horgan, Baldwin, Tucker, & Frid, 2008) to be able to make sense of the information gathered. Please see the template in Figure 3.3.

The CCPNR assessment process that we have developed has nine stages, which we will attempt to describe in further detail:

1) Introduction to the service and pre-assessment information gathering
2) Pre-assessment formulation
3) Meeting the family
4) Initial formulation and team discussion
5) Hypothesis testing with detailed assessments
6) Detailed formulation and team discussion
7) Feedback, collaborative sense-making and goal setting with children and families
8) Report writing and agreement
9) Feedback and collaborative sense-making to those supporting them

1. Introduction to the service and pre-assessment information gathering

Due to the complexity of the assessment process and the number of clinicians involved, families have highlighted the importance of one coordinator who is their main contact for the team. Once the referral has been accepted and allocated, the coordinator contacts the family by telephone, introduces him or herself, describes the service and team and explains what will happen.

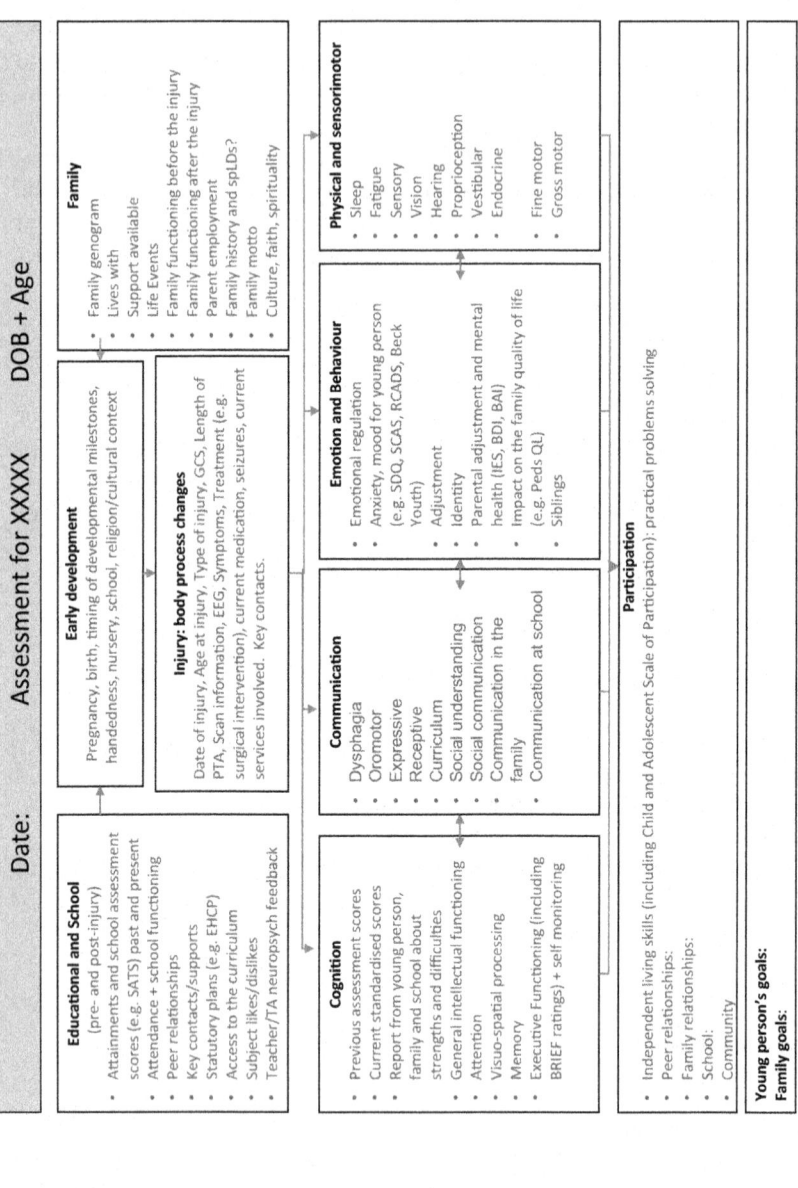

Date: Assessment for XXXX   DOB + Age

Educational and School
(pre- and post-injury)
- Attainments and school assessment scores (e.g. SATS) past and present
- Attendance + school functioning
- Peer relationships
- Key contacts/supports
- Statutory plans (e.g. EHCP)
- Access to the curriculum
- Subject likes/dislikes
- Teacher/TA neuropsych feedback

Early development
Pregnancy, birth, timing of developmental milestones, handedness, nursery, school, religion/cultural context

Family
- Family genogram
- Lives with
- Support available
- Life Events
- Family functioning before the injury
- Family functioning after the injury
- Parent employment
- Family history and spLDs?
- Family motto
- Culture, faith, spirituality

Injury: body process changes
Date of injury. Age at injury. Type of injury, GCS, Length of PTA, Scan information, EEG, Symptoms, Treatment (e.g. surgical intervention), current medication, seizures, current services involved. Key contacts.

Cognition
- Previous assessment scores
- Current standardised scores
- Report from young person, family and school about strengths and difficulties
- General intellectual functioning
- Attention
- Visuo-spatial processing
- Memory
- Executive Functioning (including BRIEF ratings) + self monitoring

Communication
- Dysphagia
- Oromotor
- Expressive
- Receptive
- Curriculum
- Social understanding
- Social communication
- Communication in the family
- Communication at school

Emotion and Behaviour
- Emotional regulation
- Anxiety, mood for young person (e.g. SDQ, SCAS, RCADS, Beck Youth)
- Adjustment
- Identity
- Parental adjustment and mental health (IES, BDI, BAI)
- Impact on the family quality of life (e.g. Peds QL)
- Siblings

Physical and sensorimotor
- Sleep
- Fatigue
- Sensory
- Vision
- Hearing
- Proprioception
- Vestibular
- Endocrine
- Fine motor
- Gross motor

Participation
- Independent living skills (including Child and Adolescent Scale of Participation): practical problems solving
- Peer relationships:
- Family relationships:
- School:
- Community

Young person's goals:
Family goals:

Figure 3.3 The CCPNR interdisciplinary formulation and planning framework based upon the ICF-CY, WHO (2007); McDougall et al. (2008)

We are learning to get a sense of what the brain injury means to the young person and his or her family early on. As outlined by the CORe model, it can be the case that even attending a rehabilitation service appointment or talking with a "brain injury professional" can be so threat activating that it is difficult to process what is being said. We have previously described the usefulness of taking a "long view", working slowly over time to meet with the family where they are and to begin a process of developing reflective capacity in the system (Gracey et al., 2015).

We are also learning the importance of early expectation management regarding (a) the pace of community neurorehabilitation in comparison to hospital rehabilitation and (b) the nature of our approach in that we work with those supporting the young person to deliver rehabilitation in their everyday lives. Without making this clear at the beginning, families can be disappointed that they do not have, for example, three sessions of speech and language therapy "delivered to" their child every week. As a community service, we explain our goal of developing a shared understanding and that this takes time in terms of gathering information and making sense of it all. We explain our understanding of the better outcomes when those supporting the CYP can deliver interventions that are integrated into their everyday lives, thus maximising their participation.

At this point, the coordinator establishes which services have been involved and who is currently supporting the CYP and his or her family. Permission to contact other professionals is sought verbally and then sent in the post with a stamped addressed envelope along with baseline screens for the following:

(i)   The CYP's emotional and behavioural well-being with the Strengths and Difficulties Questionnaire (Goodman, Meltzer, & Bailey, 1998) parent and self-report (depending on the age of the CYP);

(ii)   The CYP's executive functioning skills with the Behavioural Regulation Inventory of Executive Function (Gioia, Isquith, Guy, & Kenworthy, 2000) parent and self-report;

(iii) The CYPs levels of participation with the Child and Adolescent Scale of Participation (Bedell, 2009) parent and self-report (again age dependent);

(iv)   The family's quality of life with the PedsQL Impact on the family questionnaire (Varni, Sherman, Burwinkle, Dickenson, & Dixon, 2004); and

(v)   The family needs questionnaire (Marwitz, 2000).

If we are already aware of specific strengths or difficulties that we would like to screen for at this point, we add measures for these. Sometimes it is helpful to get the scores from Resiliency Scales, the Children's Communication Checklist, the La Trobe communication questionnaire or the Sensory Profile Measure in advance, but there are other times when it is more helpful to do these in person with the CYP and his or her family. There is also a limit as to how many questionnaires we can ask them to complete at once.

Parents are usually able to signpost who is the best person to contact at school (e.g. special educational needs coordinator, schoolteacher, teaching or learning support assistant) in order to gain an initial impression of their presenting needs at school and how they were functioning before the injury. This person is contacted and requested to share school records (e.g. Cognitive Abilities Tests, Standard Attainment Tests, National Curriculum scores) from before the injury where possible. Copies of any previous (pre- and post-injury) education assessments and education and health care plans are requested.

The school contact is also sent the BRIEF, the SDQ, the Children's Communication Checklist (Bishop, 2006) and the Neuropsychological Processing Concerns Checklist for School-Aged Children & Youth (Miller, 2007). Where possible, a school observation is carried out. This helps to begin a relationship with key teaching staff and ascertain their understanding of the CYP's strengths and needs, and their appraisals of any presenting problems.

We are interested in school attendance and participation. In seeking to better understand factors associated with the diversity of ways in which a family might want or be able to work with the service, recent analysis of our service data suggests a significant association between low school attendance and the high level of indirect intervention (not with the CYP) required to deliver rehabilitation (Shravat, Wagner, & Gracey, 2016). The service uses this kind of information to begin to understand the types of service that we might need to provide.

An early developmental history is sought from community records through the GP or paediatrician. Acute hospital records are acquired and followed up where specialist expertise is required. The lead consultant paediatric neurologist for neurorehabilitation in the hospital attends team clinical discussions and is an important link for accessing and sharing more detailed aspects of the medical and acute care history. Electronic copies of scans are gathered and explained where possible. We've found that young people often like to be able to go through these images and be a part of peer education sessions that enable their friends to understand what has happened.

2. Pre-assessment formulation

All pre-assessment information is collated in the ICF framework (Figure 3.3) and presented to the wider interdisciplinary team to begin to formulate and plan the assessments required to test hypotheses and gain a comprehensive understanding of the impact of the injury on the child and their family. An assessment timetable is constructed, and the family is sent a visual assessment timetable with photos of who they will meet and when.

3. Meeting the family

The first contact with the family is always with the coordinator and where possible, this is the clinician who is most likely to be the most involved with any ongoing intervention. As part of the welcome and introduction to the service, the family is offered tea (or another refreshment) and then invited to work with the team member(s) to develop a family genogram. Our specialist teacher has inspired us to start by supporting the young person to draw out his or her family system on a flipchart (or in another way that maximises the child's participation).

We have found that this process reduces anxiety levels, helps us to get an impression of the CYP's functional difficulties and gets the whole family talking. It allows us to get to know the family more before asking them to tell us about what has happened. We ask the family members for their family "motto" to get a sense of family identity, what keeps them going and their overarching approach to life before beginning to think about the resonance between the effects of the injury within this specific family system, how it was functioning and how things are presenting now.

Clinicians reading will know that the presentation of the story of what happened provides much information about what the family understand, how they are coping and the level of impact on them and their CYP. It is often at this point that we start to become more aware of any parental mental health difficulties (most commonly symptoms of post-traumatic stress, depression and anxiety). We retain a position of curiosity and sense-making while trying to understand the core phenomena for the family. We recognise that it is often an emerging account that sparks ideas to interrogate the other information we have. Where possible, we externalise the difficulties to separate them from the child and relate this to information we have gathered about the injury. We normalise and provide psychoeducation where possible.

We then divide the session so that there is time for the parents to speak about the impact on them while initial standardised assessment with the child begins. It has been interesting to learn that many parents say they wished they had known the likely level of impact on their relationships in advance of discharge from hospital. This part of the assessment is an opportunity for parents to talk freely about the experience of the injury for them, the ambiguous loss (Boss, 2000) and their hopes and goals for intervention. It allows them to describe in full the difficulties they face and to make sense of these in the context of the story of the injury so far. Given the literature about the better outcomes for parent delivered rehabilitation, we are eager to prioritise this throughout the process of assessment.

By the end of the first meeting with the family, we aim to have an overview of the CYP's strengths and the difficulties they face. We try to begin to understand (and hypothesise) what the presenting problems might be and for whom they are problematic. We aim to have identified hopes and goals for intervention. Finally, we will have also identified and formulated potential complexity in the system (such as significant ambivalence about rehabilitation or problematic differences in perspective between key individuals or agencies) that might have implications for progressing with assessment, shared understanding and rehabilitation.

4. Initial formulation

The ICF framework is updated and presented to the team to plan the specialist psychometric, practical and qualitative assessments to follow. This is an opportunity for the coordinator to receive supervision from the team. Hypotheses are made with plans as to how to assess these. For example, executive difficulties highlighted by the BRIEF and by parents in the first meeting may not be reported by the child. Indeed, standardised measures may not capture the functional day-to-day difficulty they face but a practical cooking task or building a construction toy might help understand the areas of executive difficulty that make everyday tasks challenging. We have filmed tasks where it is helpful to have multiple perspectives to consider.

5. Hypothesis testing with detailed assessments

Based on the information collated so far, individual clinicians carry out their assessments with the CYP and where necessary, further assessment is carried out with the parents. If a child has already had an assessment, we try to repeat the assessment with the same tests so that we can track their trajectory of their scores. We have found the Crawford and Garthwaite (2007) Regbuild programme a valuable statistical tool to help us make sense of the significance of any change in scores over time. We take a formulation-driven approach to the assessments, holding a hierarchical organisation of functions in mind to include consideration of the sensory and physical functioning of the CYP before any of the higher language and cognitive functions, academic attainment and emotional well-being. As psychologists, we feel privileged to be able to be a part of such a comprehensive assessment with our CCPNR colleagues. A hearty dialogue can arise between professionals within the team who might each prioritise different discourses such as behaviour at school, different psychometric test scores, perception of threat or underpinning information about neurobiological functioning. Such dialogue can help drive the interpretation of scans, reports from school and neuropsychological test scores. It helps to enrich the understanding of what's happening in real-life situations and contribute to understanding the effects of brain-behaviour processes.

Throughout the assessments, we take opportunities for informal, dynamic assessments. If a child is struggling with a task, we will score the level they were able to achieve but then work with the child to discover compensatory strategies that are helpful (e.g. what cues help them to cope with their difficulty, how can they learn to cope with difficult tasks independently). At this point, we are testing out what kinds of interventions might be helpful. Would they respond well to goal management type structures to help them cope with the six elements task on the Behavioural Assessment of the Dysexecutive Syndrome? Would an alarm set on their watch/phone enable them to manage the metacognitive demands of that type of task? If they are struggling with the fine motor demands of writing, can they use voice recognition or is their ability to type on a keypad better than their oromotor skills?

Qualitative observations are as important as scores on standardised tests. As we do our assessments as individual team members, we regularly feed back to the CYP, family (and team) as to what is going well, what is more difficult and the things we are finding helpful. We are constantly thickening the narrative of the ways the injury does and does not seem to be having an impact and the strategies that we are finding helpful. Informal assessment is often equally if not more important. An example of this was a young boy whose family described him as "unable to speak". The assessment included standardised language assessments and anxiety screens with the speech and language therapist and the psychologist due to concerns about the damage to his left temporal lobe. His language scores were all very low, but our understanding shifted dramatically when he shouted, "Hey, you!" down the corridor to his mother. It is a great opportunity to be able to reflect on the story when a different narrative is presented. In this instance, the "hey, you" could be flagged in the corridor to build up the subordinate story of him speaking is easier. His "ability to speak" in different circumstances could be developed. He is now studying at university.

TEAM WORKING

The unity of the team is a vital component to the assessment process as the CYP and family narrative is thickened. A CYP might tell the psychologist, "My mum cries a lot", and might tell the occupational therapist, "My dad doesn't want me to go to school; he doesn't think any of us (girls) should go to school". It is only by bringing this information together that understanding of what is happening for the child at home can begin. We find the informality and fun of the cooking tasks or practical craft tasks times when CYP are more likely to be able to disclose this kind of sensitive family information. We then have to be sensitive and agree with the CYP as to how we feed this information back. The weekly team meeting has time dedicated to sharing this information in order to update our formulations using the ICF framework. This allows us as individual professionals to check in with each other and make sense of and manage new information.

The CCPNR team identity is, therefore, very important. It has been essential that the development of the team is owned by the individual professionals that are part of it. This cohesion and thinking have been the foundation of the service, and we use the weekly team meetings to share ideas from the literature, our practice, the CYP and families to help us evolve.

The process of bearing witness to people's often traumatic stories is a humbling and powerful process. As team members, we are learning to understand each other's clinical and personal comfort zones, and when to seek additional supervision. There is a recognition of the need to look after each other and support team members' well-being when exposed to so much stress and pain. Every week, we have a shared healthy team activity to ground us before we start the team meeting. Team members take turns to lead a "team healthy activity" (which might include singing, mindfulness meditation, Tai Chi or an inspiring article). The chair for the team meeting rotates, enabling co-ownership of the team process. We seek to formulate our own responses in a safe environment using different models when helpful (e.g. psychodynamic principles, the Y-shaped model, Gracey et al., 2009).

As well as meeting with the clinical lead on a monthly basis, individual team members have specialist external supervision to support them in their roles, spanning profession-specific identity and identity as a neuropsychological rehabilitation practitioner.

A NOTE ABOUT SAFEGUARDING

When a CYP or their family member discloses information that concerns us, we share our concerns with the person who has disclosed this immediately. Often, they are not aware of the level of risk associated with their injury or their child's injury. An example of this might be a teenage boy with a significant frontal lobe injury who likes to climb on the roof or a child with significant response inhibition difficulties being left to look after a younger sibling. Our assessment includes a comprehensive risk assessment, and this is ongoing throughout our contact with the CYP and family. Often, the family would benefit from locality level support (e.g. respite, family support worker) but sometimes we refer to the child in need team or the safeguarding team where necessary. As much as possible, we try to bring social care into the process of developing a shared understanding and we recognise that the service would benefit from having a social worker in the team. It is difficult for social services to understand the risks associated with paediatric brain injury, and we have needed significant support from our local safeguarding board to be able to support social care with the specialist understanding to help meet CYP's and the family's needs.

6. Detailed formulation

Once all the assessments have been completed, the team updates the ICF framework to share its assessment information. If there are remaining questions, we seek to answer these through further liaison or assessment where necessary and can invite the CYP and family back to the service for feedback. There are times when we have found it more helpful to use formulation frameworks to make sense of specific presenting difficulties (please see the chapter on formulation).

7. Feedback, collaborative sense-making and goal setting

If the child has the level of functioning to cope, we present an accessible version of the ICF on PowerPoint with a projector to feedback our understanding of all the information we have gathered with them and their family. This is an interactive editing process where we are checking our assessment findings so that we have a shared understanding that is written in the language of the CYP and family. We find this to be an intervention in itself, as it allows us to formulate together and prompt further dialogue with the family.

If, for example, throughout the assessment we have been normalising the impact on language and verbal memory from left temporal lobe damage, the experience of hallucinations due to PTA and lack of sleep and normalising the anxiety this can cause for CYP and families, then the feedback of all the information allows us to consolidate a shared understanding and engage in appropriate intervention. We recognise that this is often the first time that the family have told their story and heard it presented to them. We are aware that this co-creation of the story is very important, and we are sensitive to the language used and the framing of "problems" in a way that makes sense of them and gives power to the CYP and family.

Not only is shared sense-making of the child's injury with the family emotionally challenging, but it can be cognitively demanding for CYP. We find different ways of presenting the information with sensitivity to the CYP and family adjustment and strengths. We often use more accessible visuals to talk about strengths and difficulties (see Figures 3.4 and 3.5).

Once a shared understanding has been attained, it allows us to address goals for intervention. We aim to foster co-ownership of these goals in order to draft a rehabilitation plan with clear expectations of who is going to do what.

8. Report writing and agreement

Having agreed the key information with the CYP and family during the feedback session, we write up our interdisciplinary report and send this in draft for agreement before sharing with other professionals. This includes the ICF framework and has a summary page on the front with what has happened, the assessment findings and the plan for our involvement as a service.

Often the experience of coming to assessment carries significant challenges for a family. For example, they might be learning that the "miracle recovery" they were told about in hospital a year ago has turned into a daily nightmare

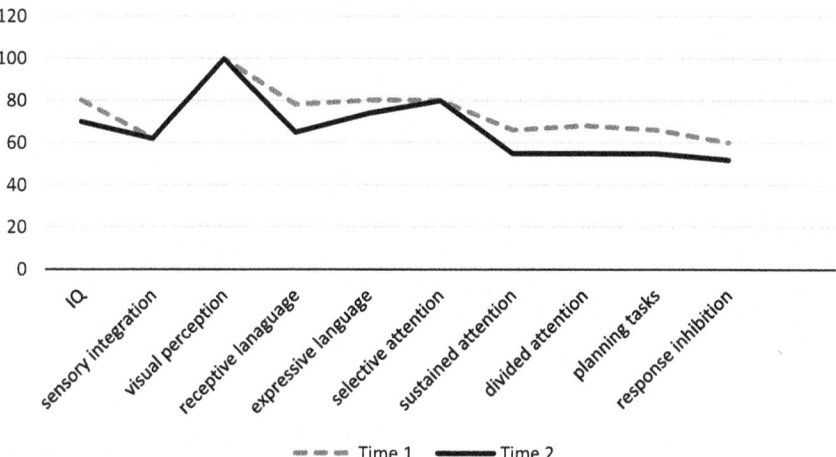

Figure 3.4 Visual presentation of standardised assessment scores

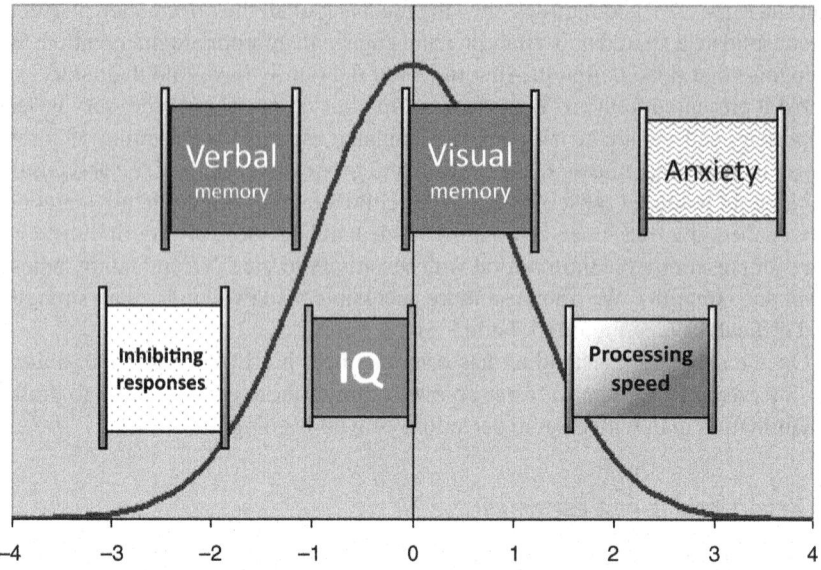

Figure 3.5 Assessment scores presented with standard deviation curve

of arguments, problem behaviours and issues at school with friendships and attainment. A narrative style covering letter recognising the efforts made by the family to attend, and the positive qualities they demonstrated in tolerating the challenge may be included. The wider report is then structured developmentally (starting with sensory and physical functioning through to higher language and cognitive skills, academic attainment, social participation, emotional well-being and family functioning). The neuropsychological literature seems to have many unhelpful descriptions such as "impairment" and "dysfunction", which we actively try to avoid. We report the child's performance on standardised assessments according to the different ranges in which a CYP has scored and keep the scores in the appendix. Due to the different ranges used by different tests (and some strong interdisciplinary discussion!), we have agreed to use the same language for the different ranges across tests according to the standard deviation from the mean (e.g. scaled scores between 8–12 represent the "average range").

We write these reports primarily for parents and the professionals supporting the child in keeping with the notion that for the assessment to be useful, parents and those supporting the child need to have this understanding of their strengths and needs. For younger children, we often write shorter separate reports, but for older, higher functioning CYP, we write the report for them in their language in support of their transition to adulthood.

9. Feedback and collaborative sense-making to those supporting the child and family

Once the CYP and family are happy with the report, we encourage them to co-present our shared understanding of what has happened and the impact of the injury to those supporting them in the key contexts (e.g. school, church, football team). We offer different ways to do this (e.g. by video, PowerPoint) and find this empowering for the CYP and family. Sometimes they want to do this with the wider family before telling their story to those at school, church or community. We find the first place they want to share the information with is school or college. The coordinator brings all of the assessment information together, and the CYP and family often want to bring photos to be able to tell the story of what has happened. We can then give feedback on what the assessment showed in terms of their strengths, the areas that they are finding difficult and the strategies that have been found helpful. This is done by the CYP and parents as much as possible, giving them the power of what information they want to share so that the people supporting them know how to help them.

TRANSITIONS

The process of assessment and intervention for CYP with ABI would not be complete without thinking about what they will need to cope with the significant developmental and psychosocial milestones ahead. As we have outlined in our developmental model of brain injury (Figure 3.1.) and principles for assessment and rehabilitation (Box 3.1.), we try to keep in mind the downstream needs of the young person as they approach key transitions. Analysis of our service data indicates that there is a higher rate of referral for CYP at the age of 11 years old, which is the time of the transition between primary and secondary school in the UK and the onset of puberty.

When required, we work with schools and families and other services to understand what the new environment will bring with the knowledge that the narratives shared in the new environment will be paramount for successful transition. We are fortunate to work alongside the Child Brain Injury Trust Family Support officer in providing information and support in school, including (where appropriate) work with the young person's friends or peers. This process applies for later transitions to further or higher education and transition from the child brain injury service to adult services.

Consistent with the legalities of transition to adulthood, consent is sought after turning 16, and new discussion will be had with the CYP and family about preferences for who attends sessions, enabling the young person to take more of an active role.

We are fortunate to have close links with the adult community brain injury team in Cambridgeshire, which promotes discussion about the best service pathways for young people beyond school leaving age. We are able to continue working with children up to the age of 19 if they are in education. However, if the young person has a clear vocational route that he or she wants to follow (rather than staying on at school), it may be more appropriate for the young person to work with the occupational therapist in the adult service who has more expertise in vocational rehabilitation and related statutory processes. When it comes to leaving the service beyond age 16, we work to extend the understanding that has been developed with the CCPNR into the young person's new contexts. Often, young people will begin to take more of a role in "owning" the narrative, consistent with their own developmental stage, making choices about what to say to whom and learning about systems such as disability officers or learning supports in higher education settings.

Reflections

All models are wrong, but some are useful (George Box, 1976)

We have developed this process of assessment over the past nine years, and it continues to evolve. We recognise that it can be a lengthy process, but we find that CYP and their families need this time to be able to have an understanding that will enable the best for their developmental trajectory and quality of life. By applying the principles of the CORe model, we hope to allocate resources appropriately. Sometimes the most complex situations do not require multiple appointments with the IDT. There are times when relationship building with family or services less intensively over time is best conducted by the coordinator, thus improving efficiency and reducing further possible service disruption. In this situation, the wider team becomes a reflecting team for the coordinator, allowing them to retain a meta-position in the development and exploration of family and service stories.

We are dedicated to continuing to evolve and support the development of specialist community neurorehabilitation services across the UK. Although we have not conducted a full economic analysis of the impact of the service, we have witnessed considerable financial cost savings for commissioners to have this level of specialist service following CYP ABI. When we have compared and costed up the journeys of children who have accessed the CCPNR with those who have not, we find the latter experience increased distress associated with services not understanding or effectively meeting their specific needs. Increased service costs are attributable to use of multiple inappropriate service referrals initially, with the potential of requiring highly specialist inpatient services where deterioration of mental health and social vulnerability occurs (Desarathi, Grace, Kelly, & Forsyth, 2011).

The service development has been an ongoing co-creation between the different team members and the CYP and families we have met in the process. We value the feedback we get from CYP and families and have tried to edit the process in line with this as much as possible. In this spirit, and in that of this book, we present this chapter as a stepping off point to start wider conversations about assessing and meeting the needs of children and families following ABI. It is a work in progress, and we welcome questions and thoughts from those reading this. Please do not hesitate to contact Suzanna at suzanna.watson@nhs.net.

References

Bedell, G. (2009). Further validation of the child and adolescent scale of participation (CASP). *Developmental Neurorehabilitation*, *12*, 342–351.

Beers, S. R., Wisniewski, S. R., Garcia-Filion, P., Tian, Y., Hahner, T., Berger, R. P., . . . Adelson, P. A. (2012). Validity of a pediatric version of the glasgow outcome scale – extended. *Journal of Neurotrauma*, *29*(6), 1126–1139.

Ben-Yishay, Y., Ratook, J., Lakin, P., Piasetsky, E. G., Ross, B., Silver, S., et al. (1985). Neuropsychologic rehabilitation: Quest for a holistic approach. *Seminars in Neurology*, *5*, 252–259.

Bishop, D. V. M. (2006). *CCC-2; Children's communication checklist-2, United States edition, manual*. San Antonio, TX: Pearson.

Boss, P. (2000). *Ambiguous loss: Learning to live with unresolved grief*. Cambridge: Harvard University Press.

Bowen, C., Yeates, G., & Palmer, S. (2014). *A relational approach to rehabilitation*. London: Karnac.

Box, G. E. P. (1976). Science and statistics. *Journal of the American Statistical Association*, *71*, 791–799. doi:10.1080/01621459.1976.10480949

Braga, L., Da Paz, A. C., & Ylvisaker, M. (2010). Direct clinician-delivered versus indirect family-supported rehabilitation of children with traumatic brain injury: A randomized controlled trial. *Brain Injury*, *19*(10), 819–831.

Butler, R. W. (2007). Cognitive rehabilitation. In S. J. Hunter & J. Donders (Eds.), *Paediatric neuropsychological intervention* (pp. 444–464). New York: Cambridge University Press.

Butler, R. W., Copeland, D. R., Fairclough, D. L., Mulhern, R. K., Katz, E. R., Kazak, A. E., . . . Sahler, O. J. Z. (2008). A multicenter, randomized clinical trial of a cognitive remediation program for childhood survivors of a pediatric malignancy. *Journal of Consulting and Clinical Psychology*, *76*(3), 367–378.

Byard, K., Fine, H., & Reed, J. (2011). Taking a developmental and systemic perspective on neuropsychological rehabilitation with children with brain injury and their families. *Clinical Child Psychology and Psychiatry*, *16*(2), 165–184.

Coetzer, R. (2008). Holistic neuro-rehabilitation in the community: Is identity a key issue? *Neuropsychological Rehabilitation*, *18*(5–6), 766–783.

Couchman, M., Rossiter, L., Colaco, T., & Forsyth, R. (2001). A practical outcome scale for paediatric head injury. *Archives of Disease in Childhood*, *8*(2), 120–124.

Crawford, J. R., & Garthwaite, P. H. (2007). Using regression equations built from summary data in the neuropsychological assessment of the individual case. *Neuropsychology*, *21*, 611–620.

Desarathi, M., Grace, J., Kelly, T., & Forsyth, R. (2011). Utilization of mental health services by survivors of severe paediatric traumatic brain injury: A population-based study. *Child: Care, Health and Development*, *37*(3), 418–421.

Dunn, D. S., Ehde, D. M., & Wegener, S. T. (2016). The foundational principles as psychological lodestars: Theoretical inspiration and empirical direction in rehabilitation psychology. *Rehabilitation Psychology*, *61*, 1–6.

Eyres, S., Carey, A., Gilworth, G., Neumann, V., & Tennant, A. (2005). Construct validity and reliability of the Rivermead post-concussion symptoms questionnaire. *Clinical Rehabilitation, 19*(8), 878–887.

Gioia, G., Isquith, P. K., Guy, S. C., & Kenworthy, L. (2000). Reviewed by Baron, I. S. "Test review: Behavior rating inventory of executive function". *Child Neuropsychology, 6*(3), 235–238.

Goodman, R., Meltzer, H., & Bailey, V. (1998). The strengths and difficulties questionnaire: A pilot study on the validity of the self-report version. *European Child & Adolescent Psychiatry, 7*, 125–130.

Gracey, F., Evans, J. J., & Malley, D. (2009). Capturing process and outcome in complex rehabilitation interventions: A "Y-shaped" model. *Neuropsychological Rehabilitation, 19*(6), 867–890.

Gracey, F., Olsen, G., Austin, L., Watson, S., & Malley, D. (2015). Integrating psychological therapy into interdisciplinary neuropsychological rehabilitation of the brain injured child. In J. Reed, K. Byard, & H. Fine (Eds.), *Neuropsychological rehabilitation of childhood brain injury: A practical guide* (pp. 197–215). London: Palgrave Macmillan.

Gracey, F., Watson, S., McHugh, M., Swan, A., Humphrey, A., & Adlam, A-L. R. (2014). Age at injury, emotional problems and executive functioning in understanding disrupted social relationships following childhood ABI. *Journal of Social Care and Neurodisability, 5*(3), 160–170.

Hobfoll, S. E., Watson, P., Bell, C. C., Bryant, R. A., Brymer, M. J., Friedman, M. J., . . . Ursano, R. J. (2007). Five essential elements of immediate and mid term mass trauma intervention: Empirical evidence. *Psychiatry, 70*(4), 283–315.

Kaufman, J. N., Lahey, S., & Slomine, B. S. (2017). Pediatric rehabilitation psychology: Rehabilitating a moving target. *Rehabilitation Psychology, 62*(3), 223–226.

Lewis, M., & Todd, R. (2007). The self-regulating brain: Cortical-subcortical feedback and the development of intelligent action. *Cognitive Development, 22*, 406–430.

Limond, J., Cormack, M., & Adlam, A-L. R. (2014). A model for paediatric cognitive interventions: Considering the role of development and maturation in rehabilitation planning. *The Clinical Neuropsychologist, 28*(2), 181–198.

Luria, L. R. (1973). *The working brain: An introduction to neuropsychology*. Pennsylvania, PA: Basic Books.

Marwitz, J. (2000). The family needs questionnaire. *The Centre for Outcome Measurement in Brain Injury*. Retrieved from http://www.tbims.org/fnq/fnqref.html

Master, C. L., Gioia, G. A., Leddy, J. J., & Grady, M. F. (2012). Importance of "Return to learn" in pediatric and adolescent concussion. *Pediatric Ann, 41*(9), 1–6.

McDougall, J., Horgan, K., Baldwin, P., Tucker, M. A., & Frid, P. (2008). Employing the international classification of functioning, disability and health to enhance services for children and youth with chronic physical health conditions and disabilities. *Paediatrics & Child Health, 13*(3), 173–178.

Miller, D. C. (2007). Neuropsychological processing concerns checklist for children and youth (3rd ed.). In *Essentials of school neuropsychological assessment* (2nd ed.). Hickory Creek, TX: KIDS.

Ponsford, J. L., Spitz, G., & McKenzie, D. (2016). Using post-traumatic amnesia to predict outcome after traumatic brain injury. *Journal of Neurotrauma, 33*(11), 997–1004.

Prigatano, G. (1999). *Principles of neuropsychological rehabilitation*. New York: Oxford University Press.

Rocca, A., Wallen, M., & Batchelor, J. (2008). The Westmead post-traumatic amneisa scale for children (WPTAS-C) aged 4 and 5 years old. *Brain Impairment*, *9*(1), 14–21.

Roscigno, C. I., & Swanson, K. M. (2011). Parents' experiences following children's moderate to severe traumatic brain injury: A clash of cultures. *Qualitative Health Research*, *21*(10), 1413–1426.

Roscigno, C. I., Swanson, K. M., Vavilala, M. S., & Solchany, J. (2011). Children's longing for everydayness: Life following traumatic brain injury in the USA. *Brain Injury*, *25*(9), 882–894.

Schlaggar, B. L., Brown, T. T., Lugar, H. M., Visscher, K. M., Miezin, F. M., & Petersen, S. E. (2002). Functional neuroanatomical differences between adults and school-age children in the processing of single words. *Science*, *296*(5572), 1476–1479.

Shravat, G., Wagner, A. P., & Gracey, F. (2016). *Painting a picture of possible clinical pathways to address the diversity of needs following acquired brain injury in children.* NIHR CLAHRC Showcase Event, Cambourne, December. Retrieved from www.clahrc-eoe.nihr.ac.uk/

Thomas-Unsworth, S., & Tucker, P. (2012). *Autonomy in young people following brain injury: A qualitative study of the perceptions of parents.* Poster Presentation at The Ninth World Congress on Brain Injury International Brain Injury Association Edinburgh. Brain Injury, Abstracts, 156.

Tonks, J., Yates, P., Williams, W. H., Frampton, I., & Slater, A. (2010). Peer-relationship difficulties in children with brain injuries: Comparisons with children in mental health services and healthy controls. *Neuropsychological Rehabilitation*, *20*(6), 922–935.

Turner-Stokes, L., Nyein, K., Turner-Stokes, T., Gatehouse, C. (1999, August 13). The UK FIM+FAM: Development and evaluation. Functional assessment measure. *Clin Rehabil*, (4), 277–287.

Varni, J. W., Sherman, S. A., Burwinkle, T. M., Dickenson, P. E., & Dixon, P. (2004). The PedsQL family impact module: Preliminary reliability and validity. *Health Quality of Life Outcomes*, *2*, 55.

Watson, S. (2016). *What do children with brain injuries want?* Conference poster presented at the First International Paediatric Brain Injury Symposium in Liverpool.

Wilson, B. A., Gracey, F., Evans, J. J., & Bateman, A. (2009). *Neuropsychological rehabilitation: Theory, models, therapy and outcome.* Cambridge: Cambridge University Press.

World Health Organization. (2007). *International classification of functioning, disability and health – child and youth version.* Geneva, Switzerland: World Health Organization.

Yeates, K. O., Taylor, H. G., Walz, N. C., Stancin, T., & Wade, S. L. (2010). The family environment as a moderator of psychosocial outcomes following traumatic brain injury in young children. *Neuropsychology*, *24*, 345–356.

Ylvisaker, M. (2003). Context-sensitive cognitive rehabilitation after brain injury: Theory and practice. *Brain Impairment*, *4*(1), 1–16.

Ylvisaker, M., & Feeney, T. (2000). Reconstruction of identity after brain injury. *Brain Impairment*, *1*(1), 12–28.

Chapter 4

Using biopsychosocial formulations in paediatric neurorehabilitation

Jenny Jim and Heather Liddiard

This chapter describes biopsychosocial formulations that Jenny and Heather developed specifically to guide rehabilitation of children and young people (CYP) with an acquired brain injury (ABI).

Jenny and Heather are clinical psychologists with extensive experience working across all tiers of CAMHS and tertiary level one national and specialist multidisciplinary inpatient intensive neurorehabilitation services. Collectively their experience covers much of the lifespan. Jenny specialises in paediatric services (0–18 years old) and Heather in adult services. These services are rare and designed to meet the needs of CYP that have the most complex needs following a severe/moderate-severe ABI. The needs of these CYP cannot otherwise be adequately resourced in their local community services (British Society for Rehabilitation Medicine, 2015).

Rehabilitation of CYP is inherently an intensely personal journey – no brain injury can possibly be identical, much less the impact upon an individual's own sense of their lives and values. The ultimate goal of improving an *individual's* quality of life is underpinned by piecing together, thoughtfully, a picture that explores who the *individual* was pre-injury, what happened to them and how this has affected them across *all* relevant parts of their lives. Whilst this translates for psychologists rather matter-of-factly as employing a process of assessment, formulation and intervention, what is paramount as a therapeutic target for clinicians is to get to a very human position of being able to mentalise (Fonagy, Gergely, Jurist, & Target, 2002) what it is like to be that CYP, their family and members of their systems. How else can clinicians truly "help"?

Formulation is a vehicle for delineating what this "help" may look like based upon a recognition of the heterogeneity of impacts from an acquired brain injury. Whilst a diagnosis is necessary (and helpful) in of itself it is not sufficient to predict what the main issues are for an individual in context, as well as the resources they bring to the rehabilitation process.

The formulation models described next have potential to be applicable across community, residential and inpatient rehabilitation settings (both paediatric and adult). Differences we foresee in use will reflect pertinent commissioning and stakeholder priorities. For instance, the remit of the service will impact on what is being asked of the clinician, by whom and time afforded to the task. Possible interventions will depend on the range of other professionals in the team and wider support network. Clinicians' decision making will then guide the purpose for what is shared, how it is shared and with whom.

Fragmentation of services for this population can discourage a coherent contemporaneous narrative to accompany a CYP through their lifespan. It is hoped that handing over formulations at key transition points (between support services and community settings) will emphasise the centrality of a compassionate understanding of the brain injury, within a comprehensive understanding of the individual in context.

CYP with severe injuries are commonly living with a complex range of difficulties encompassing medical, physical, sensory, cognitive, communicative, behavioural, social and emotional needs. Being able to understand and contextualise needs using an explanatory framework is essential in ensuring we target current key needs, as well as anticipate transition needs (both practical and psychological).

Formulation drawing upon interpersonal, biological, social and cultural factors has been a core skill of clinical psychologists since the 1950s (the British Psychology Society, 2011). Key features of a generic psychological formulation have been distilled as

- A summary of an individual's core problems,
- Suggestions of how difficulties relate to one another,
- Theory-based explanations of how the difficulties developed and how they are maintained,
- Indicating a theory-based intervention plan and
- Being open to revision – i.e. "re-formulation" (Johnstone & Dallos, 2006).

Formulation models can be based on a particular theory or therapeutic approach such as behavioural (Pavlov, 1849–1936; Skinner, 1904–1990), personal construct theory (Kelly & Maher, 1969), cognitive behavioural therapy (Beck, 1976, 1979), narrative (White & Epston, 1990), psychodynamic (e.g. Freud, 1856–1939) and systemic schools, such as structural (Minuchin, 1974), strategic (Haley, 1977), Milan (Selvini-Palazzoli, Boscolo, Cecchin, & Prata, 1978, 1980) and post-Milan (e.g. Anderson & Goolishian, 1986). Newer approaches include third wave cognitive behavioural therapy (CBT) (e.g. ACT; Hayes, Luoma, Bond, Masuda, & Lillis, 2006), Mindfulness-based CBT (Segal, Williams, & Teasdale, 2013)), social constructionist and critical approaches.

During the course of clinical practice, the authors became aware of the need to extend and develop specific formulation models for CYP with ABI within an inpatient rehabilitation setting. This is in line with Byard, Fine, and Reed (2011) PEDS model which emphasises the psychosocial context. A remaining challenge for us as clinicians was to operationalise our observations into an explicit formulation template to summarise the large amounts of clinical information necessary to guide multidisciplinary practice. We wanted to not only include results of assessment (clinical and neuropsychological) but also to provide an explanatory interactive framework for issues of concern and their relationship to risk, inclusion of key stakeholder roles, possible interventions, evaluation and clinician self-reflexivity.

The process of developing these models was not explicitly focussed on an extensive review and critique of existing formulations. Rather they are an adaptation of the clinicians' existing knowledge that developed through a wish to improve routine clinical practice. The focus therefore was on having systematic tools that built upon one another logically to provide framework for pre-formulation/assessment, formulation and intervention/evaluation.

Several complimentary models developed organically ("SPECS", "SNAP" and "NIF-TY"), which are all embedded in a theoretically pluralistic framework. They are hierarchical in their complexity (starting from pre-formulation information gathering frameworks to a fully integrated formulation) and designed for different professional audiences.

Principles that are embedded in the models are that of

- Dynamic systems and the centrality of a neuro-biopsychosocial perspective;
- The recognition of circular and bidirectional effects across factors;
- The need to consider both risk and resiliency factors to typical child development as well as those pertinent to ABI;
- Using a multi-layered, multi-contextual approach;
- Recognising the importance of intergenerational transmission on coping and attachment;
- Taking into account developmental trajectories;
- Recognising the need to empower parents and CYP affected by brain injury; and
- Placing the CYP's voice and personhood at the centre (Kitwood, 1997).

Theories of family life cycle (Carter & McGoldrick, 1989) and ecological systems theory (Bronfenbrenner, 1979) that acknowledge wider systems and systemic contexts were also influential in our thinking.

In brief, the models seek to recognise the interplay of environmental influences on the brain and of emotional well-being and the brain. Whilst the models have a basic common architecture, they are designed to capture the uniqueness of any one system.

The models will be presented in order of ascending complexity, with the simplest level accessible for all clinicians/workers to the most complex for those with more professional training.

SPECS

SPECS (Jim & Norton, 2014, 2015a, 2015b, 2015c, 2015d, Jim, 2017) is an acronym for key psychosocial factors that we know are important in optimising the quality of life for CYP with acquired brain injury. The letters pertain to the following:

- S = Social
- P = Physical
- E = Emotional
- C = Cognitive
- S = Spiritual

This model was first developed as a core framework for a psychosocial training package for staff that aims to operationalise the concept of "psychosocial care" so that it can be used in everyday practice. SPECS is also a play on the words "spectacles" and "spectrum" – it is about both seeing brain injury more clearly by looking at the different domains and acknowledging that each CYP is made up of their own diverse spectrum. In practice, the domains are colour coded analogous to white light being dispersed by a prism.

The SPECS model encourages a holistic/contextualised perspective on rehabilitation. It also encourages staff and clinicians to think about their own SPECS needs, thereby having a normalising and non-pathologising approach. By doing this, the interplay between clinician and CYP is acknowledged encouraging reflective practice.

The SPECS model is illustrated in Figure 4.1.

> Effective holistic care will take into account all of the following needs of the children. Ideally, these needs would be assessed and addressed throughout their care: from acute admission, throughout their hospital stay, whilst in intensive rehabilitation, on discharge and by community services.

An initial SPECS profile can be obtained from the referring service and an updated SPECS profile could be passed to the services the CYP is consequently discharged to. It aims to give a thumbnail sketch of the CYP in context and highlight any clear areas of clinical priority. In each box, there is room to write both strengths and needs.

Importantly, clinicians themselves are asked to complete their own SPECS to understand the resonances with the people they work with. Of particular importance (due to its frequent neglect) is allowing clinicians to think about the use of "self" in their work, with specific reference to spirituality, faith, cultural or religious beliefs. These beliefs can influence all aspects of rehabilitation from acute to rehabilitation settings via expectations of help, recovery and involvement.

A template with prompts for strengths and needs with possible examples for each domain is shown in Figure 4.2.

SPECS has been particularly helpful when working with professionals from a variety of backgrounds with less experience of psychosocial formulation and knowledge of brain injury.

Cognitive

Intellectual and cognitive (thinking) skills underpin the way we make sense of the world around us. Many of our children's ability to read, write, remember, problem solve and pay attention will be less than before (but this can change over time as the child heals but also through active intervention). Rehabilitation and therapy aims to build upon children's thinking skills and help them re-learn/cope.

Emotional

It is normal for our children to have a range of feelings. Injuries can make them prone to mood swings that are more intense due to a combination of the brain injury and the emotionally traumatising event. They may have difficulty labelling and understanding their feelings. Being mentally healthy is extremely important in our sense of self-esteem and belonging in society.

Spiritual

This domain covers many aspects important to a sense of personal identity. Children and/or their families may belong to spiritual, religious, cultural, faith or ethnic groups. These can give a sense of belonging which can be comforting. Injury can challenge our beliefs and sense of who we are. Many difficult questions can arise such as 'why me?' and 'what does this mean for me?'.

Physical

Physical needs may include drinking, eating, exercising and managing personal hygiene. Our children can be totally dependent on support from family and carers to meet their physical needs either temporarily or permanently. They may also have to use a range of equipment.

Social

Being able to interact and communicate successfully with others (family, friends, teachers, etc.) is an important part of our life. Injuries may change our ability to communicate with others (verbally and non-verbally) and will be challenging for our children to adjust to. You'll have to be creative in thinking about ways in which to help the child participate fully in their lives.

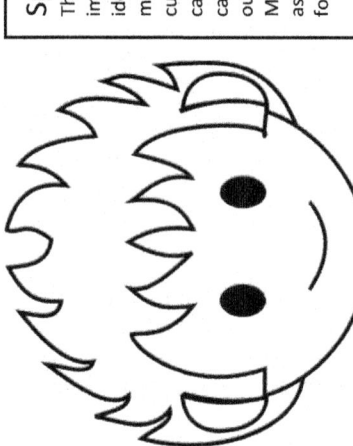

Figure 4.1 The SPECS model

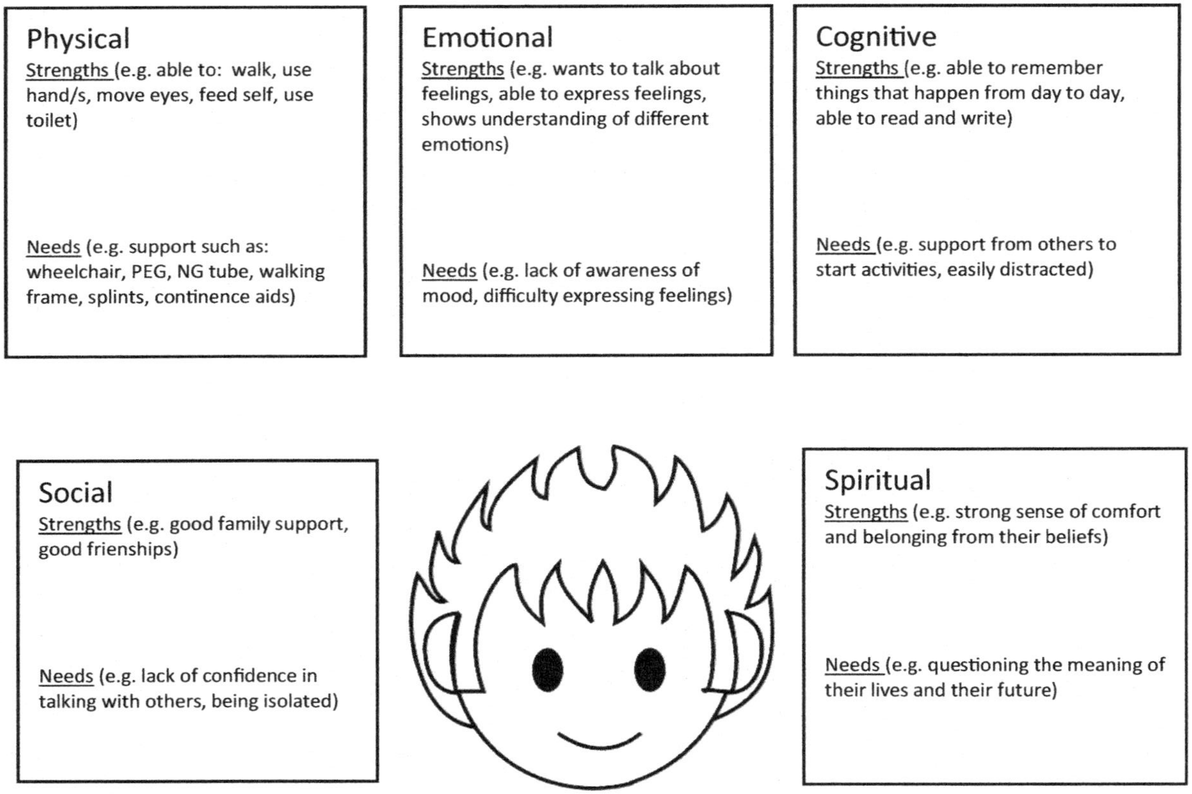

Physical

<u>Strengths</u> (e.g. able to: walk, use hand/s, move eyes, feed self, use toilet)

<u>Needs</u> (e.g. support such as: wheelchair, PEG, NG tube, walking frame, splints, continence aids)

Emotional

<u>Strengths</u> (e.g. wants to talk about feelings, able to express feelings, shows understanding of different emotions)

<u>Needs</u> (e.g. lack of awareness of mood, difficulty expressing feelings)

Cognitive

<u>Strengths</u> (e.g. able to remember things that happen from day to day, able to read and write)

<u>Needs</u> (e.g. support from others to start activities, easily distracted)

Social

<u>Strengths</u> (e.g. good family support, good friendships)

<u>Needs</u> (e.g. lack of confidence in talking with others, being isolated)

Spiritual

<u>Strengths</u> (e.g. strong sense of comfort and belonging from their beliefs)

<u>Needs</u> (e.g. questioning the meaning of their lives and their future)

Figure 4.2 A SPECS profile: strengths and needs

The SNAP

The SNAP is an acronym for the Systematic Neuropsychological Assessment Profile. Adapted by Jim for clinical use in 2014 (and extended by Liddiard & Jim, 2015a, 2015b, 2015c, 2015d) from the model developed by the Cambridge Centre for Paediatric Neuropsychological Rehabilitation (CCPNR), it is a profile that allows the systematic mapping of an individual's neuropsychological skills (either formally tested and/or from observation) over time and to contribute to a biopsychosocial formulation and interventions. Therefore, it is most beneficial when used in a multidisciplinary team that has access to occupational therapy and psychology.

"SNAP" also refers to an abridged version of the word "snapshot" as it is meant to be a picture of the CYP and their system at a particular point in time. It builds upon the general overview afforded by SPECS and incorporates core information about the CYP, and sets them alongside the acquired brain injury and its neuropsychological and functional impact at that time. It then prompts the team to think of proposed goals (i.e. Goal Attainment Scaling [GAS]) and further actions needed to be undertaken by the multidisciplinary team or team around the child (TAC).

The SNAP is illustrated in Figure 4.3.

The SNAP is amended/repeated in line with further information from ongoing standardised and unstandardised assessment. A key advantage of the SNAP it that it ensures coverage of relevant domains. Furthermore, it encourages clinicians to look for relationships across the domains and to reflect on whether there can be novel interpretations/understandings of observed behaviour that are useful to understanding how to meet the CYP and family's needs.

The NIF-TY

The NIF-TY is an acronym for the Neuropsychological Integrated Formulation profile (Jim & Liddiard, 2016a, 2016b) It facilitates a transtheoretical neurobiopsychosocial formulation and represents the most complex of the models presented. Designed to integrate information from SPECS and the SNAP, the NIF-TY holds a greater complexity of data and acts as a springboard for the incorporation of a wide range of theoretical and therapeutic approaches.

Key features of the NIF-TY are as follows:

- It allows the impact of the brain injury to be explicitly acknowledged through the entirety of the person's biopsychosocial world
- It is multifactorial and multisystemic
- It is developmental (primary and secondary impacts)
- It is valuing of a strengths-based empowering approach
- It is explicit enough as to have predictive qualities
- It is detailed enough to give rise to objective goal setting

The NIF-TY is illustrated in Figure 4.4.

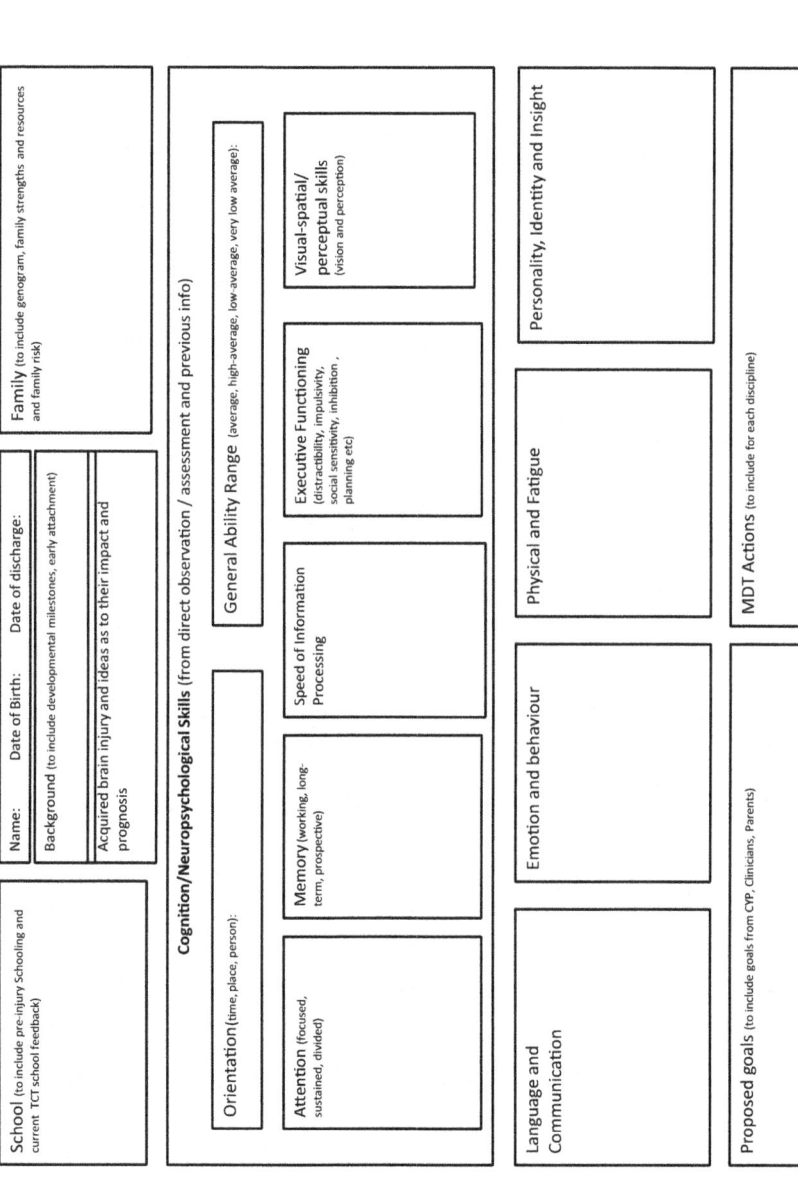

Figure 4.3 The SNAP model: The Systematic Neuropsychological Assessment Profile

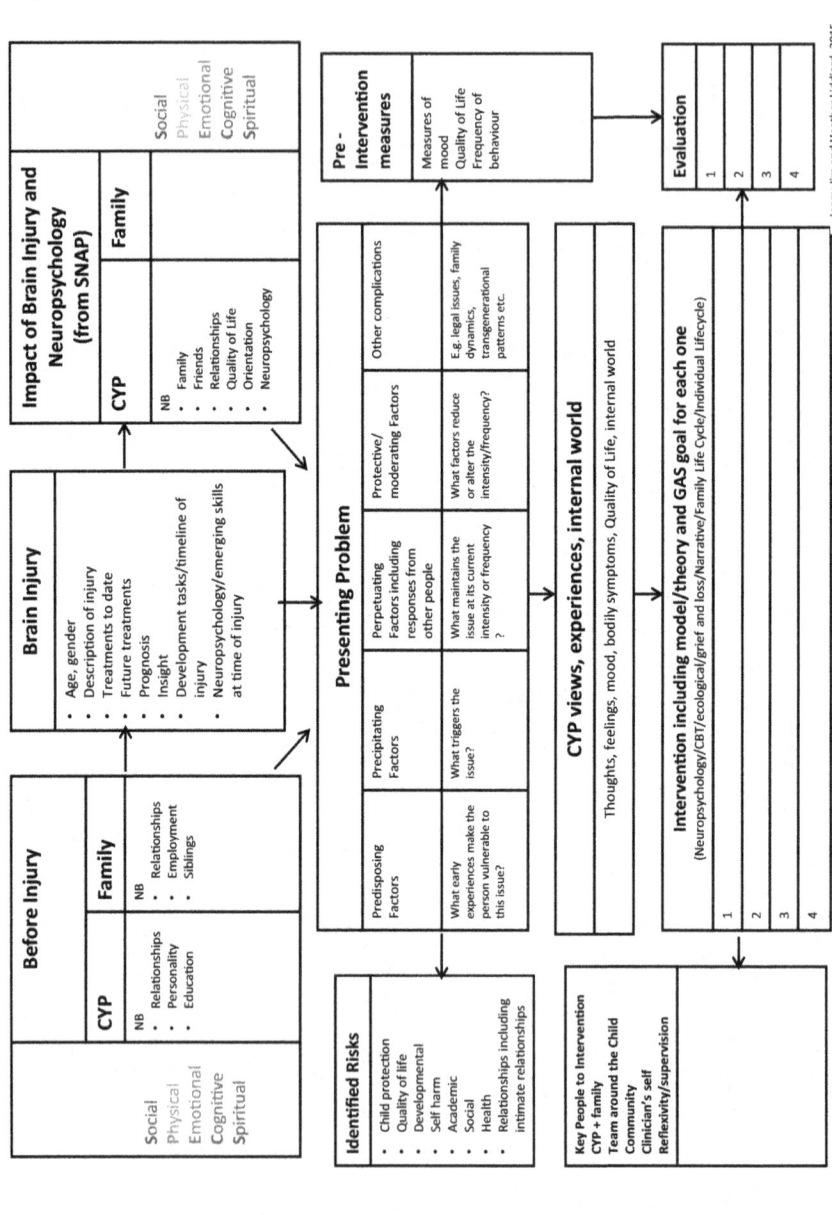

Figure 4.4 NIF-TY: The Neuropsychological Integrated Formulation profile

Jenny Jim and Heather Liddiard, 2015

The NIF-TY is a pragmatic tool potentially tangible to all members of a multi-disciplinary team and provides an integrated model to understand, intervene and evaluate clinical approaches. It allows the development of a conceptual rationale for both direct and indirect working across the multidisciplinary team and other supporting networks, therefore, having utility for individual, parent, family, couple and staff work in brain injury.

Whilst the NIF-TY is developed through information via MDT discussions and meeting with the CYP and family; construction and ownership sits with the clinical psychologist as their primary reference document guiding intervention. This rightly raises questions in relation to sharing the interpretations and decisions around the course of action proposed. This is a continuous checking-out process and subsequently will be modified through feedback. Superficially this may be misinterpreted to reflect an expert position, aligned with a medical/diagnostic model; it is, in fact, based on an intention for respecting person-centred approaches that takes into account what a particular individual or team can hold on to and their priorities at any given point in time. Meaning-making to facilitate progress is the primary goal.

For instance, the presenting problem and intervention boxes in the NIF-TY will allow clinicians to consider a range of presentations (both common and less frequent) following ABI. The NIF-TY allows the clinician to identify specific areas of work such as trauma-related intervention; it is then down to the clinician to choose which theoretical presentation-specific approach to use – e.g. CBT for trauma or EMDR. They will then use the model chosen in the way it has been evidenced. The NIF-TY is a considered triage decision-making tool. As such, the NIF-TY can be used for myriad CYP and family concerns as wide-ranging as cognitive impairment and remediation, pain management to marital breakdown.

The NIF-TY in practice

We aim to illustrate how we use the models to gather and interpret clinical information. In doing this, we reflected on our dilemmas about what would be the most helpful, ethical and, indeed, practical approach to sharing how the tool is implemented.

Gaining consent was not solely the issue. It became clear that whilst different formulations had been shared in stages with families, they had rarely been presented in such a format. Whilst the understandings within the formulation are collaborative, we realised the NIF-TY is primarily a tool for clinicians. Its very nature and purpose are to organise an overwhelming amount of complex information. The NIF-TY's key advantage to clinicians can paradoxically mean that it is rarely appropriate to share in its entirety to families.

Working in a post-acute context there are a number of additional issues that make sharing the NIF-TY difficult. The families are post-crisis or actively experiencing post-traumatic symptoms, their daily routines are still in flux resulting in limitations (at times adaptive) around processing the situation.

Given this families are often focussed on their immediate needs; parents often talk about their sense of perspective being restricted to hour-by-hour fragments.

In this psychological context, it has rarely felt appropriate to ask them to take on board such information presented in this way. Whilst we acknowledge criticisms relating to paternalism may be levied at our stance, we feel strongly it is the clinician's responsibility to use their judgement to sensitively co-construct an understanding over time and within the safety of a solid therapeutic relationship.

The following example (Figure 4.5) is an amalgamation of recurring themes we face in our everyday practice. It is hoped that clinicians will gain a fuller sense of the NIF-TY's potential utility. Reading the NIF-TY mirrors the clinical process of its construction; thus, it is designed to be read left to right, progressing from the top to bottom of the page. The process of formulation begins with distilling the content generated from both SPECS and SNAP. This populates the NIF-TY with the key information that you will see on the top layer of the model.

The layer that follows (Figure 4.6) focusses on the clinical priorities, which are then broken down using the generic 5 Ps model. Most pertinent is the box that follows this (Figure 4.7), which concentrates on the mentalising of the CYP.

This information can be integrated by the clinician (drawing upon their knowledge, skills and practice) to make decisions regarding key levels of psychological intervention. Such interventions should relate to wider rehabilitation goals. The formulation prompts the clinician to consider objective methods of evaluation and to identify key people as partners to the success of these interventions. There is also a place to consider risk issues. Alongside these processes the formulation provides a space for clinicians to reflect on their feelings and experiences.

As such the NIF-TY is much more than simply a formulation diagram. It allows information from assessment and pre-formulation, formulation and interventions and evaluations of any input to be synthesised. As such it prompts clinicians to think reflexively regarding appropriate outcome measures at the beginning of any intervention. Often, ways of evaluation are only considered after psychological work has begun/is complete. This may mean that creative ways of measuring change may be missed.

In this way, the NIF-TY prompts clinicians to consider the question, early on in their work, "How can we tell if there has been a change?" The NIF-TY also helps the clinician to think about a range of outcome measures. These might include the following:

•   Changes in the frequency, intensity or duration of challenging behaviour
•   Evaluations via video recording
•   Using standardised and unstandardised questionnaires for childhood or parental mood states

Dilemmas in sharing formulations

Whilst SPECS, SNAP and NIF-TY have proved invaluable in clinical psychological practice with people across different life stages, we have faced dilemmas in creating the conditions whereby using these models becomes truly a

Before Injury		
	CYP	Family
Social Physical Emotional Cognitive Spiritual	S – shy, stable peer group, bullying prior to injury P – small for age E – close relationship with mum C – above average in most subjects S – belief in academic identity	S – feeling of isolation P – needs met E – insular coping C – able to integrate info about diagnosis S – Muslim faith – beliefs about disability and optimism around recovery

CYP and Brain Injury
Thirteen year old female, adolescence Intimate relationships, independence, developing identify. Emerging self-regulation and executive functioning. Short history of nausea and vomiting. Brain tumour – posterior fossa. Cerebellar mutism post surgery. Chemotherapy and radiotherapy. In hospital for months, ops ++. Severe brain injury. Prognosis unclear. CYP shows insight into impact of injury.

Impact of Brain Injury and Neuropsychology (from SNAP)		
	CYP	Family
Social Physical Emotional Cognitive Spiritual	S – more exuberant P – wheelchair, sever ataxia and weakness in left side E – more needy, less regulated C – attention, executive functioning, processing speed, SLT difficulties S – challenge to identity	S – isolated + P – living in different places E – exhausted coping C – felt unprepared S – kept their faith in full recovery

Figure 4.5 NIF-TY: pre-injury, developmental stage, brain injury and impact post-injury

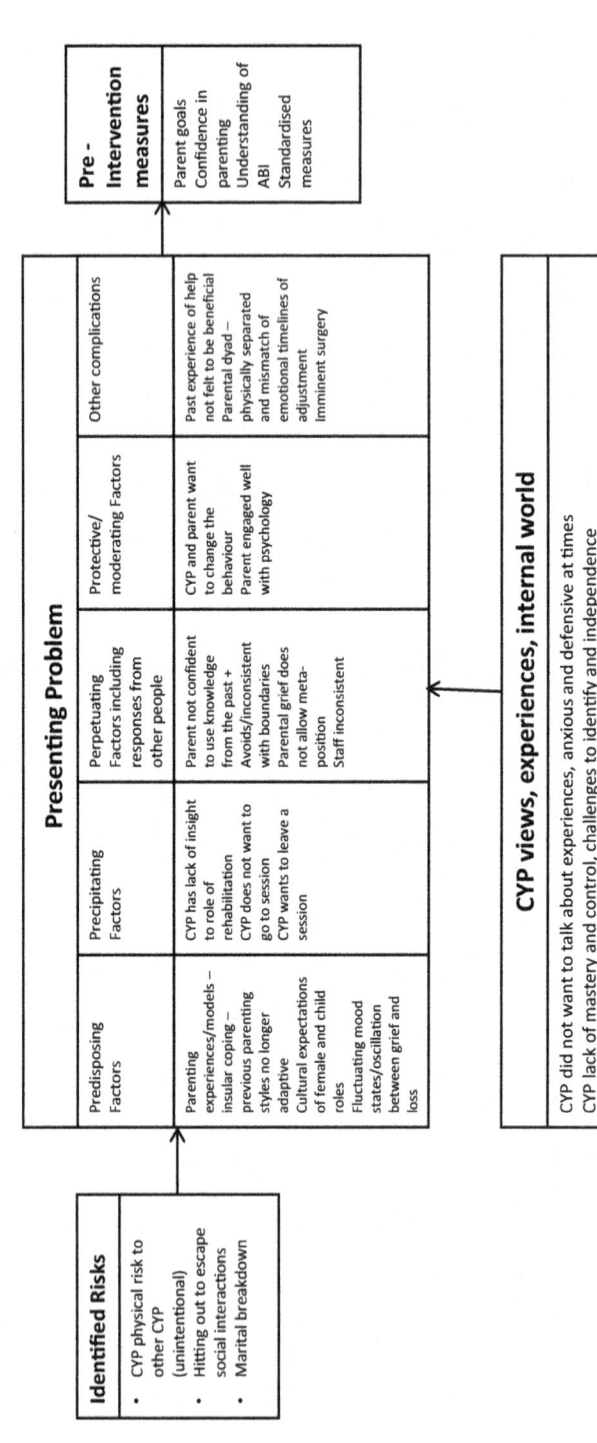

Figure 4.6 NIF-TY: presenting problem, risks, measures and CYP's view

Identified Risks

- CYP physical risk to other CYP (unintentional)
- Hitting out to escape social interactions
- Marital breakdown

Pre - Intervention measures

Parent goals
Confidence in parenting
Understanding of ABI
Standardised measures

Presenting Problem

Predisposing Factors	Precipitating Factors	Perpetuating Factors including responses from other people	Protective/ moderating Factors	Other complications
Parenting experiences/models – insular coping – previous parenting styles no longer adaptive Cultural expectations of female and child roles Fluctuating mood states/oscillation between grief and loss	CYP has lack of insight to role of rehabilitation CYP does not want to go to session CYP wants to leave a session	Parent not confident to use knowledge from the past + Avoids/inconsistent with boundaries Parental grief does not allow meta-position Staff inconsistent	CYP and parent want to change the behaviour Parent engaged well with psychology	Past experience of help not felt to be beneficial Parental dyad – physically separated and mismatch of emotional timelines of adjustment Imminent surgery

CYP views, experiences, internal world

CYP did not want to talk about experiences, anxious and defensive at times
CYP lack of mastery and control, challenges to identify and independence

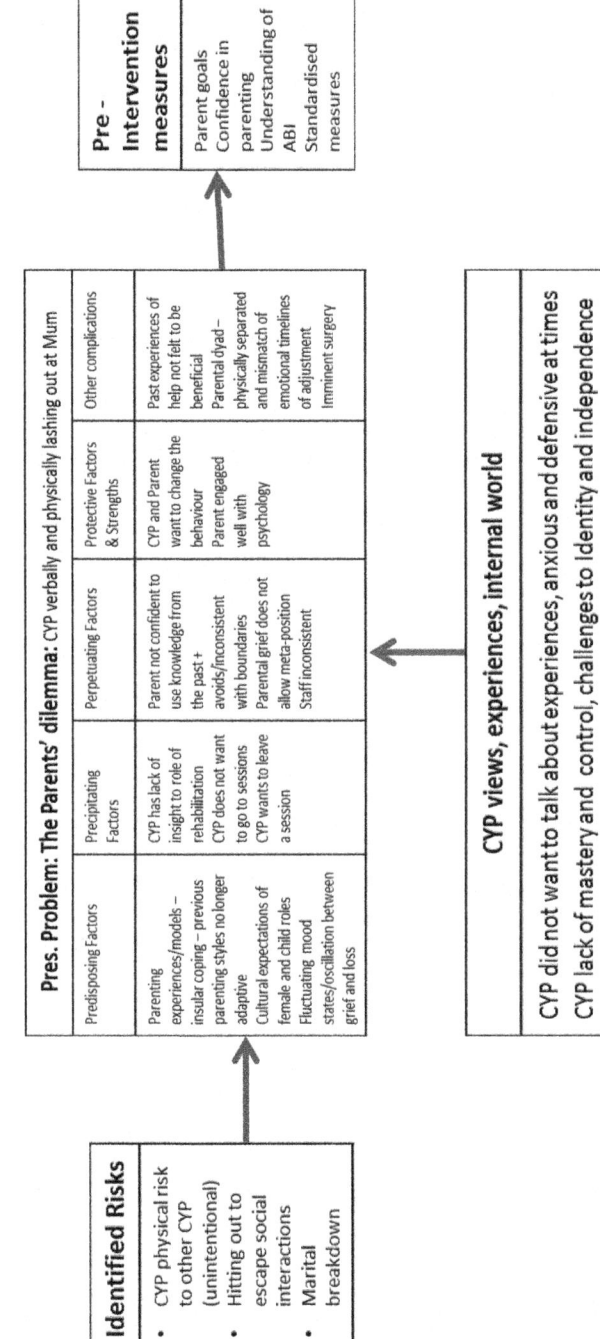

Figure 4.7 NIF-TY: intervention and evaluation

multidisciplinary team activity. We have encountered challenges in making these models meaningful to other professionals and hence there have been difficulties in implementing the interventions within systems. Without this, it is not possible to evaluate the formulation and reformulate when necessary.

Implementation and clinical process

The NIF-TY is not a tool that can be used independently from the knowledge gained from clinical training. Theory-driven enquiry underpins the clinical process of how information is gathered, the models drawn upon and, consequently, the therapist's aims/stance. To illustrate using another example, the diagram that follows (Figure 4.8) represents these interactive processes in relation to a family's concerns around parenting post-ABI.

Whereas assessment, formulation and intervention exist in other professions, these tend to be less embedded in a psychosocial context, and as a consequence, the models can seem overwhelming. At times, we have also wondered if this way of thinking is seen as the responsibility of psychologists.

Sharing formulations to all relevant audiences is equally as important as having a robust formulation itself. In our clinical practice, it has been challenging to make this meaningful enough to the agents of change (including CYP, their families and staff) in the systems we work in.

Paradoxically, the strength of these models relies on time for a systematic assessment period; however, we have found there is often a pressure to intervene without a robust formulation.

Summary

We have presented three models that sit within a hierarchical assessment process. These have grown organically through our clinical practice using our training and knowledge. Superficially, the models may appear simplistic in their nature; however, they require considerable skills and interpretation to use them to their fullest extent.

Evaluations

SPECS, SNAP and NIF-TY prove their utility in our daily clinical practice and for supervisory discussions. They help us to answer questions such as the following: "What are the important things for that person and their family?" "What is the role for us as clinicians?" "What tests would be suitable for this person at this point in time?" "What domains have not been sufficiently assessed?" And, "What are the risks for this person at discharge?"

All three models have been validated at a number of levels including during clinical practice and supervision, internal training, neuropsychology and clinical training courses, national and international conferences. They have been

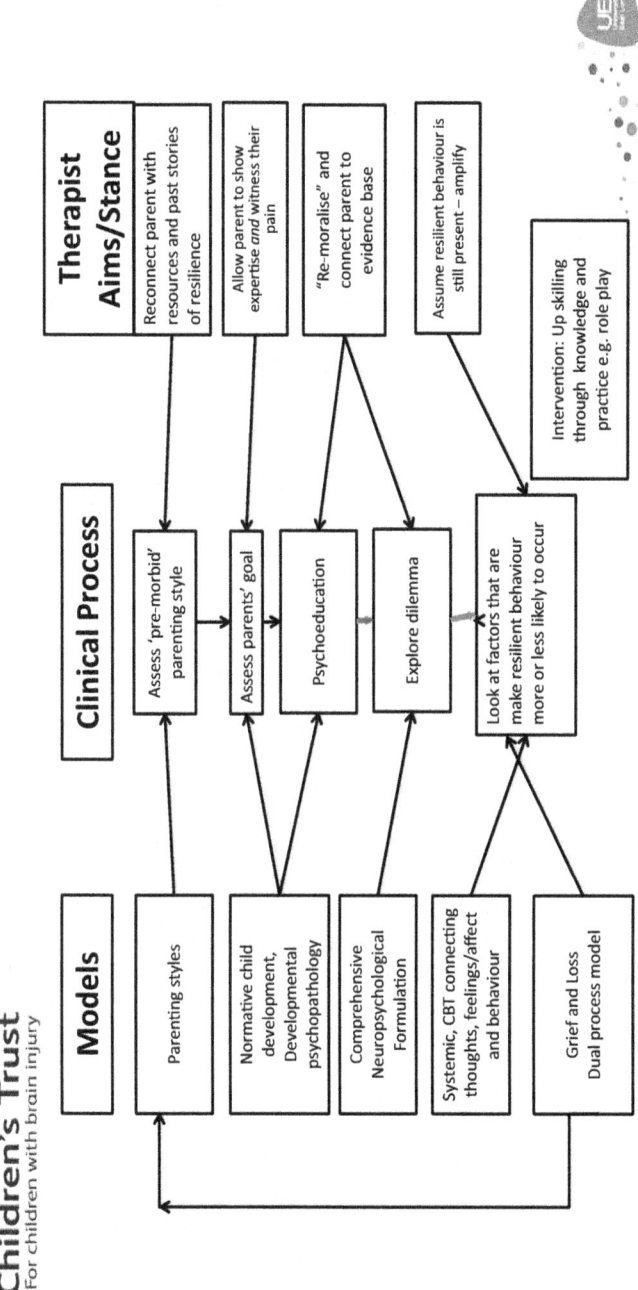

Figure 4.8 Diagram of the clinical process underlying formulation and goal setting

positively received though these models are not evaluated empirically. We anticipate that it may be helpful if we were to ask leaders in the field to review their content and utility.

We have presented our interpretation of a "biopsychosocial approach"; however, we know this might not align to the use of this term to other contexts. We are aware this approach has been critiqued (please see Pilgrim, 2015).

Specialist rehabilitation services play a vital role in maximising recovery and supporting safe transitions back to community services (British Society for Rehabilitation Medicine, 2015). Although the models described earlier in no way have been measured in terms of financial savings, it is hoped that they optimise the "slinky models of rehabilitation" (British Society of Rehabilitation Medicine, 2003) with CYP moving from rehab to other services with a coherent formulation and intervention plan that transfers with them. In such a way, it is envisaged that this reduces time and resources in the receiving service.

Reflections

We have psychological and practical reflections from using SPECS, SNAP and NIF-TY. Firstly, we acknowledge the importance of our own cultural, social context and the political contexts that influence the services we can provide.

Embedding these models as a routine way of working is a challenge exacerbated by working in a national and specialist service, as we need to liaise with a multitude of referring and receiving organisations. As a consequence, it takes time to build up a shared understanding of the approach, and there is often a lack of organisational memory.

Future directions

Empirical testing of these models would identify the mediators of outcome and allow one to make conclusions regarding the variance any particular risk or resiliency factor may account for in terms of overall outcome. In this way, clinicians could benefit from potentially a more algorithmic but personalised approach.

However, routine clinical practice does not make this very practicable, though we acknowledge a path-analytic approach or other such statistical modelling approach could be very beneficial.

Conclusions

We hope that the SPECS, SNAP and NIF-TY illustrate the benefits of a comprehensive biopsychosocial formulation with clinical and neuropsychology at its heart. By using this hierarchical approach, we are able to draw upon the diverse evidence bases to guide clinical intervention and evaluation across multiple systems and across the lifespan.

References

Anderson, H., & Goolishian, H. A. (1986). Problem determined systems: Towards transformation in family therapy. *Journal of Strategic & Systemic Therapist, 5*(4), 1–13.

Beck, A. T. (1976). *Cognitive therapy and emotional disorders*. New York: International University Press.

Beck, A. T., Rush, A. J., Shaw, B. F., & Emery, G. (1979). *Cognitive therapy of depression*. New York: Guildford Press.

British Society of Rehabilitation Medicine. (2003). *Rehabilitation following acquired brain injury: National clinical guidelines*. London: Royal College of Physicians.

Bronfenbrenner, U. (1979). *The ecology of human development: Experiments by nature and design*. Cambridge, MA: Harvard University Press.

Byard, K., Fine, H., & Reed, J. (2011). Taking a developmental and systemic perspective on neuropsychological rehabilitation with children with brain injury and their families. *Clinical Child Psychology & Psychiatry, 16*(2), 165–184.

Carter, B., & McGoldrick, M. (1989). *The expanded family life cycle: Individual, family and social perspectives* (3rd ed.). Boston: Pearson.

Fonagy, P., Gergely, G., Jurist, E., & Target, M. (2002). *Affect regulation, mentalization, and the development of the self*. New York: Other Press.

Haley, J. (1977). Toward a theory of pathological systems. In P. Watzlawick & J. Weakland (Eds.), *The interactional view: Studies at the mental research institute* (pp. 11–27). New York: W.W. Norton & Company.

Hayes, S. C., Luoma, J. B., Bond, F. W., Masuda, A., & Lillis, J. (2006). Acceptance and commitment therapy: Model, processes and outcomes. *Behaviour Research and Therapy, 44*(1), 1–25.

Jim, J. (2015). *Empowering parents to be parents in post-acute neurorehabilitation for severe acquired brain injury*. The first international conference on paediatric acquired brain injury: Supporting young people and their families to maximise good outcomes and quality of life. International Paediatric Brain Injury Symposium (IPBIS). Liverpool.

Jim, J. (2017). *"SPECS": A psychosocial training package for staff working in paediatric acquired brain injury*. National Paediatric Brain Injury Conference. The Children's Trust. BMA House, London.

Jim, J., & Liddiard, H. (2016a). *The "NIF-TY": The neuropsychological integrated formulation model for use in paediatric and adult acquired brain injury*. 28th annual meeting. Challenge the boundaries – international conference on cerebral palsy and other childhood onset disabilities, 2016. European Academy for Childhood Disability (EACD), Copenhagen, Denmark.

Jim, J., & Liddiard, H. (2016b). *The "NIF-TY": The neuropsychological integrated formulation model for use in paediatric and adult acquired brain injury*. 11th world congress on brain injury: Brain injury from cell to society. International Brain Injury Association (IBIA), The Hague, The Netherlands.

Jim, J., & Liddiard, H. (2016b). *The "NIF-TY": The neuropsychological integrated formulation model for use in paediatric and adult acquired brain injury*. National Paediatric Brain Injury Conference, 2017. The Children's Trust. BMA House, London.

Jim, J., & Norton, B. (2014). *"SPECS": A psychosocial training package for staff working in paediatric acquired brain injury*. Paediatric Seminar of the Association of Brain Injury Lawyers, ABIL, London.

Jim, J., & Norton, B. (2015a). *"SPECS": A psychosocial training package for staff working in paediatric acquired brain injury*. Division of Neuropsychology annual conference. Complex challenges in neuro-rehabilitation. British Psychological Society, Division of Neuropsychology, (BPS, DoN). London.

Jim, J., & Norton, B. (2015b). *"SPECS": A psychosocial training package for staff working in paediatric acquired brain injury*. 27th annual meeting. New ways, new moves – neuroplasticity, physical activity and nutrition, new technologies, cognition, perception and movement. European Academy for Childhood Disability (EACD), Copenhagen, Denmark.

Jim, J., & Norton, B. (2015c). *"SPECS": A psychosocial training package for staff working in paediatric acquired brain injury*. 13th Congress of European Forum for Research in Rehabilitation: Being, doing and participating. European Forum for Research in Rehabilitation (EFRR), Helskini, Finland.

Jim, J., & Norton, B. (2015d). *"SPECS": A psychosocial training package for staff working in paediatric acquired brain injury*. 11th World congress on brain injury: Brain injury from cell to society, 2016. International Brain Injury Association (IBIA), The Hague, The Netherlands.

Johnstone, L., & Dallos, R. (2006). Introduction to formulation. In L. Johnstone & R. Dallos (Eds.), *Formulation in psychology and psychotherapy: Making sense of people's problems* (pp. 1–16). London and New York: Routledge.

Kelly, G., & Maher, B. A. (1969). *Clinical psychology and personality: The selected papers of George Kelly*. New York: John Wiley & Sons.

Kitwood, T. (1997). *Dementia reconsidered: The person comes first*. Buckingham and Philadelphia: Open University Press.

Liddiard, H., & Jim, J. (2015a). *The "SNAP" 1 and 2: Post-acute systematic neuropsychological assessment profiles for paediatric and adult severe acquired brain injury*. Division of neuropsychology annual conference: Complex challenges in neuro-rehabilitation. British Psychological Society, Division of Neuropsychology, (BPS, DoN), London.

Liddiard, H., & Jim, J. (2015b). *The "SNAP" 1 and 2: Post-acute systematic neuropsychological assessment profiles for paediatric and adult severe acquired brain injury*. 28th annual meeting: Challenge the boundaries – international conference on cerebral palsy and other childhood onset disabilities, 2016. European Academy for Childhood Disability (EACD), Copenhagen, Denmark.

Liddiard, H., & Jim, J. (2015c). *The "SNAP" 1 and 2: Post-acute systematic neuropsychological assessment profiles for paediatric and adult severe acquired brain injury*. 11th world congress on brain injury: Brain injury from cell to society, 2016. International Brain Injury Association (IBIA), The Hague, The Netherlands.

Liddiard, H., & Jim, J. (2015d). *The "SNAP" 1 and 2: Post-acute systematic neuropsychological assessment profiles for paediatric and adult severe acquired brain injury*. New perspectives in paediatric rehabilitation, 2016. Society for Rehabilitation Research (SRR). Royal Hospital for Neuro-Disability Putney, London.

Minuchin, S. (1974). *Families and family therapy*. Boston: Harvard University Press.

Pilgrim, D. (2015). The biopsychosocial model in health research: Its strengths and limitations for critical realists. *Journal of Critical Realism*, (14), 164–180.

Segal, Z., Willliams, J. M. G., & Teasdale, J. D. (2013). *Mindfulness-based cognitive therapy for depression: A new approach to preventing relapse* (2nd ed.). New York: Guilford Press.

Selvini-Palazzoli, M., Boscolo, L., Cecchin, G., & Prata, G. (1978). *Paradox and counter-paradox: A new model in the therapy of the family in schizophrenic transaction*. New York: Jason Aronson.

Selvini-Palazzoli, M., Boscolo, L., Cecchin, G., & Prata, G. (1980). Hypothesizing-circularity-neutrality: Three guidelines for the conductor of the session. *Family Process*, *19*, 3–12.

White, M., & Epston, D. (1990). *Narrative means to therapeutic ends*. New York: W.W. Norton & Company.

Web resources

The British Psychology Society (BPS). (2011). *Good practice guidelines on the use of psychological formulation*. Division of Clinical Psychology, British Psychological Society (DCP, BPS). Retrieved August 2017, from www.bps.org.uk/system/files/Public%20 files/DCP/cat-842.pdf

British Society for Rehabilitation Medicine (BSRM). (2015). *Specialised neuro-rehabilitation services standards. Specialist neuro-rehabilitation services: Providing for patients with complex rehabilitation needs*. Retrieved August 2017, from www. bsrm.org.uk/downloads/specialised-neurorehabiliation-service-standards-7-30-4-2015-forweb.pdf

Innovations in psychological therapy

Chapter 5

Narrative-inspired interview with the brain

Jenny Jim

This chapter invites you to listen in on a therapeutic interview between the brain (B) and a narrative therapist (T). It compresses some key therapeutic aspects of the narrative process into one stylised episode. The appendix allows you to see how T has interpreted questions suggested by White (2007) as characteristic of narrative interviewing.

Context: The brain, B, is an adolescent seeking help with feelings of loss and despair following injury 12 months prior. B sustained a moderate brain injury and is currently living at home and attending sixth form. To others, B's injury is not visible, as they have no outward scars.

T: Please tell me what is troubling you and what you hope I can help with?

B: *I was in an accident and am damaged and feel damaged . . . I won't ever get better.*

T: What happened?

B: *I was in a car accident. I was busy directing my body to college, and we got hit on a zebra crossing. Now I can't think straight. I can't keep up with my friends. I feel in a constant . . . fog. I can't explain it.*

T: I am so sorry to hear that. So you have been in an accident and now you feel you are damaged and that you will never recover from this. That sounds very painful. What troubles you the most?

B: *That I will never get better, I am damaged, I am not 'me' anymore.*

T: Hmmm, how difficult for you. If you can, do tell me a bit more so I really understand where you are coming from.

B: *It's not easy for me to say. My mum and best mate keep saying I should feel lucky to be alive. I get annoyed and angry, sometimes I shout – I can't use words like I could before the accident. I know what I want to say but can't say it.*

T: I see, not only is it hard emotionally but it's also just harder to express yourself overall? And it seems linked to frustrations that people close to you don't real-ise where you're coming from?

B: *Yes, everyone says how 'lucky' I am, but I don't feel it. I want to be who I was before. No one understands. All I see is black. I'll never get better.*

T: I wonder if we can capture what you are saying distinctly perhaps by giving it a name? What could we call this feeling of "never getting better . . . being damaged"?

B: *The Doom?*

T: That's very evocative. Are you happy for us to talk about "The Doom" and for it to refer to what makes you the most upset and what you want help with?

B: *OK*

T: So, if I can ask more about "The Doom" – when is the "The Doom" most likely to be around?

B: *It's always around. Even when I am out with my friends, it can be worse then, because it reminds me that I'm not the same as them anymore. I don't have as many friends; they don't like hanging around with me. "The Doom" makes me feel sick and angry.*

T: Before "The Doom" was around, what had you hoped for yourself – your ambitions?

B: *I wanted to develop just like other brains, to keep getting better, faster, denser. Now all my connections are broken. The scientists say that I have 'diffuse axonal injury' – it basically means all the work I have put into making information highways has been for nothing. My neurones are broken, and I have a whole part of me missing, which the doctors took out because it was so damaged. The Doom is here now – I am forever changed. I'm not me, and I'll be damaged forever.*

T: It sounds like "The Doom" has a very engulfing effect on the way you think about your ambitions and what your future can be. Tell me, if you can, how do you think it has affected other parts of your life?

B: *Well, I can't control myself like I used to. I know that is part of my damage too, but when I feel "The Doom", I think "What's the point in trying?" and then I get embarrassed about not being able to control myself. It's as if my HQ's control panel doesn't work anymore. I have to stay away from other brains as I know they will see me as defective too, and I can't trust myself to know what to say or not blurt something out I don't mean.*

T: I can see that you are saying that the damage has made emotions and behaviour hard to control, plus "The Doom" then gets in on the act and brings thoughts of "What's the point?" – I guess this connects to the idea that you will never get better? I am also hearing that because of this combination of the damage and "The Doom" that your life is more limited in terms of hanging out with others.

B: *Yep*

T: I am hearing very strongly a very dominant idea from you that "you will never get better" – is that right?

B: *Yes (cries).*

T: How painful. Do you know where you got that idea or story from?

B: *Everybody knows that once brains are damaged, they never get better. We never grow any new neurones, not cell bodies, nothing. What chance do I have?*

T: When you say "everybody" can you tell me anybody in particular?

B: *Well, we all know about the brain of Phineas Gage and his disastrous decline. All the books I read are all about deficits and what brains can't do anymore. In fact, I think scientists delight in finding something new that injured brains can't do. It's twisted.*

T: I see what you mean. Connecting those stories about injured brains has maybe given "The Doom" quite a bit of power.

How do you feel about the power of "The Doom" on your life?

B: *It's so sad for me (cries). I hate myself.*

T: It is OK with you that it has such a strong effect? It sounds like you have enough to cope with beside "The Doom" making you feel worse.

B: *No, it's not OK, but I feel helpless; my limbic system is just red hot all the time, and I can't put the brakes on it anymore. I want everything to work together like it used to. Now I have to spend so much time trying to recover and work against "The Doom".*

T: Why do you think it's not OK that "The Doom" affects you like this?

B: *I guess the more I focus on what "The Doom" wants me to then the more I'll feel like I can't do anything to get better, and I'll keep staying away from other brains, which I don't want to do. I want to be myself again.*

T: So, I can see from this that you have hopes for yourself and what you want to be and do.

B: *I guess you must be right.*

T: I'm interested in trying to explore this more with you. I know it might be hard, but tell me when there was a time, however small, when "The Doom" didn't stop you from doing something you wanted or perhaps learning something new?

B: *That's a hard one.*

T: What rehabilitation sessions have you had recently?

B: *Physio and SLT.*

T: Can you think of anything new you have learnt or made progress with?

B: *Well, my physio says my balance is improving, and I can signal to my body to walk on the treadmill for 5 minutes now. Before, I couldn't even make my body walk.*

T: Wow, that is pretty amazing. You have gone from having no ability to make your body walk to walking on a treadmill for 5 minutes?! Tell more about this.

B: *I guess I have gone from not being able to activate these areas of my motor cortex to being able to.*

T: But how? Tell me. It doesn't just happen! What did you have to do?

B: *It started with helping my body practise transfers to the bath and toilet. Then I got more muscle tone and balance to stand my body with two people supporting it.*

T: Goodness me. This has been a long journey needing a lot of persistence and stamina.

B: *Sometimes I thought I would never be able to do anything. I thought I would always need people supporting my body. "The Doom" – it was so strong some days that I just stayed in bed crying.*

T: But what I am hearing is that "The Doom" could not have been that powerful all of the time; otherwise, how would you have got to where you are now?
I am excited because you have told me about a time when you learnt something new. Changes must have happened to allow you to control your body. It was a time when "The Doom" didn't control the situation and it had no power.

B: *True (smiles).*

T: I guess this is a sort of "Anti-Doom" – what would you call it?

B: *Hmmm, I feel it is like a new light went on, and I could see where I needed to make the new connections and reach out. Like a light switch or torch?*

T: How evocative, "The Torch"?

B: *Yes.*

T: When "The Torch" is around, what does it allow you to do?

B: *It lets me 'try' and not just give up.*

T: So it sounds like you have hope when "The Torch" is around? . . . Hope about achieving something and changing?

B: *I feel I can do things. That's right. I also feel better seeing other Brains. It's funny, but at those times, I really believe what I am going through is just temporary.*

T: "The Torch" certainly seems to change a lot about what you think about yourself, being social and putting things in perspective.
Is it OK for you that "The Torch" has this power?

B: *Sure, I wish it was around all the time.*

T: So, you would prefer if "The Torch" was *on* all of the time because . . .?

B: *Because I could get on with doing my rehab and not getting stuck in dark thoughts. I might see other Brains more, and that always makes me feel better. It also challenges me and gives me inspiration.*

T: Now that we realise "The Torch" exists, when else have you experienced it as being on?

B: *I think it must be on every time I learn something new, when I managed to go out and the rare times when I feel happy again.*

T: So, it's always been there, but we've only just noticed today?

B: *Yes, just like "The Doom".*

T: I guess we both didn't know about "The Torch" until today – I am wondering if there are others who *wouldn't* be surprised about the times the "The Torch" exists?

B: *I guess my sister is always talking about what I have achieved and how I am getting better. She must have paid more attention to what "The Torch" brings.*

T: What do you think she knows about you, which means she wasnt surprised that you can use The Torch's light?

B: *I guess she knows I am a fighter.*

T: She knows you are a fighter and that you will make the most of when "The Torch" is around . . . how does that make you feel about yourself now?

B: *It makes me feel stronger and not hopeless like before. I may be damaged, but I shouldn't keep putting myself down thinking I won't ever change because I have.*

T: If you were to invest more in "The Torch" and less in "The Doom", where do you think that would get you?

B: *I might get closer to my goals without so many hiccups and bad days. I might have more friends again and spend less energy battling with 'The Doom'.*

T: What could you do or think that would help you listen more to "The Torch" and less to "The Doom"?

B: *I could speak to my sister more. I could think more about the things I have achieved rather than the things I lost, though that would be hard. I may have to discipline myself somehow and write a diary.*

T: I agree it won't be easy as "The Doom" has gotten so much power in the past. What seems to switch "The Torch" on?

B: *It's more likely to be on when my sister is with me and when I have slept enough.*

T: So do you need to see if you can make more of those times happen? Also, it might be good to think more about what flicks the "on" button for "The Torch".

B: *That sounds good.*

T: I'm interested also in giving you some time to think about what our conversation about "The Torch" now makes you feel about yourself?

B: *I feel stronger. And though I know I will always be living with the damage, I also know I can change.*

T: That feels very powerful to me.

If we think together about where the "The Doom" and "The Torch" come from . . . "The Doom" connects to a very strong idea for you "that Brains never recover" but "The Torch" must resist connecting to this idea? Do you know what could be another idea that powers the "The Torch"?

B: *My therapists talk about plasticity. I never believed them because it seemed so hard to make any progress, and I guess I ignore the new connections I was making, as they were nowhere near as elaborate as the ones I used to have.*

T: So yes, you are right; there is an idea of plasticity which concerns how easy it is for you to make connections. We think this is the basis of new learning and new ways of doing things. Like your example of walking again.

B: *But I thought the cells were dead?*

T: You are right in the main, for most of the neurones you have that have their cell bodies affected, they do die off, but for the ones which still have intact cell bodies they make new branches.

For some specific areas of the Brain, you may be surprised to know that new neurones are born.

B: *Really?*

T: Yes, but this is only very limited – but as neurogenesis, as they call it, does happen people feel there may be a way to use this to help in the future.

We shouldn't be unrealistic about this, as this technology needs to be developed, but I am telling you as it might help make a different story about how amazing damaged Brains are?

B: *My neurones are still able to grow new branches; some areas even grow new neurones and maybe in the future, scientists may even be able to grow more neurones.*

T: How does that make you feel about "never getting better and being damaged"?

B: *I guess it means I can get better in ways I didn't realise. That while some parts are damaged, some are also getting better and not totally dead.*

T: When you think about what you just said, how does it make you feel?

B: *I feel things can change.*

T: Do you think you may have flicked the switch on "The Torch"?

B: *Yes (smiles), yes 'The Torch' is on.*

T: So, thinking about a new way of talking about what you are going through gives you a way to switch 'on' "The Torch". What else could you do?

B: *Listen to my sister more?*

T: Yep, and you also mentioned writing a diary earlier?

B: *True. Also, hanging out with friends . . . that's still hard, but if I am not going to be like this forever then things will change?*

T: I don't see why not.

We do need to be careful about "The Doom" trying to steal its power back too. Perhaps we could think about how to manage those times when we meet again.

B: *Yes, it's still very strong.*

T: For now, let's give "The Torch" more power by devoting our thinking time to it – who can we tell about it, give it more airtime?

B: *My mum, best mate and sister?*

T: Great thinking, let's work out how you might want to do that. Let's get planning.

Reference

White, M. (2007). *Maps of narrative practice*. New York, NY: W. W. Norton.

Chapter 6

Child-centred play therapy for trauma

From non-verbal to narrative expression

Anne Fullalove

This chapter will describe how child-centred play therapy can provide a safe emotional space for children to process the psychological trauma associated with an acquired brain injury (ABI) through the practice example of a 5-year old boy.

It will describe his therapeutic journey through the following:

- Non-verbal expression via sensory materials
- Metaphorical expression through small world figures
- Verbalisation and the creation of a document about his real-life experience

I will outline the theoretical underpinnings of the approach, including sensory and narrative elements, referencing models that attempt to describe the play therapy change process and drawing upon evidence from play therapy research and neuroscience. My background is that I am a play therapist, filial therapist, video interaction guidance supervisor and advisory teacher, with 30 years of experience working with children with additional needs and their families. I now work in private practice, following my post as play therapist within the psychosocial team at the Children's Trust, a residential rehabilitation centre for children with ABI. I am an associate tutor in the BSc Hons programme in Child Health and Well Being at Edge Hill University, West Lancashire.

Child-centred play therapy

Child-centred play therapy derives largely from the work of Carl Rogers, a humanist psychotherapist (1902–1987) who believed that individuals have an inherent drive towards health and that given a supportive and facilitative environment, they will find their own effective solutions to their difficulties and challenges. He called this process, "self-actualisation".

Rogers (1967) identified three core conditions that need to be embodied by the therapist, which he described as congruence (authenticity), unconditional positive regard (acceptance) and empathy (the ability to feel the inner experience of the client, and to communicate these feelings with compassion). Axline (1947) applied these Rogerian principles to her work with children. In this approach, the child is considered to hold the expertise, deciding which issues to explore rather than relying on the therapist to name problems or develop solutions.

Wilson, Kendrick and Ryan (2001) describes child-centred play therapy as a process of developing reparative relationship experiences between therapists and children, using play as the predominant means of communication. In the words of Landreth (2002, p. 16),

> Play is to the child what verbalization is to the adult. It is a medium for expressing feelings, exploring relationships, and self-fulfilment . . . toys are used like words by children, and play is their language.

Play therapy capitalises on the fact that play uses non-verbal symbols and is the natural way in which children develop new understandings, investigate areas of conflict and practice new emotional and social skills without the higher cognitive and abstract processes, such as self-reflection and discussion that are necessary in other approaches. Thus, symbolic expression and the safety of a strong therapeutic relationship are key factors central to the child-centred play therapy approach.

Research evidence for play therapy

Bratton, Ray, Rhine and Jones (2005), in their meta-analytic review of treatment outcomes, evidenced that play therapy is a developmentally sensitive approach that produces significant change across a variety of childhood emotional and behavioural problems. Cozolino (2006) stated that the experiences of a young child are stored in neural networks and connections of the brain, and not yet in language. This means that play at the sensorimotor and metaphorical level is particularly important for this age group.

Scaer (2014) and Steele and Malchiodi (2012), recognised that to heal from trauma, a secure therapeutic relationship may be the most important factor. Cozolino (2010) stated that neural integration is supported by the Rogers (1980) core conditions of empathy, unconditional positive regard and congruence, as they describe the ideal interpersonal relationship.

Although there is an evidence gap for the effectiveness of play therapy for children with acquired brain injury, Jones and Landreth (2002) provided much evidence for positive emotional outcomes for children with chronic illness who have accessed individual play therapy interventions. Studies by Ray, Schottelkorb and Tsai (2007), and Baggerly and Bratton (2010) support the value of play therapy for children having to undergo similarly prolonged medical procedures.

Narrative play therapy

Narrative play therapy is an intervention adapted for children from the narrative therapy approach of White and Epston (1990). Children play out stories that enable them to explore situations from an imaginative standpoint of alternative identities and perspectives, providing a sense of distance from problematic experience. The stories represent aspects of experience of high saliency for the child, as well as conveying powerfully experienced emotional responses. This is achieved with the sensitive responding of the therapist who pays close attention and sensitively reflects back to the client any material that reveals a thematic connection until new meanings emerge and a narrative is produced and recorded.

Narrative play therapy is an area of practice that does not have an established research base. However, research supports the emotional benefits of creating a clear and organised account of a traumatic experience (Pennebaker & Seagal, 1999). Studies by Brewin, Dalgleish and Joseph, (1996) and Van der Kolk and Fisler (1995) agree that the representation of the self through narrative is essential to recover from trauma and re-establish a strong sense of personal identity.

Sensory approaches within play therapy

Sensory materials such as sand, water, clay and slime are often appealing to children, offering an accessible way for the child to explore, problem solve and experience control over the environment. They have no prescriptive structure, which releases the child from any perceived pressure to perform, succeed or please. The child can create sensory images (somatic metaphors) through his or her choice of materials and interaction with them. They also offer opportunities for cognitively undemanding attunement experiences with the therapist through facial expressions, gesture and shared discovery.

Schore (2003) stated that trauma memory existing in pre-symbolic form can be resistant to representation even through metaphorical play, so the therapist needs to provide opportunity for the child to work at the sensorimotor level before they can advance to more mature representations through symbolic play and the higher cognitive task of verbalisation.

Badenoch (2008) stated that sensory responses in the body encourage connections between the lower brain (instincts), limbic brain (emotions) and the cortex (cognition), thus promoting vertical integration. There are an increasing number of studies available to evidence that working at a sensorimotor level can activate neural network changes. Sensory and motor play can help build a more resilient nervous system when the stress regulation systems in the lower brain are forming or have been impacted by trauma, as these networks cannot be accessed by language. (Gaskell, 2008; Perry, 2009; Levine & Kline, 2007).

The emergence of themes and the process of change

In play therapy, children communicate emotional difficulties and process traumatic events by recreating experiences through symbolic play. These symbolic preoccupations will eventually develop into themes, inner emotional dynamics consistently expressed through play. The development of therapeutic themes, along with behaviours within the context of the therapeutic relationship, can be monitored over time to describe a healing process of change within the child.

The child-centred nature of the therapy ensures that the unfolding of each child's process is unique to them. Given that themes can reflect confusion or an internal struggle for understanding by the child, they can emerge in an incoherent way. This may seem to imply that a convergence of comparative experience cannot easily be established. However, theorists have identified commonalities in the change process for children in play therapy. Cochran, Nordling and Cochran (2010) attributed this to the fact that children share universal developmental challenges, as well as having common needs such as the desire for self-expression, achieving self-control, forming positive relationships with others and experiencing feelings of competence. Within the therapeutic space, children also all share the challenge of developing a relationship of trust and emotional safety with the therapist.

Models of change encompass these factors and in general describe a progression from exploring the physical therapy space and resources, establishing trust and boundaries with the therapist, expressing feelings related to their personal challenges, working through issues related to attachment and connection with others and developing increased self-efficacy and competence.

Traumatised children exhibit some play behaviours that are different from other children (Terr, 1981, 1983). These include higher levels of repetitive play, negative affect, play avoidance or disruptions and aggression. Theorists have developed tools for mapping the course of patterns of change for these children, such as the Trauma Play Scale (Findling, Bratton, & Henson, 2006), which can further support the therapist's detailed process notes taken immediately following a session. Immediate post-sessional note taking and regular analysis of these is essential for tracking progress, providing insights that can also inform the focus of responses back to the child in future sessions. It is impossible to reflect everything the child presents and what the therapist chooses to focus on and communicate can powerfully reinforce the value of the child's expression (O'Connor, 2000).

Assessment

Assessment for play therapy follows referral from parents or the multi-professional team. The play therapist considers all diagnostic reports and meets with colleagues, parents or carers to ascertain need. To fully benefit from play therapy, children will evidence a level of sufficient cognitive functioning to enable them to form a therapeutic alliance and be able to work symbolically through metaphor. The approach is explained to the child at a level consistent with their understanding. Parental consent is sought and assent given by the children. Assent is always reassessed at the beginning of each session, and children can leave at any time.

Goal setting

Due to the child-centred nature of play therapy, objectives centre upon the development of the child's inner capacities and coping strategies. It is a typical experience of children to be given constant instruction as they learn to develop skills across the developmental spectrum, and their success is often evaluated by others. This can also be true in a psychotherapeutic context. As Rogers (1951, p. 152) stated, "The locus of evaluation is outside".

Because of their significant impairments, and with so many therapeutic demands upon the children with ABI within the rehabilitation setting, there is perhaps an even greater need to offer a space for children to interact at a self-determined level of challenge. These children often have high levels of dependence upon others due to their physical impairments, as well as increased emotional vulnerability as they struggle to re-establish their sense of self. Play therapy goals aiming to restore a sense of environmental control back to the child that could later be generalised into their daily life (Councill, 2006) seem particularly relevant in this context.

Practice example: Jackson and the mouse who hid in the cheese

Jackson was 5 years old when he sustained a hypoxic brain injury through a near drowning incident. This resulted in widespread challenges to his communication, cognition, motor planning and co-ordination skills. Jackson had been a shy child before his injury, and the complex interplay of his difficulties and his personality initially impacted on ascertaining his strengths and areas of difficulty.

Jackson was presenting as predominantly non-verbal to professionals within the setting but would talk to his family. He was demonstrating high levels of anxiety, lack of engagement in sessions, regular enuresis with no medical basis and a refusal to talk or hear about his trauma. Because of this, his family felt that they were unable to move forward. They welcomed an opportunity for Jackson to process his experience that was not reliant upon verbal expression. His emotional vulnerability was protected by using a graded approach whereby his mother was initially present and with clear emphasis that he had control of how he used the play space.

Jackson's narrative journey began on a non-verbal, sensory play level, corresponding to Erikson's (1972) autosphere stage and Jennings's (1990) embodiment stage, in which a child focusses on early physical experiences of exploring the body self and gaining movement confidence. Jackson was exclusively preoccupied with exploring materials such as stretchy, rubber toys of different shapes and textures that responded very flexibly to pulling, squeezing and throwing, yet retaining their structural integrity.

Interaction with these materials provides resistance within the body, activating the proprioceptive sense. As well as potentially having a soothing, regulatory effect on the nervous system, this sense can help a child gain important information about the position of the body in space (Warner, Cook, & Koomar, 2011). This preoccupation with sensory activity also related to Chazan's (2002) profile of the extremely anxious and isolated player, as did his brief and repetitive interactions with me.

Over several sessions, Jackson's explorations intensified and became more vigorous, with increasing levels of laughter as he began to squeeze and throw the toys with all his strength. As well as potentially working on regulatory processes and gaining body confidence, he also used this play to begin inviting shared attention and relationship with me through looking, pointing and laughing.

I responded by reflecting on Jackson's gesture, touch, movement and vocalisations, naming his experiences and perceived affects. Rothschild (2000) emphasised the importance of the therapist attuning to the child's physical impulses, sensations and emotional responses. Van der Kolk (1996) described this attention as a kind of attuned servitude, with the exclusive aim of helping the child to befriend and trust their inner felt experience, facilitating self-acceptance and expression.

In reviews at this stage, I reported that Jackson was using the time to engage in sensory activity, which appeared to be meaningful for him. He was slowly building a relationship through increasingly shared exploration, becoming less anxious and isolated within the sessions.

Eventually, Jackson's somatic expressions were interspersed with narrative fragments of symbolic play with small world characters. He began to comment on his play scenarios, at the level of play activity consistent with Erikson's (1972) microsphere and Jennings's (1990) projection stage, in which the child uses miniature toys for real objects, offering opportunities for thematic exploration.

For Jackson, this play involved characters falling, being buried or disappearing, followed by discovery and rescue. The first fall appeared accidental, as a prince fell through the unstable floor of the castle's turret. Jackson was visibly shocked by this, displaying frozen posture, open mouth and a flushing of the face, indicating a deep resonance for him. I focussed on the metaphor, reflecting on the feelings of shock and fear that the "character" may have been feeling, and wondered aloud what would happen next.

Within the safety of symbolic distance, Jackson resolved this scenario. The prince was rescued and thus began a preoccupation within the theme of safety and failed protection, with a specific focus on creating boundaries to keep characters out of danger. He reworked the narrative of the fall and rescue over many more sessions. Each time, there were subtle developments and resolutions in the action. This post-traumatic play repetition showed progression, suggesting processing of his real experience at a metaphorical level.

Another prominent feature was Jackson's play preoccupation with a small rubber mouse and rubber cheese with holes winding through it. This play displayed a level of focus and concentration that indicated it had great significance to him. The mouse would often hide in the cheese and re-appear, and would sometimes journey away from the cheese, to be buried in the sand or fall down the tower and be rescued.

The journey can be lengthy before a child arrives at clear narrative exposition, and it can be a challenge for the therapist who is witnessing sensory and symbolic stages of expression to understand what is happening. Interpretive or therapeutic questions constantly arise about the child's motivation behind their play behaviour, the symbolic representation of the materials, along with any affect or emotion attached to the action. The child may be conveying something about self, or another person. The action may be an aspect of reality or a state of mind or may represent perspectives they are holding. Interpretation in child-centred play therapy is, therefore, approached with caution.

I felt that the mouse could be a self-object for Jackson, but as he was choosing symbolic representation to express himself, I respected his choice to remain within the metaphor. Discussions in external supervision supported me in trusting his process and refraining from making overt links to Jackson about his real experiences, which could have been incorrect or too intrusive at this stage for him.

After several weeks of working together (two to three sessions weekly), narrative fragments and isolated moments of interaction gradually lengthened into verbalised sequences, such as the following, which revealed that Jackson was beginning to consider a variety of perspectives around this metaphorical trauma:

> The prince has fallen down the tower. He is stuck. It is very dark, and he can't see. There is a door with a gate on it. He can't stand up or get out. But there are some gaps he can see through. There are people out there. They are fighting. He is looking for someone to find him, but they are all fighting. And there are a lot of dead people. Some of the dead people are not dead. Some people have got to the top of the tower. They are trying to get him but there are no stairs. They don't know how to get up the tower and go down it.

Jackson's journey towards narrative exposition through somatic metaphor in his sensory play, and now symbolic re-enactment, had revealed aspects of his feelings and experience. He now began to play out narrative sequences increasingly representative of his trauma, such as children having accidents and undergoing rehabilitation experiences in medical settings. Jackson was also beginning to tell me small details about his family and friends from home.

I met regularly with Jackson's parents throughout the intervention, and they supported Jackson in bringing in photographs of important people in his life, as well as photographs depicting special times he had enjoyed in the past. He began to create a book to contain them, with simple captions developed spontaneously, with me as his scribe. I respected his need to focus on the content he wanted to include, which consisted of his family relationships, favourite toys, films and places. Gradually, Jackson approached more recent life events and began to talk about the people at the rehabilitation centre, whose photographs he also included.

In general, Jackson was showing reduced anxiety and was also interacting more in other rehabilitation sessions. Within the play therapy room, I often saw changes in behavioural presentation as well as progress across the range of skills before they were generalised into other contexts. In the play therapy space, children could challenge themselves to explore, take risks and progress in a playful way.

Three weeks before Jackson was due to leave, he filled a small bowl with water. He slowly rolled the small mouse over and over in it before taking it out, wrapping it in a tissue and stroking it very gently. I reflected that it looked like the mouse had been going around and around in the water, and it needed some careful looking after now. He nodded thoughtfully. I told him I could see that he was really thinking about that, and it felt very important. He looked at me and nodded before suddenly jumping up and having an energetic throwing session with what he now called the "squishy toys". This interruption and physical expression seemed to allow Jackson to discharge strong feelings and remain in control of the pace of his process.

Thus, Jackson tiptoed towards the events leading up to his time at the rehabilitation centre. Cockle and Allan (1996) describe how a child moves gradually closer to their most painful preoccupations as if in a kind of spiral pattern, which they describe as "circumambulation". The protection of the symbolic play over time brings them eventual resolution of painful feelings at a pace they can cope with.

As his time for leaving approached, Jackson invited his mother into sessions to share his progress in the book. In one session, he took out the mouse to show her. As he did this, he quietly told her that he wanted to "know what had happened", so he could put it in his book. When he did so, the page had a large sad face in the middle of it, with the words

> one day I was playing in the sea, but I fell down under the sea and I really hurt myself. I had to go to hospital to get better. I was asleep for a really long time and it was very sad.

Jackson was then able to complete the book, including simple facts about subsequent events, as well as thoughts about going home. The book reflected aspects of his relationships, life experience and character, which had remained consistent and reinforced a sense of continuity, as well as referencing his changed capacities and hopes for the future.

By this time, Jackson was walking more solidly, with more confidence. He was no longer troubled with enuresis and would ask to go to the toilet when needed. Although still quietly expressed, he was talking in all his rehabilitation sessions. He could access resources with confidence, attempt to problem solve with his use of materials and ask for assistance when required. These behaviours are consistent with Cochran's (2010) final mastery stage in his process of change model. Jackson's parents also reported a feeling of significant relief that they could all now talk about the accident.

Outcomes

Jackson made a good start in beginning to process his experiences through play therapy. In future, he may be able to engage in more directive therapeutic approaches to help him develop further understanding about his brain injury, his changed capacities and work on strategies to help him cope with differences in his abilities and relationships.

At this setting, I witnessed the unfolding of many different narrative journeys, some more developed than others, with children with a wide range of abilities.

All parents, and those children who could verbalise, wished to continue with this approach on return to their home community. In post-intervention satisfaction surveys, every parent reported that the service had been of significant benefit for their child and would highly recommend it to other families.

Discussion

Other creative arts therapies, such as music therapy, art psychotherapy and drama-therapy, also provide therapeutic support for children and young people with complex needs, such as those with ABI. These approaches focus on one art form as the main modality for the work, whereas in play therapy, the child and therapist use a wide range of expressive media, depending on the child's needs from moment to moment.

Stacey (2008, p. 220) stated that human expression represents "multi-layered and multi-sensorial experiences". Play therapy provides a particularly rich breadth of communicative resourcing to facilitate this for young children who have not yet developed verbal fluency, or for those with an ABI who have experienced a regression in communication and other skills. It combines expressive play with elements of the other creative art therapies, offering opportunities for sensory exploration and expression with a wide range of materials, symbolic re-enactment through small world toys and puppets, artistic and musical expression and socio-dramatic expression through role play.

The play therapy room offers a meaningful space for children to creatively respond to their trauma and to the unpredictability of the unfamiliar, medicalised environment. The unchanging presentation of the play therapy room, with the appeal of its toys and creative materials, can provide a sense of normality and comfort to the child. The consistent positioning and accessibility of materials alleviates anxiety for children who may experience memory loss, altered verbal and physical capacity and brain injury–related fatigue.

As the child chooses their own level of activity and engagement within sessions, burdens caused by external pressures to perform are all reduced and challenging behaviours. If emotional dysregulation occurs, the play therapy space provides safe containment for more intense levels of expression. In a busy rehabilitation environment, wherein families and workers are attempting to contain emotional expression to achieve focus on important functional rehabilitation goals, the play therapy room provides a much-needed space in which children can safely locate their distress, which can often be expressed physically.

Play therapy can be extremely advantageous for children with an ABI because it is developmentally appropriate, and the child can determine his or her own level of interaction and challenge. This offers a high level of emotional safety from which to begin their healing process.

The processes of play within a therapeutic relationship create an ideal neu-robiological environment for integration and growth, which can change the brain in a positive way. Trauma memories can, therefore, be reworked at both a metaphorical and a neurobiological level. Even very short-term work can be helpful and, depending upon the extent of the brain injury and time available, new verbal and written narratives can also be developed.

Play therapy is unique in that play is an intrinsically rewarding experience. The experience of joy within the therapeutic relationship further aids healing from trauma with "therapeutic moments of mutually shared joy", being perhaps "one of the greater emotional gifts that psychotherapy can ever provide" (Panksepp & Biven, 2012, p. 467).

References

Axline, V. M. (1947). *Play therapy: The inner dynamics of childhood* (Carl R. Rogers, Intro.). Boston: Houghton Mifflin.

Badenoch, B. (2008). *Being a Brian-wise therapist: A practical guide to interpersonal neurobiology*. New York: W.W. Norton & Company.

Baggerly, J., & Bratton, S. (2010). Building a firm foundation in play therapy research: Response to Phillips. *International Journal of Play Therapy*, *19*(1), 26–38.

Bratton, S., Ray, D., Rhine, T., & Jones, L. (2005). The efficacy of play therapy with children: A meta-analytic review of treatment outcomes. *Professional Psychology: Research and Practice*, *36*(4), 376–390.

Brewin, C. R., Dalgleish, T., & Joseph, S. (1996). A dual representation theory of posttraumatic stress disorder. *Psychological Review*, *103*, 670–686.

Chazan, S. (2002). *Profiles of play: Assessing and observing structure and process in play therapy*. London: Jessica Kingsley Publishers.

Cochran, N. H., Nordling, W. J., & Cochran, J. L. (2010). *Child- centred play therapy: A practical guide to developing therapeutic relationships with children*. New York: John Wiley & Sons.

Cockle, S. M., & Allan, J. A. (1996). Nigredo and albedo: From darkness to light in the play therapy of a sexually abused girl. *International Journal of Play Therapy*, *5*(1), 31.

Councill, T. (2006). *Tracy's kids art therapy program training manual*. Washington, DC: Lombardi Pediatric Center Art Therapy Program.

Cozolino, L. (2006). *The neuroscience of human relationships*. New York: W.W. Norton & Company.

Cozolino, L. (2010). *The neuroscience of psycotherapy: Healing the social brain*. New York: W.W. Norton & Company.

Erikson, E. H. (1972). In Chazan, S. (2002). *Profiles of play: Assessing and observing structure and process in play therapy*. London: Jessica Kingsley Publishers.

Findling, J. H., Bratton, S. C., & Henson, R. K. (2006). Development of the trauma play scale: An observation-based assessment of the impact of trauma on play therapy behaviors of young children. *International Journal of Play Therapy*, *15*, 7–36.

Gaskell, R. (2008). *Neuroscience and play therapy*. New York: Association for Play Therapy Mining.

Jennings, S. (1990). *Dramatherapy with families: Groups and Individuals*. London: Jessica Kingsley.

Jones, E. M., & Landreth, G. (2002). The efficacy of individual play therapy for chronically ill children. *International Journal of Play Therapy*, *11*(1), 117–140.

Landreth, G. L. (2002). *Play therapy: The art of the relationship*. New York: Brunner-Routledge.

Levine, P. A., & Kline, M. (2007). *Trauma through a child's eyes*. Berkeley, CA: North Atlantic Books.

Malchiodi, C. A. (Ed.). (2005). *Expressive therapies*. London: The Guildford Press.

O'Connor, K. J. (2000). The play therapy primer. John Wiley & Sons. In J. Panksepp & L. Biven (2012). *The archaeology of the mind: Neuroevolutionary origins of human emotions*. New York: W.W. Norton & Company.

Pennebaker, J., & Seagal, J. D. (1999). Forming a story: The health benefits of narrative. *Journal of Clinical Psychology 55*, 1243–1254.

Perry, B. (2009). Examining child maltreatment through a neurodevelopmental lens: Clinical applications of the neurosequential model of therapeutics. *Journal of Loss and Trauma, 14*(2014), 240–255.

Ray, S., Schottelkorb, A., & Tsai, M. (2007). Play therapy with children exhibiting symptoms of attention deficit hyperactivity disorder. *International Journal of Play Therapy*, 16(2), 95–111.

Rogers, C. R. (1951). *Client-centered therapy: Its current practice, implications, and theory, with chapters*. Boston: Houghton Mifflin.

Rogers, C. R. (1967). *On becoming a person: A therapist's view of psychotherapy: By Carl R. Rogers*. London: Constable.

Rogers, C. R. (1980). *A way of being*. Boston: Houghton Mifflin.

Rothschild, B. (2000). *The body remembers*. New York: W.W. Norton & Company.

Scaer, R. (2014). *The body bears the burden: Trauma, dissociation and disease* (3rd ed.). New York: Routledge.

Schore, A. (2003). *Affect regulation and repair of the self*. New York: W.W. Norton & Company.

Stacey, J. (2008). The therapeutic relationship in creative arts psychotherapy. In S. Haugh & S. Paul (Eds.), *The Therapeutic Relationship: Perspectives and Themes* (pp. 217–229). Monmouth, Wales: PCSS Books, 18.

Steele, W., & Malchiodi, C. A. (2012). *Trauma-informed practices with children and adolescents*. New York: Routledge.

Terr, L. C. (1981). Forbidden games: Post-traumatic child's play. *Journal of the American Academy of Child Psychiatry*, (20), 741–760.

Terr, L. C. (1983). Play therapy and psychic trauma: A preliminary report. In C. Schaefer & K. O'Connor (Eds.), *Handbook of play therapy* (pp. 308–319). New York: John Wiley & Sons.

Van der Kolk, B. (1996). "The black hole of trauma", "The body keeps the score: Approaches to the psychobiology of post traumatic stress disorder". In B. Van der Kolk, A. McFarlane, & L. Weisaeth (Eds.), *Traumatic stress*. New York: The Guildford Press.

Van der Kolk, B. A., & Fisler, R. (1995). Dissociation and the fragmentary nature of traumatic memories: Overview and exploratory study. *Journal of Traumatic Stress, 8*, 505–525.

Warner, E., Cook, A., & Koomar, J. (2011). *SMART: Sensory motor arousal regulation treatment: A manual for therapists working with children and adolescents. A "Bottom-Up" Approach to Treatment and Complex Trauma*. Brookline, MA: The Trauma Centre at JRI.

White, M., & Epston, D. (1990). *Narrative means to therapeutic ends*. New York: W.W. Norton & Company.

Wilson, K., Kendrick, P., & Ryan, V. (2001). *Play therapy: A non-directive approach for children and adolescents*. London: Bailliere Tindall.

Chapter 7

Structured narrative therapy for children with acquired brain injury and severe communication difficulties

Alison Perkins

If left unchallenged, an acquired brain injury (ABI) imposes its own preferred narrative of omnipotence and a desire to invade all boundaries. Unsatisfied with changing the child's experience of the world, ABI reaches further to change the children's perception of how they individually think and feel in response to the world (Wolfe et al., 2014).

Consequently, ABI has an unparalleled power to derail the developmental process behind the injured children's concept of who they are and their own identities (Lloyd et al., 2015). Rehabilitation interventions need to attend to children's developing identity as well as their functional skills (Ownsworth & Clare, 2006).

My own workplace, the Children's Trust, provides residential multidisciplinary rehabilitation for children and teenagers in the months following a severe ABI. In this setting I have gradually developed a structured narrative intervention which invites the injured child into family communication and education over his or her brain injury and needs whilst also attending to the child's identity. I have used it with young people aged 7 to 19 years. The therapy is a structured adaptation of a narrative intervention developed by Michael White (White, 2005) for children who have experienced extreme trauma and loss. It uses the protection and positive identity construction offered by White's narrative intervention within a structured approach to accommodate the child's acquired cognitive difficulties.

Through this structured narrative approach, the injured children take control in learning about their situation and in communicating over this with their families. Usually, I offer structured narrative therapy (SNT) to children with sufficient physical, sensory and communication skills to direct and control their own exploration into their situation. This work is described elsewhere (Perkins, 2015), along with an illustrative practice example. This chapter gives a brief overview of SNT. It then describes how we adapted the SNT for Theo, a child whose ABI resulted in severe communication and physical difficulties that reduced his control.

Practical application of structured narrative therapy

SNT is a gentle, child-centred approach that helps a child gain information about their situation and acquired needs, and to establish communication with their family over these. The intervention acknowledges the potential threat from the ABI on the child's developing identity (Gracey, Evans, & Malley, 2009) and aims to set a more positive trajectory for this. Within the therapy, the child creates an autobiographical document that represents their past, present and future. Initially, the child and therapist create a document of several empty chapters covering the child's lifespan in chronological sequence. The child knows that they own this document and will take it away with them when therapy ends. The child then takes full control in building the autobiographical contents, dipping in and out of different chapters as they wish.

Documents often contain photographs, pictures and the child's dictated text. It can be built using a computer; however, a paper copy is often utilised to maximise the child's physical control over how it is accessed and shared. The child builds their autobiographical story, choosing events and relationships that are important to them. Children often start by building their early lives, using these as "safe places to stand" (White, 2005) at a distance to their recent injury. As they work together, the therapist listens out for skills and resources that the child has used in the past. Resources that resonate with the child are thickened and woven through their past to create positive stories of skill and mastery.

Children often use these stories as the springboard by which to explore the recent events surrounding their injury, rehabilitation and future. The stories become subordinate stories of skills and mastery by which the child has managed adversity (White, 2005). Most children invite family members into sessions to witness their autobiographical document and to work on sections together. During these shared sessions, the therapist models how to maximise the child's control. The therapist constantly monitors the child's attachment to their document, and reattends to its safety, accessibility and positive stories if the child starts to disengage. When undertaking SNT with a child, parallel work is always carried out with family members before, during and after the narrative work. The focus of this family work is to ensure that they understand the model and therapeutic approach, to prepare them for their important role within the therapy, to reflect on their experience of the therapy and to monitor the emotional regulation of the family and child since this is foundational to the narrative work.

Rationale for using SNT

It is well documented that individuals with an ABI need to gain insight into their acquired needs to improve their long-term independence and quality of life (Caplan et al., 2016). Within paediatric ABI, all goals and interventions should be selected according to a developmental framework that considers the child's existing capacities, as illustrated by the Paediatric Neurocognitive Intervention (PNI), which guides the selection of neurocognitive interventions (Limond et al., 2014). I use a similar developmental framework (Figure 7.1) to guide my selection of interventions over helping the child develop insight into their injury and needs. My framework is provisional and references the PNI (Limond et al., 2014), as well as neuropsychological models of insight (Gracey, Longworth, & Psaila,

HIGHEST RESOURCES

Level 5: Child gains independence in rehabilitation: anticipation of needs, flexible and proactive strategies

- Child starts to adapt own strategies to suit current or anticipated context, including seeking social support and advocating for own needs
- Child starts to show anticipatory self-awareness of difficulties and learns to apply pre-emptive strategies
- Child spontaneously shows emergent awareness of needs and learns to apply key strategies with support
- Family communication and problem solving over difficulties becomes flexible
- Family roles become more flexible and adaptive to increased independence of injured child

Level 4: Child gains intellectual and emergent awareness of situation, acquired needs, strategies

- ☐ Child fully oriented to journey (level 2), and can tolerate reflection of strengths, acquired needs, coping strategies, problem solving
- ☐ Child tolerates or requests extended, explicit brain injury education
- ☐ Child has sufficient emotional and metacognitive skills to benefit from Cognitive Behaviour Therapy
- ☐ Child can participate in the creation of information for others over situation and needs (eg family, school, peers)
- ☐ Child starts to shows emergent self-awareness of needs within daily routine and intensive practice of skills
- ☐ Family have made meaning of events surrounding ABI, family communication over situation has become open and emotionally authentic, able to look to future

Level 3: Child under takes intensive practice of core skills

- Child tolerates intensive practice of key strategies and skills (physical, self-help, cognitive, educational) delivered across contexts by teachers, therapists or parents
- Child understands their need for intensive practice of key rehabilitation strategies (this will differ across physical, educational, cognitive, social domains)
- Child has understanding of 'practice – improvement' link
- Family communication and problem solving over situation becomes routine and involves injured child

Level 2: Child learns key information and daily rehabilitation skills

- Child experiences daily rehabilitation routine-Fully supported, all contexts, natural supports
- Child gains cohesive, factual understanding of their situation (injury, rehabilitation needs, strategies, and dischargeplans) as foundation for intellectual self-awareness
- Parent - child communication over situation and needs is established, including simple problem solving and planning
- Child has sufficient tolerance of threat to identity implied by daily rehabilitation and use of aids

Level 1: Child experiencing significant emotional dysregulation due to:

- ☐ Acute emotional distress (e.g. acute identity threat, mental health symptoms, poor advocacy, poor attachments, very poor quality of life)
- ☐ Acute family stressors causing systemic dysregulation
- ☐ Child is uninformed over situation or daily routine due to poor availability of information, or poor access due to sensory or cognitive impairments
- ☐ Acute behavioural dysregulation (challenging behaviour, self-harm)
- ☐ Acute medical needs (e.g. acute fatigue, epilepsy, pain, muscle tone invasive medical procedures)
- ☐ Cognitive: post traumatic amnesia, low arousal, low awareness

LOWEST RESOURCES

Figure 7.1 Provisional developmental model of capacities required to develop insight

2016), Krasny-Pacini et al. 2015), developmental models of self-awareness (Harter, 2012) and systemic family resources for managing adversity (Walsh, 2012). It guides me when to offer SNT. Similar to the PNI, the table represents a hierarchical pyramid of the child's capacities as these increase from lower levels to higher levels. It is, therefore, intended to be read from base to tip, to show this developmental progression.

Within this developmental framework, SNT is a Level 2 intervention. It aims to help a child gain factual information about his or her situation and to safely communicate with the child's family over this. SNT is selected once the child gains sufficient emotional and behavioural regulation through the use of Level 1 interventions, such as orientation, positive behaviour support, regulatory family work, medical interventions, environmental interventions or therapeutic interventions offering non-directive containment. SNT can pave the way towards higher level interventions, such as family problem-solving interventions (Wade & Hung, 2015), structured family interventions (Gan, Gargaro, Kreutzer, Boschen, & Wright, 2010) or cognitive behaviour therapy (Waldron, Casserly, & O'Sullivan, 2013).

The aims of SNT

This hierarchical framework defines the following aims for structured narrative therapy:

- For the child to gain information over his or her injury and rehabilitation needs. The level of detail is determined by the child to avoid emotional dysregulation.
- To establish communication between child and his or her family over the child's acquired needs, in which the child holds an empowered and central position. This can be expanded to include the child's teachers and peers, whilst preventing the child from becoming marginalised from this communication (Yeates, Henwood, Gracey, & Evans, 2007).
- Protecting the child's identity to manage the implicit threat within rehabilitation and to pave the way towards positive identity development as child matures.

The therapy takes a narrative, post-modernist position on identity construction that proposes multiple representations of self-development in different contexts. It assumes that some self-representations have the flexibility and durability to exist across time and contexts to give an authentic "essence of self" (Harter, 2012).

The ABI has propelled the child into a context of disempowerment and dependency. This implicates a dominant story involving self-representations of "passivity", "damage" and "needing to be fixed by others". SNT invites the child to look across their past and to select skills and resources that feel important and re-emerge across different times and contexts. The child and therapist thicken these authentic self-representations into positive stories of identity, giving them detail and highlighting their endurance and flexibility.

The document then invites the child to trace how they have used these skills and resources to manage their recent injury and early recovery. By doing this, the final document presents the development of positive and authentic self-representations which have the endurance and flexibility to be used in the face of acute adversity. The final document also symbolises the child's empowered decision to explore some of the recent events that threaten their identity.

Most children become very proud of their document. This is why empowering the child to take control over the discovery and discussion about their situation is so critical to SNT. For this reason, the therapist usually works with the child first to establish his or her control and then expands outwards to include the family.

How to establish Theo's control, whose ABI resulted in severe communication difficulties, posed a lot of challenges as described next.

Adapting SNT for Theo: a practice example

Theo, aged 11, lived at home with his parents and two younger siblings, Daniel and Emily. He was academic, gentle natured and slightly shy; however, made some close friends over his first term at secondary school. At Christmas, he became unwell, lost consciousness and was admitted to hospital with meningoencephalitis, which caused a severe brain injury. Investigations showed widespread inflammation throughout his brain, involving both grey matter and the white connective tissue. Theo remained in hospital for three months. He then stayed in our rehabilitation unit for six months with his mother, Grace, before returning to live at home.

On his arrival to us, Theo was wheelchair bound and unable to communicate or handle objects functionally. As the inflammation in his brain reduced, his gross motor skills recovered such that he could walk, run and climb. Certain contexts became meaningful: he could listen to a storybook, ride a tricycle and eat a meal. Outside of these settings, he lost his functional skills and was drawn into repetitive sensory responses. He understood some spoken language but could not communicate his needs, which frequently led to acute distress. We hypothesised that he experienced highly fragmented cognition, reflecting widespread disruption to his brain circuitry. I worked with Grace and the team to reduce his agitation, develop meaningful contexts to promote his skills and optimise his communication.

Six weeks before discharge, we observed Theo's attention and processing improve, although his motor and verbal apraxia continued to preclude formal assessments. He demonstrated more cognitive skills in a wider range of contexts. He could now sit and attend in class and show recognition of numbers and text using simple multiple choice. He could understand and retain simple spoken language. He could read, understand and retain simple passages of text, one or two sentences in length. He also started to join in reciprocal social games, such as hide-and-seek. He started to approach others to meet his needs. He remained unable to speak but if calm, he could indicate yes or no to simple questions using body language. He started to use a simple press button communication device. He remained unable to use everyday objects functionally; for example, he could not turn the pages of a book, use a pen, point to named objects or pictures or build with Lego. Consequently, he required full support during his personal care.

Grace celebrated this sudden improvement in Theo's skills, but it prompted her to consider Theo's understanding of his situation. She had occasionally given a short explanation of his illness to orient him to our setting but could never tell whether he found it meaningful. She stopped altogether when his cognition suddenly improved, since her own experience of learning about his illness had been traumatic. She wanted Theo to have an understanding of his illness and needs, and to advocate within his discharge plans. However, she was unsure what he wanted to know, and Theo was unable to spontaneously ask. I negotiated with Grace that maximising Theo's control in learning about his situation would show us what he wanted to know and prevent us from overwhelming his coping strategies.

Grace set the following two goals within a Goal Attainment Scaling (GAS) approach:

Goal 1: To provide Theo with a means by which he can initiate and control what he learns about his situation

Goal 2: To increase Theo's knowledge about his illness, his rehabilitation and discharge home

Theo's improved skills had helped him gain emotional regulation. This allowed me to offer SNT to achieve Grace's goals. I explained the usual process in which the child builds an autobiographical document to represent their skills and resources, and then explores how they used these resources to survive their experience of brain injury. This approach appealed to Grace, and we planned how to adapt the SNT to accommodate Theo's cognitive, communication and functional difficulties.

We decided to offer Theo an initial version of his autobiography. This would show him our offer to learn more about his situation, create a reading context that he understood and support his cognition. We would also offer enjoyable games to give him the option to refuse his autobiography. Theo would then direct how his autobiography developed. We created the initial autobiography with the guidance of Theo's team, using clear photographs and simple text that he could process, reason with and retain with repetition.

We presented his story in a predictable, chronological sequence of colour coded chapters: "Theo and his family", "growing up", his illness, hospitalisation, rehabilitation at Tadworth, return home and return to school. The early sections on his family and childhood would enable Theo to develop positive stories of identity (Morgan, 2000) and provide a "safe place to stand" at a distance to trauma (White, 2005). The later sections gave limited but accurate information of his illness and hospitalisation that Grace knew Theo could tolerate. We planned our roles within the therapy. Grace would regulate Theo's emotions and facilitate his communication. She was a secure attachment figure, and he habitually looked to her to interpret his behavioural signals, gain reassurance or share his joys. I would provide a structure, which gave Theo choice, control and safety in which to explore his situation.

It was particularly important to explore Grace's expectations over the pace and outcome of the therapy. To empower Theo, we would need to invest time in developing his positive stories and allow him to determine the limits of what he wanted to learn about his situation. This placed uncertainty over Grace's GAS goal to increase Theo's knowledge about his situation. We identified this as a potential source of adult frustration and discussed how to protect the therapy process from this and how to continue progress towards this goal after Theo's discharge. We discussed the practicalities of how to facilitate Theo's engagement or withdrawal from activities and topics. We placed a colour-coded "contents" page in his document to help him guide us. His speech therapist added "stop"/"keep going" and a "how I am feeling" tool to his communication aid.

Together, we took great care to ensure that Theo was led by his own needs when working on his autobiography and not by our agenda. The physical set up and social context never assumed that he would choose to work on his autobiography, and it never elevated the status of this work. His autobiography was laid out alongside two of his favourite games. All were equally accessible, and we were equally content to partner him in a game or in working on his book. He was never directed towards his autobiography but was invited to scan and freely choose his activity, and to change his choice at any time. In all but one session, Theo spent most of the time working on his autobiography. Occasionally, he finished with a game.

The intervention involved eight shared sessions with Grace and Theo over four weeks, each lasting 30 to 40 minutes. I also met with Grace alone on five occasions to create the document, to plan, review and evaluate the therapy, and to reflect on her experience of it. Within the shared sessions Theo used a mixture of gesture, expression, vocalisation and his communicator to show us which pages to look at and read to him. Grace and I carefully observed Theo's non-verbal responses to pinpoint areas of importance, curiosity or concern for him. He returned with pleasure to certain areas of text, and we interpreted this as potential positive stories in need of thickening. We offered Theo choices based upon our joint knowledge of him to gain more detail or identify areas of concern. Theo gave explicit consent before any new medical information was offered. After each session, I updated his autobiography with the key ideas that were most meaningful to him. In this way, Theo took control over developing the contents of his autobiography.

Theo developed three significant positive stories (PS) of identity which weaved through the chapters of his document. These positive stories are described in Table 7.1.

Theo often used his PS as a way to visit more difficult topics, such as his illness and future schooling. Table 7.2 summarises my sessions with Grace and Theo.

Grace rated her two GAS goals as "achieved". Theo had learnt more of his illness, situation and discharge home, and he had a means by which to initiate and control communication over these issues.

Table 7.1 Positive story themes in Theo's document

Positive story 1 (PS1)	His importance to his family, their continual presence through the toughest times in hospital
Positive story 2 (PS2)	His continual role as older brother in caring for his siblings and his cats
Positive story 3 (PS3)	His healing body, the determination of his brain and body to recover from illness and regain physical skills

Table 7.2 Summary of therapy sessions with Grace and Theo

Session 1	This session aimed to determine Theo's engagement with the initial autobiography and to show him he had control over the session activity (autobiography vs. game). Theo readily approached the autobiography and invited us to read it with him. He reviewed the entire contents in sequence. He started to develop PS1 (family support in hospital). He looked at his nasogastric (NG) tube in one photo and gestured to indicate his memory of sensory discomfort. He agreed for me to add his information to his autobiography. Theo then chose a game, perhaps to check these were truly on offer.
Session 2	Theo showed enjoyment of holding and reviewing his autobiography. He added detail to PS1 (family support in hospital). He started PS2 (role as older brother) and considered how this continued through his rehabilitation. Through considering PS1 he reviewed his time in the acute hospital. He did not wish for more information on encephalitis.
Session 3	Theo attended to his autobiography for 40 minutes, starting at the safety of life before his illness. He added detail to PS2 (role as older brother) and PS1 (family support in hospital) as he moved through his autobiography. Whilst considering PS1, he indicated his poor knowledge and recall of his illness and consented to hear a short explanation. Theo pointed and gestured to show his recollection of having his NG tube. Guided by Theo's signs of engagement, we focussed on his memories about having his tube and its removal. This introduced a new positive story 3 (PS3) about the determination of his body and brain to recover. Theo remained highly focussed on this new positive story, and we expanded it under his guidance. Within this story, he visited the sections on his rehabilitation and discharge home. He consented for me to add a visual countdown to discharge. He quickly disengaged when we revealed the page about his future school, indicating he did not wish to think about this.
Session 4	Theo reviewed the sections associated with PS1 (family support in hospital) and PS2 (role as older brother). After thinking about these positive stories, he visited the section on his future education, and indicated he was anxious. Together we identified his main questions and he asked Grace to research answers for these. He made a plan to see photographs of potential schools in preference to visiting them in person.

(Continued)

Table 7.2 (Continued)

Session 5	Theo reviewed his whole autobiography in sequence. By thinking about PS2 (role as older brother), he visited the topic of his discharge home, particularly his change of bedroom. He rested briefly on the topic of his new school and then indicated he felt too anxious to think about this today.
Session 6	Theo reviewed the section of his stay in the acute hospital. Whilst thinking about PS3 (brain and body recovery), Theo asked Grace to describe her memories of this period. Theo traced the recovery of his skills through his rehabilitation. He then chose to hear a little about meningoencephalitis.
Session 7	Theo was keen to come to his session. Grace reported he had been visibly low in mood and less motivated in his rehabilitation that morning. Theo directed his autobiography to review the acute stages of his encephalitis. He then disengaged, indicating a need to use the toilet. Within this privacy with Grace, he became tearful. He chose to return and engaged in sensory play. After a while, he tolerated my closed questions to identify the following concerns: • I want to know more about encephalitis. • Do I still have encephalitis? • I want to know more about my brain learning new skills Under his direction, Grace and I answered these concerns. Theo indicated that he wanted to ask a medical professional, and we made a plan for this. Theo looked visibly tired but relieved. As I waved goodbye, he reapproached me, carefully interlocked his fingers with mine, made eye contact and smiled. Grace and I interpreted that he had greatly valued the session and the plan we had created. At this stage, Grace and I identified the information to offer Theo about his encephalitis. This was offered to him by a specialist brain injury nurse and written up to be offered for his autobiography.
Session 8	The last therapeutic session, held two days before Theo's discharge. Theo reviewed the topic of his discharge. We extended PS3 (his brain's recovery of skills) through the later stages of his rehabilitation, adding the photos of horse riding he had brought to evidence this. We extended this positive story into his future life at home. He did not wish to review the additional information on encephalitis. Instead, he chose to add it at the back of his autobiography in a separate section. I collated Theo's feedback on the therapy. Theo indicated he planned to take his autobiography home. We reviewed where he would keep it and with whom he would share it.

Using a 10-point Likert scale (0 = 'none', 10 = 'full'), Grace indicted the degree to which Theo's understanding and their communication over his situation had changed. Her comments show how the autobiography set a context for their communication over his situation. Her ratings are given in Table 7.3:

Table 7.3 Grace's ratings of therapy outcome using Likert scale

Item to Be Rated	Rating Taken Prior to Start of Psychotherapy	Rating Taken at Completion of Psychotherapy
Theo's overall understanding of what has happened and his current situation	3–4	8–9
Your awareness of how much he understands of what has happened and his current situation	5–6	7
How much he can initiate and control communication over his situation	1–2	10, "with autobiography in quiet setting"
How much he can indicate what he does/does not want to know about his situation	1–2	9–10 "with his autobiography It's great he can skip sections"

Theo gave his feedback by choosing one of three responses (like/not sure/do not like) to a series of questions. This is given in Table 7.4:

Reflections

Theo's feedback shows his ambivalence towards the difficult content of his journey. It also shows he felt attached to his autobiographical document, despite its challenging contents. I believe Theo's high degree of control in accessing and developing his autobiography was critical to his attachment. In its final form, the autobiography told his story of the resources he used to survive his illness and brain injury. Within its pages, Theo presents positive and authentic self-representations that have endured and adapted through acute adversity. Theo's autobiography symbolises another authentic self-representation of his courage to explore and learn about his situation, as witnessed by Grace.

Theo's dependency on us to build his document raised additional clinical and ethical dilemmas about protecting him from our own therapy goals. SNT always carries a tension between establishing the adult goals to improve the child's understanding and communication, and handing control of therapy outcome to the child. It is critical to manage this tension at all stages of the therapy to establish and maintain the child's control. This minimises the risk of the child feeling influenced by adult expectations to visit distressing information, which would support the dominant narrative of disempowerment and victimisation (White, 2005). As the therapy progressed, I became uncomfortably aware that I was relying greatly on Grace's resources to protect Theo from her own goals. On reflection, I should have identified more explicitly what to do if adult expectation had crept in to influence the therapy.

Table 7.4 Theo's ratings of therapy outcome

Question	Like	Not Sure	Not Like
How do you feel about your book?	X		
How do you feel about the section on 'You'?	X		
How do you feel about the section on 'My Illness'?		X	
How do you feel about the section on 'My Stay in Hospital'?		X	
How do you feel about the section on 'My Stay at Tadworth'?	X		
How do you feel about the section on 'Going Home'?		X	
How do you feel about the section on 'Going to School'?	X		
How do you feel about these sessions to look at your book?	X		
Do you want to take the book home?	Yes		
Do you want other people to look at the book with you when you get home?	Mum Dad Bubba Grandpa	Daniel Emily	

As with many therapeutic interventions, SNT carries the risk of the child feeling answerable to the adult expectations of the therapy. In SNT, this risk is minimised by explicitly empowering the child as much as possible, but it cannot be eliminated altogether. This inherent risk within SNT needs to be balanced against the risks of not offering the therapy. SNT allows a child to gain a greater factual understanding of their situation than an orientation script, and it establishes a context for child-centred communication through which to learn more from their family. It also attends to the developmental process behind the child's identity.

Without SNT, a child may only learn about his or her brain injury through adult-led "brain injury education" or in separate, problem-saturated contexts where his or her needs arise. These routes are an important part of rehabilitation, but they demand more resources from the child than SNT and should be implemented with this in mind.

References

Caplan, B., Bogner, J., Brenner, L., Beadle, E., Ownsworth, T., Fleming, J., & Shum, D. (2016). The impact of traumatic brain injury on self-identity: A systematic review of the evidence for self-concept changes. *Journal of Head Trauma Rehabilitation, 31*(2), E12–E25.

Gan, C., Gargaro, J., Kreutzer, J., Boschen, K., & Wright, F. (2010). Development and preliminary evaluation of a structured family system intervention for adolescents with brain injury and their families. *Brain Injury*, *24*(4), 651–663.

Gracey, F., Evans, J., & Malley, D. (2009). Capturing process and outcome in complex rehabilitation interventions: A "Y-shaped" model. *Neuropsychological Rehabilitation*, *19*(6), 867–890.

Gracey, F., Longworth, C., & Psaila, K. (2016). A provisional transdiagnostic cognitive behavioural model of post brain injury emotional adjustment. *Neuro-Disability and Psychotherapy*, *3*(2), 154–185.

Harter, S. (2012). *The construction of the self: Developmental and sociocultural foundations*. New York: Guilford Press.

Krasny-Pacini, A., Limond, J., Evans, J., Hiebel, J., Bendjelida, K., & Chevignard, M. (2015). Self-awareness assessment during cognitive rehabilitation in children with acquired brain injury: A feasibility study and proposed model of child anosognosia. *Disability and Rehabilitation*, *37*(22), 2092–2106.

Limond, J., Adlam, A., & Cormack, M. (2014). A model for pediatric neurocognitive interventions: Considering the role of development and maturation in rehabilitation planning. *The Clinical Neuropsychologist*, *28*(2), 181–198.

Lloyd, O., Ownsworth, T., Fleming, J., & Zimmer-Gembeck, M. (2015). Awareness deficits in children and adolescents after traumatic brain injury: A systematic review. *The Journal of Head Trauma Rehabilitation*, *30*(5), 311–323.

Morgan, A. (2000). *What is narrative therapy*. Adelaide: Dulwich Centre Publications.

Ownsworth, T., & Clare, L. (2006). The association between awareness deficits and rehabilitation outcome following acquired brain injury. *Clinical Psychology Review*, *26*(6), 783–795.

Perkins, A. (2015). Psychological support using narrative psychotherapy for children with brain injury. In J. Reed, K. Byard, & H. Fine (Eds.), *Neuropsychological rehabilitation of childhood brain injury: A practical guide* (pp. 215–236). New York: Springer.

Wade, S., & Hung, A. (2015). Online family problem solving for adolescent traumatic brain injury. In J. Reed, K. Byard, & H. Fine (Eds.), *Neuropsychological rehabilitation of childhood brain injury: A practical guide* (pp. 43–59). New York: Springer.

Waldron, B., Casserly, L., & O'Sullivan, C. (2013). Cognitive behavioural therapy for depression and anxiety in adults with acquired brain injury. What works for whom? *Neuropsychological Rehabilitation*, *23*(1), 64–101.

Walsh, F. (2012). Family resilience: Strengths forged through adversity. In F. Walsh (Ed.), *Normal family processes: Growing diversity and complexity* (pp. 399–427). New York: Guilford Press.

White, M. (2005). Children, trauma and subordinate story line development. *International Journal of Narrative Therapy & Community Work*, (3–4), 10–21.

Wolfe, K., Bigler, E., Dennis, M., Gerhardt, C., Rubin, K., Taylor, H. G., . . . Yeates, K. (2014). Self-awareness of peer-rated social attributes in children with traumatic brain injury. *Journal of Pediatric Psychology*, *40*(3), 272–284.

Yeates, G., Henwood, K., Gracey, F., & Evans, J. (2007). Awareness of disability after acquired brain injury and the family context. *Neuropsychological Rehabilitation*, *17*(2), 151–173.

Chapter 8

Systemic and narrative therapeutic work with families whose child has sustained a profound brain injury

Rachel Ames

Introduction

This chapter concerns working with families of children or young people (CYP) who have sustained a profound brain injury – i.e. medically described as either having a disorder of consciousness (DOC), being in a "persistent vegetative state" or as being "minimally conscious". The injury being acquired through illness or a traumatic event. The prognosis for future change is often uncertain but likely that the child will make only limited changes. This work is with families experiencing some incredibly sad and traumatic situations. Family life has often been very suddenly and irrevocably changed. Parents, siblings and other family members are experiencing the profound loss of the child they were and the task of adjusting to them as they are. This is also a time when they are often facing a significant level of uncertainty about their son or daughters' further recovery and rehabilitation. A common theme is thinking with family members about what it is reasonable to hope for in the face of such profound loss and grief.

I carried out this work in a residential service where children, young people and their families receive intensive neurorehabilitation for up to six months. Children usually come to the service following time in an acute hospital setting. These CYP have sustained such significant brain injuries that often there has been a time when it has been uncertain whether the child will survive. Some families have been prepared for their son's or daughter's death. Most have experienced their child needing intensive care in hospital for several weeks or months.

Working with families experiencing such intense grief, loss and uncertainty can be personally and professionally challenging. One of my challenges as a clinical psychologist and family therapist has been to find a way of working and of having conversations that can be helpful to families at this time. The hope is that these conversations can help in the "emotional" rehabilitation process and can help equip families for the next stage of their lives when they will often return home with their child. This chapter is about some of the conversations that I have had with families and the systemic and narrative models that I have drawn on to guide this work.

Peer supervision and co-working have been valuable in working with families facing such significant emotional challenges. Little has been written about working systemically with families whose children have sustained such significant acquired brain injuries (ABIs) and creating contexts for working or reflecting with colleagues has been particularly important in developing this service.

What is a disorder of consciousness or profound acquired brain injury?

CYP who are diagnosed with either vegetative state (VS) or minimally conscious state (MCS) will have very significant brain injuries with little ability to respond to the world around them. Many children and young people will progress through the stages of coma, VS and MCS. Some, however, will not make this progression and will remain in a "vegetative" or in a "minimally conscious state" which can persist for the rest of their lives. Some will regain consciousness but will continue to live with very significant acquired disabilities that physically and cognitively affect them and their ability to communicate.

Once a CYP has sustained a profound brain injury, assessment tools such as the Glasgow Coma Scale (GCS) can provide information about their level of consciousness. Family members can face a significant level of uncertainty about their child's prognosis. Information from scans can provide some information about the extent of the brain injury and the most likely prognosis but there is no medical certainty about how individual children will respond.

CYP with the most profound brain injuries may remain in a condition where they have little or no awareness of their environment. Consciousness is described by the Royal College of Physicians (2003) as an ambiguous term that includes both wakefulness and awareness.

The impact of a profound acquired brain injury: some of the themes and dilemmas of therapeutic work

Coming to terms with a move from the "world of the healthy" to the "world of illness" (Sontag, 1991) is one of the most difficult challenges we are likely to confront: it shifts us from the domain of the ordinary to the extraordinary, demanding a radical reorganisation of our individual, family, social and working lives. In the face of a CYP sustaining a profound ABI, this shift is huge and happens at a time when family members are often grieving for their child as he or she was and may also be experiencing their own emotional responses to the traumas that they have experienced.

My approach: drawing on systemic and narrative models

I have experienced a number of dilemmas in deciding how to work most effectively with families whose children and young people have experienced the most severe brain injuries. Within the rehabilitation service it was often easier to agree

Table 8.1 Themes and dilemmas families face when their CYP sustains a profound brain injury

Injury Related Factors	Themes and Dilemmas
The circumstances where their CYP sustained their brain injury (can include a car crash, a child being knocked down by a car, an illness or treatment for a physical condition)	• Psychological impact of traumatic experiences • Physical impact on self or others – e.g. death or injuries • If an accident involved or was caused by another family member – feelings of guilt, blame
The medical treatment that the CYP received	• Traumatic responses to this • Feelings of guilt at consenting to treatments that may have led to or to have worsened the child's brain injury • Concerns about the medical care the child received, may include concerns about medical negligence
The need for a team of professionals to be involved in caring for and supporting the CYP	• Relationship(s) to help • Advocating for son's or daughters' needs • Feeling de-skilled/loss of confidence in parenting • Potential difficulties in working relationships – this may include working with professionals who hold different opinions about the child or young person
Complex medical and neurological information about the CYP's brain injury	• Descriptions of their CYP involving very complex medical language • The need to understand the CYP's ABI and what this is likely to mean for his or her future rehabilitation and development
The child having complex acquired difficulties and very changed abilities	• Beliefs and experiences of disability • Sadness and grief at the loss of the child as they were • The need to find ways of coping • Uncertainty about the future • Not knowing what is reasonable to hope for • The emotional and practical challenges of parenting a child with very significant and complex needs

Injury Related Factors	Themes and Dilemmas
	• Loss of confidence in abilities as a parent
	• The challenges of advocating for their child's needs in community services that are often complex and can be under-resourced.
	• Meeting the needs of other children in the family
	• The impact of others' responses to the child
The need for the CYP to stay away from home for prolonged periods in hospital and then in rehabilitation settings	• Family members being separated – impact on relationship and on support
	• Challenges about meeting the needs of different family members
	• Practical implications, including the potential need to move house and financial stresses
Impact on family members' well-being and relationships	• Sadness, grief, traumatic responses and the impact of these on relationships
	• Different styles of coping
	• Increased demands on time – reduced time and emotional availability for other family relationships – including couple relationships or other children
	• Building resilience and resourcefulness
	• The need to adapt roles and responsibilities
	• Importance of communication

goals and to engage children, young people and their families in psychological work when the child or young person was more cognitively able and might be able to communicate their own needs or be able to show emotional distress.

An initial dilemma in working with families was how, whether and when to engage with people who were experiencing such significant experiences of loss and uncertainty about the future. Until recently, a great deal of what was written about illness and death focussed on deficit and pathology. Altschuler (2012) drew on systemic theory in discussing the challenges individuals and families face when confronted with illness, disability and death and ways of intervening to help people reflect on their experience and connect with their sense of competence at times of particular difficulty.

Work on family resilience suggests that

> resilience tends to be greater when the family is cohesive, relationships are mutually supportive, the organisation of the family is clear, people are able to communicate openly, there are few other stressors, caregivers have good coping skills and family beliefs are able to help people retain or regain a sense of hope.
>
> (Altschuler, 2012)

Systemic work that focusses on relationships aims to strengthen family members' abilities to cope and to build resourcefulness and resilience.

In my systemic practice, I aim to work in a collaborative way from a position of curiosity. I use systemic questions to explore family members' beliefs and experiences and work with them to develop preferred narratives. A number of systemic practitioners have particularly influenced my practice. Burnham's (1992) systemic model that conceptualises the "approach, method and techniques" provides a framework within which to work. I work within a systemic approach and draw on a range of other psychological theories to inform my work. I often share psychological models of post-traumatic stress disorder (PTSD) and of grief with family members and explore with them whether these are helpful frameworks within which to understand their emotional experiences and reactions.

My practice is generally informed by social constructionist theorists and practitioners. Anderson's (1992) social constructionist approach emphasises working within collaborative relationships that value the relational knowledges that people hold. She described her therapeutic work as creating space for new understandings or ways of relating. I also draw on narrative approaches and techniques to work with family members to develop preferred narratives of identity. I use narrative techniques such as "externalising" in therapeutic conversations to create distance between the family member and the issue that is troubling them. Narrative ideas about trauma are also valuable and include thinking about how to create a safe space from which the traumatic experiences can be discussed without leading to re-traumatisation. Carey (2014) described pain and distress as testimony to what is held precious. She also talked about the therapeutic value of seeing "responses" to trauma rather than effects.

Relational reflexivity (Burnham, 2005) and creating an opportunity to "talk about talking" are systemic techniques that privilege the exploration of what it is helpful to talk about and within what contexts. Fredman (2003) showed how she used these ideas to have conversations with family members to think together about when, whether and who it is helpful to talk to about illness and death. When family members have had such traumatic experiences and are facing very significant losses I have found "talking about talking" helpful to create a space together that is "safe" to talk about what is most helpful or what is currently bearable.

Self-reflexivity is also important in my systemic practice. I have found Pearce's (1994) coordinated management of meaning (CMM) a helpful framework for thinking about the different contexts that may be influencing my work with families. Co-working with colleagues, case discussion and supervision are all important to me. I will now share how I have utilised some of these ideas with a family I have worked with.

William and his family

An introduction

William was a 10-year-old growing up in a family with his mother and his two younger sisters. He had a diagnosis of ADHD, was a fit and healthy child and attended his local mainstream primary school. William liked to be physically active and particularly enjoyed swimming and football. William's father had separated from his mother, Jane, when he was 6; he had some contact with the children, but this wasn't consistent. William's maternal grandparents lived locally and provided regular after-school and holiday childcare. This enabled William's mother to work in her job as a hospital receptionist.

William's traumatic brain injury

William sustained a severe traumatic brain injury when he was a passenger in the car driven by his grandfather, who was legally responsible for the accident. William was in intensive care in hospital for several weeks. He was admitted for residential rehabilitation and was presenting with a disorder of consciousness. At the time of his admission, William was showing no consistent responses. He had complex medical needs and was experiencing seizures. Whilst William was receiving rehabilitation, his mother was staying with him. His grandparents were looking after his sisters. His grandparents had told them that William was receiving rehabilitation to get better.

The prognosis that Jane had been given was that William was likely to continue to have very significant acquired difficulties following his brain injury. There was a strong likelihood that he would make limited changes and the goals of rehabilitation were broadly to carrying out an assessment of his disorder of consciousness, assess and manage his seating and other equipment needs and support his medical needs, including the management of his tone, seizures and pain.

Our first meeting

My initial meeting was with Jane. At first, it was difficult to arrange a time to meet, as she wanted to be with William during all of his rehabilitation sessions and because, particularly initially, he was having a lot of seizures. As she became confident enough to leave him with the care staff, we were able to arrange a time to meet. Jane appeared emotionally flat and said she was extremely tired and wasn't able to sleep very well. She said her main concerns were her relationship with her parents following the accident. The family had been advised that they shouldn't talk about the accident, as there was an ongoing legal claim. This meant she was also not seeing her mother, with whom she had a very close relationship and had previously been a source of support for her.

Jane was feeling guilty about having had to rely so much on her parents for childcare since her separation from the children's father. She felt guilty that she had allowed William to go in the car with her father, as she now felt she should have been aware that he might have an accident due to his age. Jane had very mixed feelings about her parents, particularly her father, looking after her two daughters. Whilst she was grateful that they were able to do this, she was now worried about their ability to make judgements about their safety. Jane was also really upset about how her parents were talking about William's future recovery to the girls and telling them he would come home when he was better.

Jane didn't feel able to or didn't find it helpful to set goals for the work. She was interested in our initial conversations about how she was coping and was interested to think about this further. Jane also said that she found it helpful to have a space to think about her experiences with someone else. She said that she found it hard to stop and think during the intensity of supporting William with his rehabilitation.

Initial formulation and some systemic hypotheses

Following our initial meeting, my colleague and I began to develop some initial hypotheses about some of the dilemmas that Jane and her family were facing and were curious about how these were affecting their relationships.

Loss and grief for William as he had been before the accident and living with uncertainty about the future were having a considerable impact on Jane and her parents. We were curious about how different family members were coping and how this influenced their relationships. An initial hypothesis was that Jane was coping in a way that protected herself and her parents from her feelings of anger about the accident but that meant that she was avoiding contact with her parents, who had previously been an important source of support to her.

We were also aware that Jane had a lot more contact with health professionals and information about the likely prognosis for William. Her parents did not have this information and appeared to be coping through remaining optimistic that William would make a full recovery. The way that they shared this view with William's sisters was very distressing for Jane and meant that she felt more isolated from her parents and angry with them. We thought that conversations about what it was "reasonable to hope" for in the future for William and for their family relationships might be helpful to talk about.

We also wondered how William's sisters were coping and how the changes in their family relationships were affecting them. We wondered about how able they felt to talk about their brother and their feelings and thoughts about their experiences. We wondered if they might have developed a similar way of coping to Jane and be avoiding talking about William to "protect" her from any difficult questions and thoughts that they might have. A systemic and narrative approach that created a therapeutic space to see if the family would be interested in talking about these potential dilemmas was offered.

Further meetings with Jane

We spent the initial sessions thinking and exploring how Jane was coping and thinking about her responses to the events she had experienced. In thinking about the impact of the traumatic events, we looked at a model of PTSD, and Jane agreed it would be helpful to fill in an Impact of Events Scale. Whilst her presentation did not meet the criteria for a likely diagnosis of PTSD, this did provide a framework for thinking together about how she was coping.

Jane became aware that she was avoiding her father in an attempt to block out her memories of the accident and angry feelings towards him. We spent some time mapping out the impact of blame and guilt on Jane's relationships with her parents. Through using an externalising conversation, we were able to create some space that enabled Jane to think about "blame" and "guilt" differently and the impact of these on her and her relationships. Jane became aware that through avoiding any contact with her father she was also losing the other aspects of her relationship with him that she valued and that she was missing her relationship with her mother. We also talked about psychological theories of grief and explored how these might fit with Jane's experiences. Jane reflected on times that she did talk about William's accident and who she found it helpful to do this with.

Family meetings

Family therapy sessions with Jane and her parents were carried out with a family therapist colleague. We paid attention to creating a place that was "safe" for Jane and her parents to talk. This involved meeting separately with Jane and then her parents to discuss how we would work together and what their hopes were for a joint session. In working systemically, we took a position of curiosity and valued hearing different perspectives. To do this, we asked systemic questions and worked collaboratively with Jane and her parents.

The planning sessions with Jane and then with her parents included asking what different family members wanted from the sessions. We thought that it was important to create a clear agreed focus. This was particularly important when we were working with such intense emotions in a family who were creating distance in order to stay "safe" and to protect one another from their thoughts and feelings. We asked Jane and then her parents, "What conversations are important to have together now?" and "What difference would you like this to make for you and your children/grandchildren?" For Jane, it was to agree what contact her parents would have with the children and what information she would like shared with them about William's injury. For her parents, their priority was to meet with Jane and to talk about whatever she chose. They particularly wanted Jane to agree to them spending time with William at the rehabilitation centre but agreed that this was her decision.

In the planning sessions and then when we met together, we spent time agreeing on "emotional safety" by asking questions such as, "How will family members let us know if they don't want to talk about a particular theme?" and "How is it helpful for the others to respond at these times?" and "What if a family member becomes upset in the session?"

We also acknowledged what we weren't going to talk about. This was both because Jane only felt able to agree to a conversation that focussed on her children's relationships with their grandparents rather than her own relationship with them and because of the legal case and the advice that we couldn't discuss the details of the accident together. Throughout the family sessions, we acknowledged that the accident had had a significant emotional impact on all of the family and that this was something that they were all attempting to find ways of coping with. Jane chose to share that she had been avoiding seeing them, as she was feeling angry and upset about the accident.

Having spent time creating a context for our meeting together, we focussed on talking about family relationships between Jane's daughters and their grandparents. "What sort of relationships would you like the children to have with their grandparents?" We explored how their relationships had been previously and how they had made decisions about the amount of contact and the roles that the grandparents had with the children. We also talked about how they might change now following William's ABI and how they were changing anyway as the children grew up. Jane was able to say how much she appreciated the time her parents spent with the children but that she also hoped that they could have less of a role as "carers" in the future and more of a focus on a relationship where they enjoyed doing activities and spending time with the children. Jane also said she felt that now that her parents were getting older and following the accident, she didn't want them to take the children out. Her parents were happy to agree with this, as they were feeling very anxious and had lost confidence following the accident.

We asked Jane what her hopes were for her parents as they took on less of a childcare role with their grandchildren. Jane was able to say that she hoped that they would be able to develop and reconnect with some of their friendships and interests that they had had less time for since her divorce. She also hoped that she could spend some time with her mother without the children as they had before. Jane also hoped that they would be able to do some of the more fun activities with the children that they had enjoyed together previously.

William's siblings

In the final family session, we talked about William's injury and how Jane would like this explained to William's sisters. Jane and I had talked about this and had prepared a structure for a book together about the family and about William's brain injury for her to share with and to develop further with her daughters. Jane had agreed that she would like to talk to her parents about this book. In the session, we asked Jane questions about the book and her preferences in a way that positioned her as a competent parent. We also explored how the family had preferred to talk about William's diagnosis of ADHD and how they had helped William and his sisters understand this. This included asking Jane and his grandparents how they had gained an understanding of this diagnosis and what their thoughts were about this.

We acknowledged the current uncertainty about how William would be in future. We asked Jane what her understanding was of the prognosis for him. As they listened William's grandparents both became very upset. They said that they had both felt that it was important to be "optimistic" and to be hopeful about William's future recovery. His grandfather said he felt that he would be letting William down if he "gave up on him". We asked Jane how she felt when her father said this. Jane shared some of her own struggles with knowing what to hope for and said how lonely she felt when her parents talked as if William would recover and return to how he used to be. As therapists, we reflected on the different information that Jane and her parents had access to. Towards the end of the session, Jane agreed that she would like her parents to spend some time at the rehabilitation centre while she was there. She thought that this could help them to better understand William as he was now. Jane also said that she would like to look at the book with her daughters and that she would then like her parents to talk about this with the girls.

At the end of the session, we asked how each family member had experienced our conversations. They all thought having the initial meetings beforehand had been helpful, as they were all feeling apprehensive about meeting. They were all glad to have begun a conversation together and felt that acknowledging that they were all coping in different ways with the impact of the accident was helpful. Jane's parents said that they were pleased that we could talk about their intentions as they both felt that they were often responding in ways that Jane did not find helpful, despite trying extremely hard to support her and their grandchildren.

Reflections on the therapeutic work

The work was carried out in a way that was flexible and could develop throughout the rehabilitation period. Being able to work in this way has often been important for families whose son or daughter has a profound brain injury. It is not unusual for families to struggle to think of any goals but to agree to future meetings to follow up on themes that have emerged or to have the opportunity to reflect on the rehabilitation process. This enabled Jane and me to have initial conversations about how she was coping, to then have family sessions with her parents and within these to think about the needs of her other children. Having the planning meetings prior to the joint family sessions seemed important to create a safe space for a family that was facing such traumatic circumstances and such significant losses. Acknowledging what couldn't or wouldn't be spoken about alongside agreeing to a focus created a context for Jane and her parents to meet. Working with a colleague was also important.

Concluding thoughts and areas for future development

This chapter is an overview of some of the work that I have carried out with children, young people and their families when the child has sustained a very profound brain injury. Feedback from the families who have chosen and been able to engage in this work has tended to be very positive. Some have met for therapeutic work, others have not chosen to meet again following the initial meeting, whilst some have met for monthly "check ins" but not focussed therapeutic work.

In thinking about potential areas for future development, the need for further feedback from parents and other family members is of central importance. It would be really helpful to gain longer-term feedback from families about their experiences of the work and their ideas about any other support that in hindsight they feel it would have been helpful to receive.

It would also be helpful to have an overarching model to guide psychosocial rehabilitation interventions. Drawing on the psychological and family therapy literature and models of family resilience, including narrative practices that enable personal and relational agency. Such a model could help to target interventions for families who are most likely to face longer-term challenges.

Neurorehabilitation is goal-focussed and incorporating goals that create the opportunity to offer regular "check ins" with families seems valuable. My experience of working with families with children with profound brain injuries is that it is often difficult to identify clear goals but that when ongoing opportunities to meet are created that these are highly valued and that therapeutic conversations can emerge during the rehabilitation time.

It is also important to think about both the immediate and the longer-term needs of siblings. A range of approaches can be helpful, including workshops for parents, sibling workshops, scrapbooking (Daisley, 2014) and creating narratives using approaches such as the Tree of Life (Ncube, 2006) or an adapted version of the Beads of Life (Portnoy, Girling, & Fredman, 2015), which I have experimented with using with this client group. As there are limited community services available to support families who have a child with an ABI, it seems an important part of the rehabilitation service to offer an opportunity to think about the needs of other children in the family.

Parents may also find it helpful to develop narrative documents to share with other families facing similar circumstances. These could include messages of understanding, hope, coping, resilience and strength to parents from others at different stages in the rehabilitation process.

References

Altschuler, J. (2012). *Counselling and psychotherapy for families in times of illness and death.* Palgrave Macmillan.

Andersen, T. (1995). Reflecting processes: Acts of informing and forming: You can borrow my eyes, but you must not take them away from me! In S. Friedman (Ed.), *The reflecting team in action: Collaborative practice in family therapy.* New York: Guildford Press.

Anderson, H., & Goolishian, H. A. (1992). The client is the expert: A not-knowing approach to therapy. In S. McNamee & K. J. J. Gergen (Eds.), *Therapy as social construction*. London: Sage.

Burnham, J. (1992). Approach-method-technique: Making distinctions and creating connections. *Human Systems, 3*(1), 3–26.

Burnham, J. (2005). Relational reflexivity: A tool for socially constructing therapeutic relationships. In C. Flascos, B. Mason, & A. Perlesz (Eds.), *The space between: Experience, context and process in therapeutic relationships*. London: Karnac.

Carey, M. (2014). Narrative therapy and trauma. In S. Weatherhead & D. Todd (Eds.), *Narrative approaches to brain injury*. London: Karnac.

Cecchin, G. (1987). Hypothesizing, circularity and neutrality revisited: An invitation to curiosity. *Family Process, 26*, 405–413.

Daisley, A., Prangnell, S., & Seed, R. (2014). Helping children create positive stories about a parent's brain injury. In S. Weatherhead & D. Todd (Eds.), *Narrative approaches to brain injury*. London: Karnac.

Epston, D., & White, M. (1990). Consulting your consultants: The documentation of alternative knowledge's. In D. Epson & M. White (Eds.), *Experience, contradiction, narrative and imagination. Selected papers of Donald Epston and Michael White 1989–1991*. Adelaide: Dulwich Centre.

Fredman, G. (2003). *Death talk conversations with children and families*. London: Karnac.

Hagen, C., Danese Malkmus, M., & Durham, P. (1992). *Ranchos Los Amigos scale: Communication disorders service*. Rancho Los Amigos Hospital.

Hoffman, L. (1993). *Exchanging voices: A collaborative approach to therapy*. London: Karnac Books.

Ncube, N. (2006). The tree of life project. *International Journal of Narrative Therapy & Community Work*, (1), 3–16.

Pearce, W. B. (1994). *Interpersonal communication: Making social worlds*. New York: Harper Collins College.

Portnoy, S., Girling, I., & Fredman, G. (2015). Supporting living with cancer to tell their stories in ways that make them stronger: The beads of life approach. *Clinical Child Psychology and Psychiatry*.

Royal College of Physicians. (2003). *The vegetative state*. London: RCP.

Royal College of Physicians. (2013). *Prolonged disorders of consciousness national clinical guidelines*. London: RCP.

Teasdale, G., & Jennett, B. (1974). Assessment of coma and impaired consciousness: A practical scale. *Lancet, 2*, 81–84.

White, M. (1989). *The externalising of the problem and the reauthorizing of lives and relationships*. Selected Papers. Adelaide: Dulwich Centre.

Chapter 9

Narrative approaches for behaviour that challenges post-injury

Esther Cole

Looking back, we can't believe how far James has come. He was so poorly that even hospital staff are surprised at how well he is doing now. He now attends a school for additional needs and is well liked by his peers and teachers. We are eternally grateful for all the expert care and advice we received during this scary time.

(Emily, Mum)

The purpose

My inspiration for this book began in late 2012 in my last few months of training as a clinical psychologist on my child and adolescent mental health service (CAMHS) placement. I had the opportunity to meet a 12-year-old boy, "James", who had an acquired brain injury (ABI) from the surgical removal of a cancerous hypothalamic tumour at age 10.

James, his family and I really wanted his story to be told, and for his experiences of ABI to help other children and families. His story made me aware of how common childhood brain injury is in mainstream child (and adult) mental health services and how few therapies were available for children and families affected by this. Witnessing the changes James made using narrative approaches over a mere ten weeks was inspiring and powerful for me. A fundamental message I took away was that few children and young people (CYP) will access therapy from a specialist paediatric neuropsychologist, and that all therapists, including those in training under supervision, can consider adapting their existing therapy skills to help this group.

In this chapter, I hope to share how I applied the principles of narrative practises and adapted narrative techniques to working with behaviour that challenges others. I start by positioning myself and the work within the context of being a trainee applying these ideas. I use a series of medical and narrative visual formulations, or diagrams, of James's story. The process and stages of the narrative approach are detailed and how we can adapt narrative principles to take into account neuropsychological difficulties. I also describe James's outcomes across a two-year span.

Positioning the narrative approach: a critique

I position myself (then and now) as a clinical psychologist integrating evolving, evidence-based research, psychological approaches and theories to best serve the client, family or system. In terms of therapy orientation, I am an integrative therapist, working across all age groups, with a core training in cognitive behavioural therapy (CBT). I was not a narrative therapist by training then – neither am I now. Poststructural, social constructionist approaches like narrative therapy and traditionally realist, positivist neuroscientific approaches like neurorehabilitation, or even CBT, are usually positioned at opposite ends of a broad spectrum of philosophies and epistemologies (Weatherhead & Flaherty-Jones, 2011).

I use structural language in this work, which means I believe that human culture and psychology can be understood in terms of overarching systems or constructs that underpin how humans behave, think, perceive and feel. On the contrary, non-structuralists believe there is no one objective truth or view of reality. Instead, it is constructed, or shaped, through people and groups interacting together in a hierarchical social system, where meaning, or sense-making, is made through the use of language and discourse (Foucault, 1980).

According to Foucault (1980), certain social groups may have more power to determine how other groups are seen. For example, there is a dominant societal discourse that has often marginalised and stigmatised people with disabilities – even the word "disability" privileges an account of a group of people as incapable, with the "absence of 'ability'" (Baum & Lynngaard, 2006, p. 104). Therefore, power and truth are determined by these social hierarchies – they impact how language is used and which discourses are more dominant.

Following on from this, to my knowledge, until fairly recently, there were no documented ideas of "narrative formulation". Clinicians formulating with multiple therapeutic models coined this phraseology (Weatherhead & Flaherty-Jones, 2011; Harper & Spellman, 2014; Meehan & Guilfoyle, 2015). This is because narrative therapy is not based on prescriptive or directive interactions or interventions, which hold the therapist as the expert.

James invited his teaching assistant to therapy as an "outsider-witness" to listen to his story. In narrative therapy, it is important that the outsider-witness' acknowledgement is not applause, as this brings with it social expectations of what might be desirable or admirable. Instead, outsider-witnesses are invited to express what aspects of the story spoken to them and how it resonated with their own values. However, in the context of neurorehabilitation, it is rare that improvements in physical functioning would not be applauded – herein lays the conflict between epistemologies and philosophies between the therapies. By integrating narrative approaches with neurorehabilitation, my intention is to innovate in psychological practice, whilst holding in mind that it is very difficult to achieve the aims of traditional narrative therapy in an ABI setting.

Narrative therapy: the territories of life

ABI can permanently alter a person's sense of self and his or her identity. Before I move on to James's experience of identity change and loss of his sense of self, as well as how we worked together on this, I will explain the theory around the "territories of life" (Bruner, 1986) that underpins the techniques I used with him. In narrative practise, the metaphor of the "landscape of identity" and the "landscape of action" in the territories of life are described (Bruner, 1986). In these landscapes, some story lines may be thicker or thinner than others.

Therefore, therapeutic exchanges could be seen as a way to scaffold conversations so that clients can see the dominant and the alternative stories of their lives. Following on from Foucault, if the way we make meaning, or sense of the world, is through the exchange of language in social contexts, relationships and life experiences, even our sense of self is maintained and organised through language (White & Epston, 1990). Therefore, metaphorically, the stories which we tell ourselves, or have been told about us by others, form our identities. These stories about ourselves are linked through events in a sequence, across time, according to a plot, and in narrative therapy the "narrative" is the story line that weaves these events together (Morgan, 2000). This means we are multi-storied, and there is no one fixed version of our selves. These narratives form the "landscape of our identities" (White, 2004) and the themes composing this landscape give rise to the intentions, purposes, values and aspirations of a person. How the story is constructed has meaning for how we live our lives and the actions we take – this has been termed the "landscape of action" (White, 2004).

Built on this social constructionist philosophy, narrative therapy challenges the dominant discourse that is problematic in a person's life, leading to problem-saturated views of self. The therapist is urged to use language that empowers rather than disempowers. For example, externalising language is used so that the person is not the problem – the problem is the problem (White, 1989).

This process of deconstruction leads to the thickening and development of preferred stories and accounts of the person's life, rather than reducing the landscape of identity to problematic stories, which are limited or "thin" in description (White, 1989). Thin descriptions reduce possibilities and opportunities for the person and can define them according to deficits, which can draw negative conclusions, often expressed as truths about them.

Challenging behaviour in acquired brain injury

Adapted narrative approaches to ABI are showing much promise in the adult field (Weatherhead & Todd, 2014). However, there are only a few publications which draw on narrative approaches for children who have experienced an ABI (Byard, 2015; Byard & Gosling, 2013; Byard, Fine & Reed, 2011; Epston, Barlow, Murphy, O'Flaherty, & Webster, 2008; Erskine, 2013; Perkins, 2013; Portnoy, Girling, & Fredman, 2015; Perkins, 2015; Fredman, 1997). These demonstrate positive outcomes for the child and family within contexts of grief, loss, disability, palliation and bereavement.

Paediatric ABI can have permanent and devastating effects on the child and others around them. Children and families are faced with the complexity of adjusting to the physical, cognitive, educational, social, behavioural, occupational and emotional consequences of an ABI (Wilde et al., 2015). The risks to the child of developing psychological problems, such as anxiety and depression, are increased (Gracey et al., 2014), estimated as twice as common than the general population (Tsai et al., 2014). Behaviour that challenges others also increases, being up to four times more prevalent (depending on the severity of the ABI) than in children with non-neurological medical conditions (Schwartz et al., 2003).

Despite the increased chances of a child developing mental health and behavioural difficulties, few studies have directly addressed practical interventions for what is commonly termed as "challenging behaviour" (Woods et al., 2014). There is promise for parenting interventions (Brown, Sofronoff, Whittingham, Boyd, & McKinlay, 2013; Brown, Whittingham, Boyd, McKinlay, & Sofronoff, 2014; Woods et al., 2014) cognitive (Limond & Adlam, 2015), behavioural (Brown & Whittingham, 2015) and online problem-solving interventions (Wade & Hung, 2015), which can directly address behaviour that challenges. There is also an emerging systemic practice evidence base for working with children and families suffering the emotional and psychological consequences of traumatic brain injury (Byard, 2015; Byard et al., 2011; Helps, 2013; Ames & Jones, 2013).

James's story

Background information

James was a 12-year-old, white British boy who lived with his mother, Emily; father, Tony; and 20-year-old brother, Joseph. He met all his milestones from birth, was popular with his peers and thrived educationally. He described being physically well and having a happy, active childhood until the age of 9, when he would come home extremely tired and fall asleep.

He was diagnosed, aged 10, with a cancerous germ cell hypothalamic-pituitary tumour, for which he had both surgery and chemo-radiation. The brain injury from the surgery was severe, and he was in a coma for several weeks. Primary impacts of the brain tumour were hyperphagia or over-eating (sometimes forgetting he had eaten – sometimes a genuine hunger), blindness in one upper visual field, problems with mobility due to the invasive surgery, diabetes insipidus and extreme thirst.

James had to urinate in a container to measure urine output so that it could be balanced with fluid intake. He needed assistance with toileting, particularly due to problems reading the units. James had suffered some falls so used a wheelchair. Cognitively, an assessment showed James had problems with short-term memory, attention, concentration and using fine motor skills, such as handwriting.

The main impacts of the brain injury were behaviour that challenged others and depression. The behaviour consisted of repeatedly asking for food (every ten minutes), screaming with escalating physical and verbal aggression when he was refused more food and shouting and making threats to kill himself. The depression presented as low mood, lack of motivation, irritability, thoughts that life was not worth living and an existential sense of unfairness in the world. James was in hospital for nine months. He described nearly dying twice due to an allergic reaction to the chemotherapy. The family were initially told there was *"no hope for James"*. He was later called a *"medical miracle"* – he not only survived but was cured of the cancer.

Figure 9.1 shows James's narrative timeline. After nine months of inpatient physical and neurological rehabilitation in hospital, he went home for three months. The experience of being home was frightening and brought painful reminders of all the things he could no longer do. Like many affected by ABI, he felt a profound sense of loss and change in his identity compared to who he was (Segal, 2010), as did his family. James went to a residential neurorehabilitation unit for ten months. He described his time there as characterised by a sense of terror, full of worries and fears – being fearful of the future (wishing he had died), suffering low mood and over-eating. His weight was measured as above the 99th percentile.

Staff at the residential unit had tried different behavioural interventions to manage the over-eating. These included food charts, reward charts and scheduling positive activities. James then started some narrative work with a psychologist,

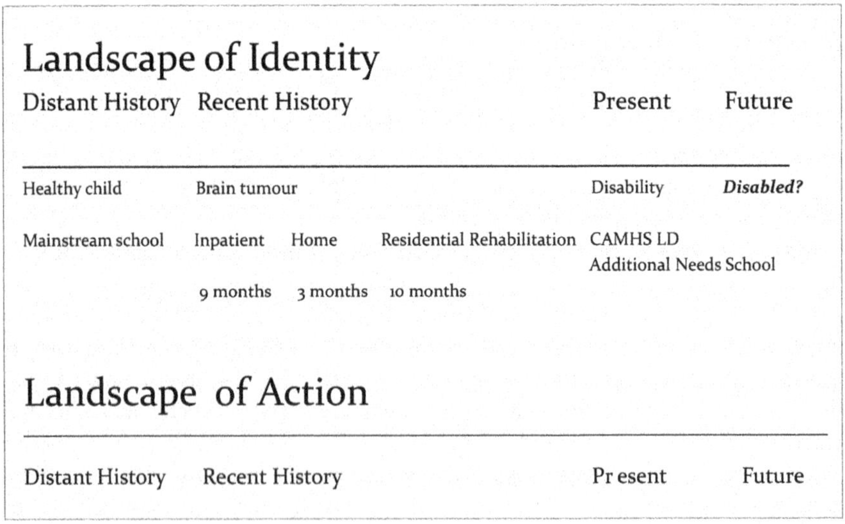

Landscape of Identity

Distant History	Recent History			Present	Future
Healthy child	Brain tumour			Disability	*Disabled?*
Mainstream school	Inpatient	Home	Residential Rehabilitation	CAMHS LD Additional Needs School	
	9 months	3 months	10 months		

Landscape of Action

Distant History	Recent History	Present	Future

Figure 9.1 Narrative timeline
Source: Adapted from White, 2004

who encouraged his parents to write material about his story for the charity and to promote his well-being, bearing witness to his progress in rehabilitation. After three months, his mood improved, and he was able to walk 25 metres. He was soon able to go home at weekends and played football from the wheelchair.

Despite the progress he had made, when James was transferred home, the depression resurfaced. Due to the dramatic change in his identity, he often maintained a "patient role" and, despite his voice breaking, sometimes spoke in a high-pitched, childlike voice. Although he could use a frame for walking, he felt safer in the wheelchair. He was transferred to a CAMHS learning disabilities team and placed in a school for additional needs for children with intellectual disabilities. James's abilities exceeded most of his peers, and classes did not always challenge him. This affected his motivation and increased his levels of boredom and requests for food.

JAMES: *I felt really happy and delighted to be home, but a little sad that I wasn't the same boy that I used to be. I was in a wheelchair, and I couldn't do the things I was able to before the cancer, and that really made me upset.*

EMILY: *When James came home for good, we were over the moon. We had had him home for a couple of nights during his time in rehab, but nothing beat the feeling of being a complete family again. Getting used to being woken up numerous times during the night took a bit of getting used to. It was like having a newborn again, but we soon got into a routine. Unfortunately though, James was still suffering from low mood, and there was nothing we could do to help him. That's when continuing with narrative work with Esther at school really helped.*

James was referred to psychology for support with "challenging behaviour". My perspective, inspired by narrative ideas, led me to think about the problem-saturated stories and the impact of the brain injury overshadowing his identity. In Figure 9.1, the words *"disability"* and *"disabled"* are in italics to emphasise the impact of language and target areas for deconstructing the dominant discourse. In narrative theory, if James can explore where these problems are not in his life, he might be able to re-author his future by thickening positive stories of self-identity and action.

Contextual, systemic neurorehabilitation formulation

Before I met James, I made a preliminary formulation of his difficulties. Figure 9.2 shows an integrative formulation of systemic, contextual neuropsychological rehabilitation adapted from the International Classification of Functioning, Disability and Health (ICF; WHO, 2002, 2007).

This captures how intra-personal (i.e. cognitive, emotional), interpersonal (i.e. family, child) and multisystemic (i.e. multi- and interdisciplinary teams) factors reciprocally contribute to the neuropsychological, psychological and social adjustment, mental health and coping of the child. In this model, there is a discrepancy

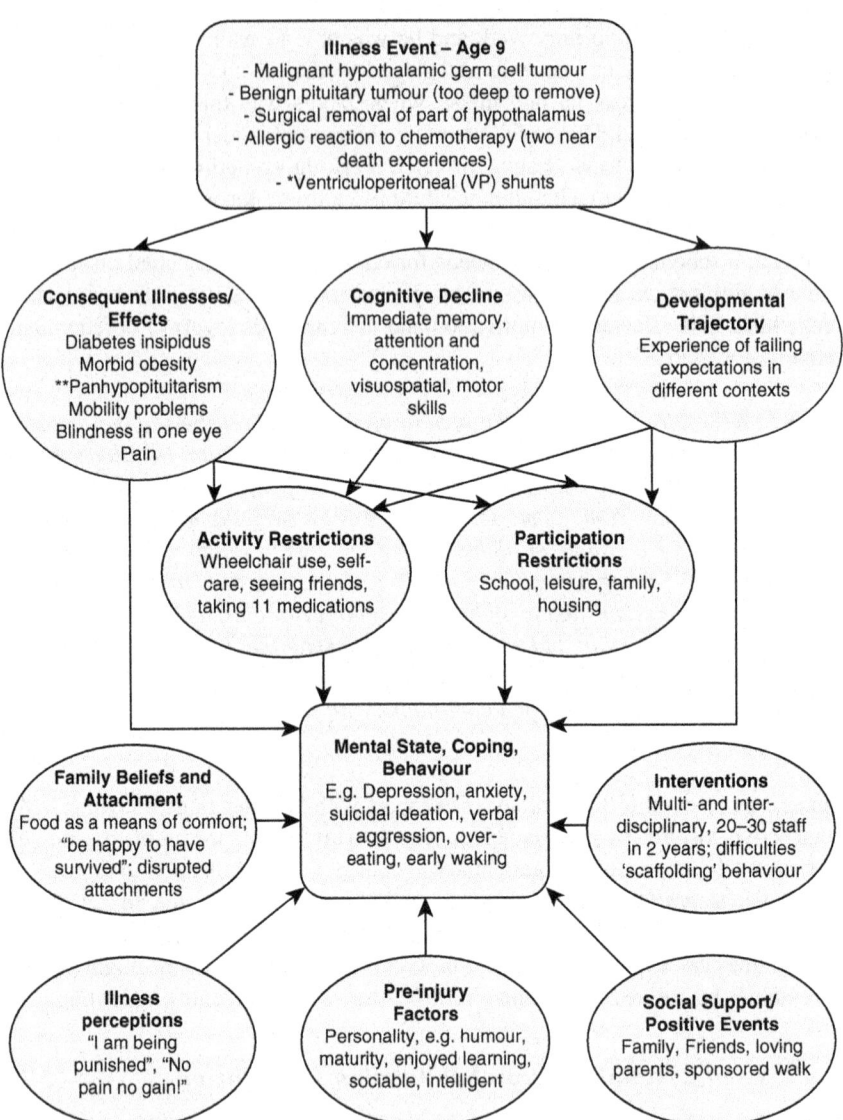

Figure 9.2 A contextual, systemic formulation of James's neuropsychological rehabilitation and psychological adjustment to ABI

Note: * Ventriculoperitoneal (VP) shunts – drains inserted into the brain to prevent the accumulation of fluid.

** Panhypopituitarism – decreased (hypo) secretion of most of the eight pituitary hormones.

in expectations between children's actual abilities and their pre-injury development. This represents a threat to their own and their family's goals, and to their own self-esteem. Other factors impacting on mental state, coping and the behaviour of the children are their opportunities for support, participation, resuming pre-injury activities and contact with peers.

The pre-injury brain, cognitive reserves and premorbid functioning also have an impact (Gracey, Olsen, Austin, Watson, & Malley, 2015). James had a good level of educational attainment, a resilient and attractive personality, positive relationships with parents and peers and high self-esteem. James's "*no pain – no gain*" mantra also bolstered his coping and resilience throughout his treatment. The family had many other protective factors, such as parental warmth and responsiveness, humour, low negative family interactions and supportive family friendships, known to buffer parental stress and support the child's rehabilitation post-injury (Wade et al., 2001).

In Figure 9.3 (Problem-Saturated Story), I illustrate a re-formulation using a narrative timeline of the territories of life that might more easily be shared with a child or family. This formulation can also be used to illustrate the child's evolving narrative and identity within the neurorehabilitation context. The arrows symbolise the conversations between James and I in therapy, moving fluidly between the past, present and future – what Michael White terms the "zigzagging nature of . . . re-authoring conversations" (White, 2004, p. 61). It is important to elicit connections to the person's values, principles, aspirations and commitments (landscape of identity), whilst linking these to the client's actions and skills over time

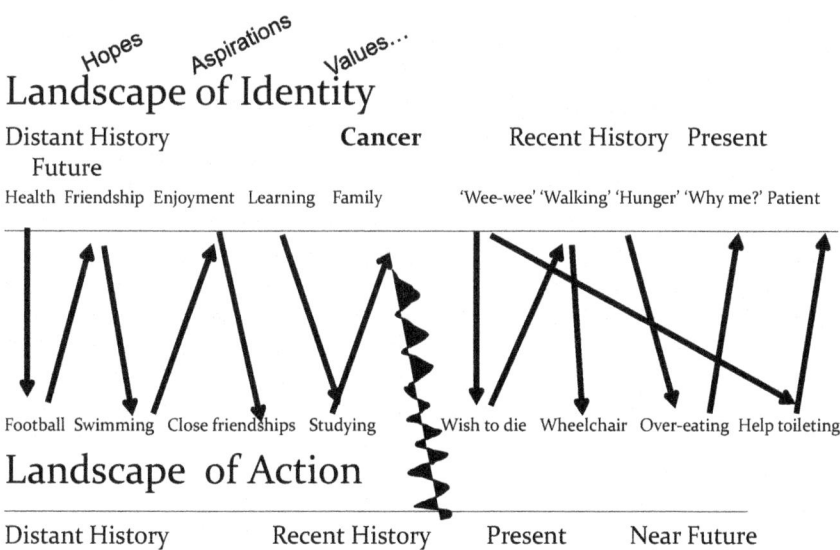

Figure 9.3 Problem-saturated story

Source: Adapted from White, 2004

(landscape of action). The lines of enquiry typically involve zigzagging between the landscapes to weave a coherent story.

Another dominant discourse, which made thin conclusions about James, was that he should be "*grateful to be alive*", rather than acknowledging that, often, James suffered, and life was painful and unbearable for him. This further darkened the territory of his preferred identity, by bringing the problem of guilt for not feeling grateful, which led him to feel he was being punished for being a "*bad person*" – and that perhaps he was a bad person in the first place, which is why the cancer came for him. This could have been an opportunity to work with the family's faith and spiritual practises. We did explore the concept of suffering in the world and how many other children, who he had met, suffered enormously. These stories seemed to create more multi-stranded beliefs and made him feel less like he was being punished.

JAMES: *I don't feel guilt or that I was a bad person. I understand now that cancer can affect anybody, and it was out of my control.*

Narrative intervention

Therapy structure

I met James for four fortnightly narrative sessions for one hour at his school. Half of each session was with his teaching assistant – who was invited by James as an "outsider-witness". I received 1.5 hours supervision. There was one review session at the end of therapy to communicate James's progress and care plan to his parents.

I sent two therapeutic letters to James and copied in members of the system to promote the formulation, shared and collaborative working. It was hoped that the wider system could co-create new stories of James's preferred identity, which included mastery, strength and empowerment. The letters served a therapeutic function: they reflected on sessions, made therapy transparent, bore witness to it and were reminders of the progress made in externalising and overcoming the problem (Epston, 1998).

The Mood and Feelings Questionnaire (Angold & Costello, 1987) was used pre- and post- therapy as a quantitative measure of change in the depression. The use of questionnaire-based outcome measures has historically been at odds with a socially constructed orientation of therapy. However, there are comprehensive arguments for combining different epistemological methods of measuring outcome (Weatherhead & Todd, 2014; Gosling, 2015).

Engagement in therapy

Before I met James, I read the article his parents had written about his experience for the charity and presented it to him. I was touched and curious about his statement: "*Oh so they do love me*" when he re-read it. I used outsider-witness practises of "de-centred sharing" (White, 2002) to engage James. This involved sharing which expressions James and his parents had used that resonated with me as an outsider-witness, actions and expressions that revealed his identity and values and how his experiences had changed me – or where they had "transported me" (White, 2002).

I explained that I had been struck by his commitment to help others when he talked about a sponsored walk he wanted to do the following year, despite needing to use a wheelchair. I noted his bravery, strength of character, determination and described him as '*heroic*', and he laughed. I said that his story had really changed my life, as it made me want to use my skills to help him and other children. I explained that I was still training, who my supervisor was and whether I could offer him some "*talking therapy sessions*".

James said he would like this. He had been feeling very upset, could not stop thinking about the cancer, treatment, missing over a year of school and things he said and did for which he felt guilt and regret. I explained that most adults did not have to go through what he had. I also reflected on how mature and articulate he came across in expressing himself. (I was hoping to bring in an alternative strand to the story of James being immature, using a high-pitched voice).

I initially offered to make a life storybook (Perkins, 2013, 2015). He declined, but thought he would benefit from talking to me. James found it difficult to write; his reading skills were good, but material needed to be in large print. He also had problems remembering things, so we agreed that I would write him letters to help him remember.

JAMES: *I can't remember not wanting to make a life storybook. I am the first to admit that I usually love talking about my journey! However, I imagine that I enjoyed talking to Esther a lot more and liked explaining my feelings. I felt happier after talking to her. The focus on writing sentences and filling pages with pictures of my story would probably have felt too much like homework.*

Process of narrative work

I used Baum and Lynngaard's (2006) stages of narrative therapy, as listed under each heading in this section, but not necessarily in a sequential order. The stages can be used fluidly as principles in the process of therapy.

Externalising the problem: language and metaphor

We identified that the problems that tricked him were "Hunger", "Why me?", "Wee-wee", and "Walking". They led to a "patient identity", which meant James believed he could not walk or go to the toilet independently. The problems brought depression, pain, anger and conflict in relationships. I brought in language and metaphor that placed these problems outside James "externalising". I asked James to draw out his problems, metaphorically describing their colour, sound, texture and other sensory qualities. This helped the problems turn into outside entities he could tangibly imagine confronting and relating to.

Mapping the influence of the problem

We then mapped the influence of the problems as shown in Figure 9.3. An example of this was "Hunger", as illustrated in the following excerpt:

> Sample narrative letter one: "*You said that Hunger asks for food – not just when you feel Hunger in your stomach – but when you have already eaten. You said that Hunger knows you had to have surgery and tricks you by telling your brain that you need food when you have already eaten. Hunger also tries to trick your parents and schoolteachers by asking them many, many times for food, when they have already said, "No!"*".

Recruitment into problem-saturated views of self

The recruitment of the self into a problem-saturated story is an aspect of narrative practise that looks at how the problem was able to dominate the person. There may be subtle benefits or explanations for the relationship between the person and the problem. This provides scope for exploration of any losses or gains to arise through overcoming the problem:

> Narrative letter one: "*At times, you give Hunger what it wants . . . because you have to deal with strong feelings like sadness and anger at what happened to you. You remember what life was like before . . . and . . . ask 'Why me?' You described how you lost the whole of Year 6 [and all your friends] . . . and how pain and suffering were in your life. Hunger gets food for you and this helps you not have to think about this as much . . .*".
>
> "*I wonder if Hunger stops 'Why Me?'. You talked about some thoughts of wanting to go back in time and start life over again. 'Wee-wee' makes you feel like this too. It seems that Hunger can control 'Why me?' and 'Wee-wee' . . .*".

Identifying unique outcomes

Examples of unique outcomes were often told by James's teaching assistant. He mentioned that when James was able to go on the climbing frame, "Walking" did not create fear. In our sessions, his teaching assistant would encourage him to use the toilet independently, and we bought a container that had large, bold markings on it so James could toilet independently. Also, when James saw his friends from his old school, Hunger was not around as much. Walking would let him go down the stairs to greet them. By having something to look forward to, James felt the problems could not occupy as much of his mind and 'Why me?' was kept at bay. Here is an example of how we deconstructed the problem of Hunger:

Narrative letter one: *"You said you can control Hunger in different ways:*

- *By thinking of the food you have just eaten and telling Hunger "I have just eaten!"*
- *By telling Hunger that it is working with your brain to trick you*
- *By letting Hunger ask parents for food only twice and letting your parents tell Hunger that he cannot have anything else to eat*
- *By asking Hunger to accept what parents and teachers say is true.* James also said by *"Trading Hunger for fruit!"*

Thickening and co-authoring new stories

Through creating more opportunities to develop preferred story lines, we enhance the young person's sense of agency so that they experience themselves as people with knowledge. At this stage in re-authoring the person's life, we want to champion the preferred story, identity and actions. For James, we co-authored new stories of a *'patient'* becoming a *"teenage boy like every other, but a bit more special!"* His teaching assistant was key to thickening his story of bravery, independence and ability. On hearing the impact on others' lives, James felt validated and this process opened up opportunities for further positive developments of his self:

Narrative letter two: *"You've told 'Walking' that you want it to stop asking for your wheelchair – you want it to spend more time with the Walking-Frame. I spoke to your Mum who said she was bringing in the Walking-Frame to school and we were very excited about this. You said you want Walking to know you have control over it and you never want it to scare you again. Over time, we think Walking won't need a frame, or a wheelchair, and your physiotherapist is doing a great job to teach Walking a lesson!"*

"So . . . it seems like we have a new story of a very brave and courageous boy who has had to battle with a lot of problems affecting his body, independence and good feelings. We are all seeing a boy who is overcoming the problems which trick his body and who is managing to succeed in living a more normal, happy life and childhood, despite everything he went through two years ago".

EMILY: *"The letters made a lot of sense. James was definitely able to control his hunger and toilet issues a lot better when distracted and still is to this day. We still find ourselves using the points made in narrative letter one with regards to his food issues".*

Consolidating and extending new stories

At this stage in therapy, we have questioned and deconstructed dominant discourses, reached a more liberating, alternative story – now we wanted to extend those positive stories into the future. Examples of this included James being enrolled into a mainstream school with his previous friends part time whilst retaining a place at his school for additional needs. He took part in more exercise and seemed to visibly be losing weight. He planned to increase his independence further with occupational therapy – e.g. learning to cook. James completed the sponsored walk. He wanted a new identity in the future as a scientist who finds a cure for cancer!

EMILY: *James seemed pretty confident after his meetings with Esther. He seemed more determined not to let his disabilities get in his way. The talking in a baby voice lessened, and he tried walking more. A cure for cancer might be out of the question as mainstream school wasn't for him, but he is still determined to help others and would like to become a teaching assistant one day.*

Table 9.1 summarises some of the elements of the narrative approach that were adapted to take into account the neuropsychological impacts of the brain injury.

Table 9.1 Narrative approach: neuropsychological adaptations

Problem	Narrative Approach	Adaptation for Brain Injury
Hyperphagia ('Hunger')	Externalisation, thickening story lines in the landscape of identity, deconstruction of 'Hunger'	Treating changes in the brain as opportunities for externalisation
Diabetes Insipidus ('Wee-wee')	Externalisation, thickening story lines in the landscape of action	As above
Cognitive difficulties	Re-storying the landscape of identity – i.e. ability not disability; outsider-witness	Short sessions, multimodal, wrote letters to aid memory
Visual difficulties	Re-storying the landscape of action	Large font used; considered placement of stimuli, awareness of impact of vision
Motor difficulties	Re-storying the landscape of action; outsider-witness	No handwriting – talking therapy; graded support with toilet use
Depression ('Why Me?')	Externalising; scaffolding, listening to personal values and strengths	Reflecting on the narratives of other peoples' health issues or mortality – i.e. other children with cancer

Outcomes

Post-therapy outcomes

After therapy, James scored 0/66 on the self-report version of the Mood and Feelings Questionnaire, indicating that the depression was no longer in his life. At his two-year follow-up, he scored 9/66 on the Mood and Feelings Questionnaire, indicating that the depression was still out of his life (the cut-off for clinical depression is 13). James had been discharged from CAMHS. Emily said there were fewer demands for food and behaviour that challenged others was rare. She thought that support from his schools and the narrative intervention (being able to talk to someone about his illness and fears, his relationship with food and taking an empowering rather than "*patient role*") had all improved his outcome. Emily also considered that James's growing maturity helped his rehabilitation, and the family was eating more healthy foods at home.

James was soon to be taking his GCSE exams and, understandably, this was causing stress and anxiety. Reflecting on the causes of James's anxiety around his exams, it became evident that consequent to the course of his illness and treatment, he had, in fact, missed the equivalent of two years of schooling. It was, therefore, agreed that James would defer his exams to give him time to work at his pace, which had a positive effect on his academic progress.

EMILY: *When I think back to how James was in 2012/2013, I am amazed at how far he has come in such a short time. We have gone from requesting food every 10 minutes (which resulted in behavioural outbursts) to being able to reason with him when he is told he can't have something. Socially, he is becoming more confident every day and attends a youth club on weekends. He is working towards being able to travel independently, though his mobility still holds him back a bit. Without the narrative work he received, I'm not sure we would be as far forward in our rehabilitation as we are now.*

Conclusions and reflections

The psychological management of behaviour that challenges, following paediatric brain injury, is a new and evolving field. This chapter guided the reader through psychological formulation, a narrative approach and outcome measurement. Cognitive behavioural, or behavioural, approaches that mainly focus on intervening with the thoughts or actions of a child, in isolation of their contexts, identities or stories, may not always benefit the young person or their family. In addition, needs may change as the young person develops and in different settings, which can be captured within a re-formulation of the problem.

The narrative approach led to consolidating and extending new stories for James, where he "traded Hunger for fruit", walked unaided without fear, toileted independently, was linked into a mainstream school and reported no depression.

Techniques which externalise the problems, identify exceptions and thicken preferred stories can empower a child's adoption of preferred identities and actions, as experts of change in their lives. Children and networks can re-author their life stories and re-write their future scripts.

It was satisfying to track James's progress over two years and invite him and his mother to reflect on their experiences of therapy with me as a trainee clinical psychologist in CAMHS. We hope that therapists, at all levels of training, are encouraged to adapt and innovate their existing therapy skills to formulate and intervene in the lives of children and young people with ABI, and their families. We have demonstrated that there can be medium- to long-term benefits of a brief, early intervention.

References

Ames, R., & Jones, C. (2013). "Think family": A staff consultation service set up within a rehabilitation centre for children with an acquired brain injury. *Context, 125*, 14–17.

Angold, A., & Costello, E. J. (1987). *Mood and feelings questionnaire (MFQ): Developmental epidemiology program*. Durham: Duke University.

Baum, S., & Lynngaard, H. (Eds.). (2006). *Intellectual disabilities: A systemic approach*. London: Karnac Books.

Brown, F. L., & Whittingham, K. (2015). A structured behavioural family intervention with parents of children with brain injury. In J. Reed, K. Byard, & H. Fine (Eds.), *Neuropsychological rehabilitation of childhood brain injury: A practical guide* (pp. 60–81). London: Palgrave Macmillan.

Brown, F. L., Sofronoff, K., Whittingham, K., Boyd, R., & McKinlay, L. (2013). A systematic review of parenting interventions for traumatic brain injury: Child and parent outcomes. *Journal of Head Trauma and Rehabilitation, 28*, 349–360.

Brown, F. L., Whittingham, K., Boyd, R., McKinlay, L., & Sofronoff, K. (2014). Improving child and parenting outcomes following pediatric acquired brain injury: A randomised controlled trial of stepping stones triple P plus acceptance and commitment therapy. *Journal of Child Psychology and Psychiatry, 55*, 1172–1183.

Bruner, J. (1986). *Actual minds, possible worlds*. Cambridge, MA: Harvard University Press.

Byard, K. (2015). A contextual, systemic perspective in child neuropsychological rehabilitation. In J. Reed, K. Byard, & H. Fine (Eds.), *Neuropsychological rehabilitation of childhood brain injury: A practical guide* (pp. 173–190). London: Palgrave Macmillan.

Byard, K., & Gosling, S. (2013). Rewriting the story of childhood brain injury: How systemic and narrative approaches help. *Context, 125*, 18–21.

Byard, K., Fine, H., & Reed, J. (2011). Taking a developmental and systemic perspective on neuropsychological rehabilitation with children with brain injury and their families. *Clinical Child Psychology and Psychiatry, 16*(2), 165–184.

Epston, D. (Ed.). (1998). *"Catching Up" with David Epston: A collection of narrative practice-based papers published between 1991 & 1996*. Adelaide: Dulwich Centre Publications.

Epston, D., Barlow, C., Murphy, M., O'Flaherty, L., & Webster, L. (2008). In memory of Hatu (Hayden) Barlow (1973–1985). In D. Epston & B. Bowen (Eds.), *Down under and up over – travels with narrative therapy*. Warrington, England: The Association of Family Therapy.

Erskine, R. (2013). Systemic thinking and neuropsychological assessment following childhood stroke related to sickle cell disease. *Context, 125*, 3–6.

Foucault, M. (1980). *Power/knowledge: Selected interviews and other writings*. New York: Pantheon Books.

Fredman, G. (1997). *Death talk: Conversations with children and families*. London: Karnac Books.

Gosling, S. (2015). Measuring outcomes for children with brain injury: Challenges and solutions. In J. Reed, K. Byard, & H. Fine (Eds.), *Neuropsychological rehabilitation of childhood brain injury: A practical guide* (pp. 191–214). London: Palgrave Macmillan.

Gracey, F., Olsen, G., Austin, L., Watson, S., & Malley, D. (2015). Integrating psychological therapy into interdisciplinary child neuropsychological rehabilitation. In J. Reed, K. Byard, & H. Fine (Eds.), *Neuropsychological rehabilitation of childhood brain injury: A practical guide* (pp. 191–214). London: Palgrave Macmillan.

Gracey, F., Watson, S., McHugh, M., Swan, A., Humphrey, A., & Adlam, A. (2014). Age at injury, emotional problems and executive functioning in understanding disrupted social relationships following childhood acquired brain injury. *Social Care and Neurodisability, 5*(3), 160–170.

Harper, D., & Spellman, D. (2014). Formulation and narrative therapy: Telling a different story. In L. Johnstone & R. Dallos (Eds.), *Formulation in psychology and psychotherapy: Making sense of people's problems*. London: Routledge.

Helps, S. (2013). Why a child's brain injury is a family affair. *Context, 125*, 10–13.

Limond, J., & Adlam, A-L. (2015). Cognitive interventions for children with brain injury. In J. Reed, K. Byard, & H. Fine (Eds.), *Neuropsychological rehabilitation of childhood brain injury: A practical guide* (pp. 82–105). London: Palgrave Macmillan.

Meehan, T., & Guilfoyle, M. (2015). Case formulation in poststructural narrative therapy. *Journal of Constructivist Psychology, 28*(1), 24–39.

Morgan, A. (2000). *What is narrative therapy? An easy-to-read introduction*. Adelaide: Dulwich Centre Publications.

Perkins, A. (2013). Adapted narrative therapy for children with severe traumatic brain injury. *Context, 125*, 7–9.

Perkins, A. (2015). Psychological support using narrative psychotherapy for children with brain injury. In J. Reed, K. Byard, & H. Fine (Eds.), *Neuropsychological rehabilitation of childhood brain injury: A practical guide* (pp. 215–234). London: Palgrave Macmillan.

Portnoy, S., Girling, I., & Fredman, G. (2015). Supporting young people living with cancer to tell their stories in ways that make them stronger: The beads of life approach. *Clinical Child Psychology and Psychiatry, 20*, 1–13.

Schwartz, L., Taylor, G., Drotar, D., Yeates, K. O., Wade, S. L., & Stancin, T. (2003). Long-term behavior problems following pediatric traumatic brain injury: Prevalence, predictors, and correlates. *Journal of Pediatric Psychology, 28*(4), 251–263.

Segal, D. (2010). Exploring the importance of identity following acquired brain injury: A review of the literature. *International Journal of Child, Youth and Family Studies, 1*, 293–314.

Tsai, M. C., Tsai, K. J., Wang, H. K., Sung, P. S., Wu, M. H., Hung, K. W., & Lin, S. H. (2014). Mood disorders after traumatic brain injury in adolescents and young adults: A nationwide population-based cohort study. *The Journal of Paediatrics, 164*(1), 136–141.

Wade, S. L., & Hung, A. (2015). Online family problem-solving for adolescent traumatic brain injury. In J. Reed, K. Byard, & H. Fine (Eds.), *Neuropsychological rehabilitation of childhood brain injury: A practical guide* (pp. 173–190). London: Palgrave Macmillan.

Wade, S. L., Borawski, E. A., Taylor, H. G., Drotar, D., Yeates, K. O., & Stancin, T. (2001). The relationship of caregiver coping to family outcomes during the initial year following paediatric traumatic injury. *Journal of Consulting and Clinical Psychology, 69*, 406–415.

Weatherhead, S., & Flaherty-Jones, G. (2011). *A pocket guide to therapy: A "How to" of the core models.* London: Sage Publications.

Weatherhead, S., & Todd, D. (2014). *Narrative approaches to brain injury.* London: Karnac Books.

White, M. (1989). *Selected papers.* Adelaide: Dulwich Centre Publications.

White, M. (2002). *Definitional ceremony and outsider-witness responses workshop.* Retrieved from www.dulwichcentre.au

White, M. (2004). Working with people who are suffering the consequences of multiple trauma: A narrative perspective. *The International Journal of Narrative Therapy and Community Work, 1*, 45–76.

White, M., & Epston, D. (1990). *Narrative means to therapeutic ends.* New York: W.W. Norton & Company.

Wilde, E., McCauley, S., Jivani, S., Hanten, G., Faber, J., & Gale, S. (2015). Neuropsychological consequences of child brain injury. In J. Reed, K. Byard, & H. Fine (Eds.), *Neuropsychological rehabilitation of childhood brain injury: A practical guide* (pp. 9–42). London: Palgrave Macmillan.

Woods, D., Catroppa, C., Godfrey, C., Giallo, R., Matthews, J., & Anderson, V. (2014). Challenging behaviours following paediatric acquired brain injury (ABI): The clinical utility for a manualised behavioural intervention programme. *Social Care and Neurodisability, 5.* doi:10.1108/SCN-03-2013-0006

World Health Organisation. (2002). *Towards a common language for functioning, disability and health: ICF international classification of functioning, disability and health.* Geneva: World Health Organisation.

World Health Organisation. (2007). *International classification of functioning, disability and health: Children & youth version: ICF-CY.* Geneva: World Health Organisation.

Chapter 10

The "Beads of Life" approach adapted for young people with an acquired brain injury

Sara Portnoy and Liz Ireland

Who we are?

Sara Portnoy is a consultant clinical psychologist who works part time at University College Hospital in London (UCLH) working with children who have a chronic illness. She manages the clinical psychologists who work with children who have a diagnosis of cancer. She also works for Life Force, a community multidisciplinary paediatric palliative care and bereavement team, which works in the London boroughs of Camden, Haringey and Islington. Sara also volunteers for the Refugee Resilience Collective, who are a group of systemic and narrative therapists who work with refugees and long-term volunteers in Northern France.

Dr. Liz Ireland is a clinical psychologist who works part time at Great Ormond Street Hospital. Liz specialises in working with children with a diagnosis of cancer, specifically children with brain tumours and their families. She previously worked with Sara on the Life Force team. Liz also works for Recolo, an independent community neurorehabilitation service for children and young people with ABI. Having completed the postgraduate diploma in paediatric and clinical neuropsychology, Liz combines her knowledge of neuropsychology with systemic ideas in her clinical work.

Sara and Liz met when Liz joined Sara working on the Life Force team. We were able to share our interests in working systemically and on drawing on an individual's resources, skills and personal contexts in order to bring about a different relationship to distress or difficulty.

The "Beads of Life" approach is relevant for working with any individual whose life is being dominated by a difficult story (e.g. illness, sudden or traumatic injury or living with loss of ability or function). It is a safe place to start to practise narrative therapy because there is a structure to the approach. We were able to share our ideas of how to adapt it to many different settings. Sara worked with teenagers and young adults in a group setting some of whom had a brain tumour. She also worked with parents whose lives were being dominated by their child having a serious illness. Liz has used the "Beads of Life" approach to work with children and young people with brain tumours and other forms of ABI, often working with individuals rather than groups and adapting the approach when needed to best meet the neuropsychological needs of the individuals.

The "Beads of Life" approach has been adapted from a programme that Sara began running in 2003 at St. Mary's hospital in London with children who were undergoing a bone marrow transplant. She has regularly used her supervision sessions to discuss how to adapt "Beads of Life" for different individuals. We have discussed using different metaphors – e.g. music tracks, wristbands, badges, buttons, and we have had numerous discussions about the "medical journey" and how to adapt that for different populations.

Introduction

In this chapter, we will first explain the theory that underlies "Beads of Life", and then we will describe how we run a "Beads of Life" one-day workshop for a group of young people. Throughout, we will describe how this can be adapted for one-to-one work and how it can be adapted for people with acquired brain injury.

At UCLH, this approach has been used with young people (aged 7–24) with a diagnosis of cancer many of whom have had a brain tumour. However, it has been adapted and used with people who have other disabilities, such as poor sight, limited verbal abilities, poor motor control and cognitive changes, such as memory or attention difficulties. As far as we are aware, there are very few descriptions of groups for children with a head injury. More frequently, there are descriptions of parenting interventions (Reed, Byard, & Fine, 2015).

When a chronic health problem such as acquired brain injury (ABI) walks into a young person's life uninvited, it generally demands to take centre stage. Medical treatments and changes in functioning can dominate the young person's life, and soon the young person can have a "thin" description or a single-stranded story about themselves. "I am a patient" can soon become the child's identity as he or she begins to forget all the other stories that make up who the person is (such as his or her interests and hobbies).

"Beads of Life" uses beads as hooks to hang stories on. It is an opportunity to bring forth rich, multi-stranded stories of those aspects of the young person's life that lie outside the influence of the chronic health problem. It is a way of getting to know them apart from their ABI.

We would like to introduce you to Emma:

> Emma was 10 years old with a tumour on her optic nerve that was treated with chemotherapy. Unfortunately, Emma experienced anaphylaxis to the treatment and despite several courses of different chemotherapy, her vision continued to deteriorate. Emma now experiences significant visual impairment and is registered as partially blind.
>
> Emma has an underlying condition called neurofibromatosis type 1. This condition, combined with the effects of chemotherapy, has meant that Emma has bone collapse in her spine. She currently uses a wheelchair due to weakness in her muscles requiring help from her parents in all aspects of daily living.

Some principles of narrative therapy
that inform "Beads of Life"

"Beads of Life" has the same theoretical roots as the "Tree of Life" approach (Ncube, 2006). The "Tree of Life" uses the tree as a metaphor to encourage children to tell the many stories of their lives. Ncube originally worked with children in Africa who had experienced loss and trauma in their families through HIV/AIDS. The children were helped to use parts of the tree as metaphorical prompts to tell the many stories in their lives – e.g. the ground that the tree is planted in represented the activities of their everyday life; the trunk represented their skills and abilities; the roots of the tree represented their stories of where they come from, including their family histories; and the branches represented their hopes and dreams for the future (Ncube, 2006).

Both methodologies are based on narrative therapy principles. Narrative therapy seeks to be a respectful non-blaming approach to counselling that centres people as experts in their own lives (Anderson & Goolishian, 1992) so that the child and his or her parents are experts in their experiences of living with a chronic health condition. Often, young people like Emma with an ABI are surrounded by doctors, nurses and physiotherapists who are all highly knowledgeable about brain injury. So putting Emma in this position of being an "expert" in how her brain tumour had affected her life was a very different experience for her.

Beads are used in many cultures. Often, they are used for adornment as well as having religious or spiritual significance – e.g. rosary beads, worry beads. Many traditional healers use beads in their work – e.g. shaking them to ward off evil spirits. The original idea of using beads to help young people tell their stories came from a social worker's teenage son who returned home with a string of beads from a wilderness weekend in Canada. Each bead symbolised an accomplishment; using his beads, he told his mother all about his weekend, the activities he participated in, what he enjoyed and felt proud of, his "preferred stories". She worked on a cancer unit for children and introduced the beads to help young people with cancer tell their own unique stories of the challenges they faced while undergoing lengthy medical treatments. She named these challenges "achievements" (Stutzer & Gove, 2000).

Developed along similar lines, the Beads of Courage Programme (Baruch, 2010) is offered in many cancer units in the US and UK. The Hearts Bead Programme is very similar to the Beads of Courage and is offered in a number of paediatric cardiac units in Australia (Redshaw, Wilson, Scarfe, & Dengler, 2011). The beads enable the child to tell the story of this unexpected episode in their lives, but both these programmes only story the medical journey and are based on different theoretical principles to "Beads of Life". "Beads of Life" is interested in the medical story as just one of the many strands of stories that make up the rich tapestry of the young people's lives.

The many stories in our lives

Narrative therapy is curious about the stories we have about our lives. These are created through linking certain events together in a particular sequence across a time period and finding a way of explaining or making sense of them. A narrative is like the thread that weaves the events together, forming a story. Some stories are rich and empowering, and others are sad and filled with problems. Children with ABI who are referred to psychologists generally come with stories filled with problems. They come with "thin descriptions" about themselves – e.g. this young girl is withdrawn, or "Bill" is refusing to do his physiotherapy. A narrative therapist wants to hear about these problem stories as well as those other incidents that are not being told in this "thin description". The stories that we tell about ourselves and the stories that others tell about us inform and shape our identity. So when 'Bill' got bored with his physiotherapy exercises, the "dominant story line" became that 'Bill' was refusing to do his physiotherapy exercises, it was easy for the incidents that fitted this story line to be told and remembered and those that do not fit often became "shy" stories and became less told.

From hearing about those times when 'Bill' had not completed his exercises as well as hearing about when it was possible for 'Bill' to do some of his physiotherapy exercises, it is then possible to alter the dominant story line. Once the dominant story line can be altered, then it was possible to alter 'Bill' relationship to that problem story. We want to help people tell their stories in ways that will make them stronger.

Getting to know the child apart from the problem

Another underlying principle is that it is important to get to know the child apart from the problem (Freeman, Epston, & Lebovits, 1997). It is particularly important if the child has experienced a traumatic event to find an emotionally safe place for the child to stand before talking about the event. The "Beads of Life" methodology encourages young people, like Emma to tell the stories which relate to how they spend their daily lives, their strengths and abilities, the important people in their lives and their hopes and dreams. Emma chose a bead for "listening to storybooks" and in the skills and abilities section, one for "being good at learning to read Braille", and "being funny". For the section called "important people", Emma chose beads for all the people in her family. One of her hopes and dreams was to write a book about her experience to help other young people who experience similar difficulties. These stories of their "preferred identity" give young people a safe place to stand before talking about their stories since the incident.

When talking about the "medical", "health" or "traumatic" story, we are interested in the effects that the trauma has had on their lives as well as being interested in a "quieter" story. This quieter story includes their responses to the trauma. Everybody, when faced with a traumatic situation, responds in a manner which minimises their exposure to trauma (White & Morgan, 2006). Some young people may cry out and complain about the injustices of experiencing a brain injury at this point in their life. Another young person may remain quiet and accept the various medical procedures in the hope that this response will mean that the horrible medical procedures will have less impact on their lives. Both of these are "responses" to the trauma but these are often untold stories. By asking about these stories of survival, it is possible to weave another strand that tells of the young persons "personal agency". We find that when young people find some personal agency, they feel less a victim of what has happened to them.

The problem is separate to the person

We are interested in separating the young person's identity from the problem for which they are seeking assistance. This is based on the idea that the person is not the problem; the problem is the problem (White, 1984). This is a practice known as externalising. So "ABI" (or any other health condition) is the problem, not the child or the family.

We try and separate the person from the problem because when the problem is no longer experienced as internal, young people are then more able to think and speak about the problem in a different way. They can think about what relationship they would like to have with the problem and about what action they would like to take against the problem, also, who else they would like on their team to help them take action.

There are complex treatment regimens and recovery associated with having an ABI, which cause young people to feel dependent on their parents. Often their education is disrupted, which can lead them to losing contact with their peers, feeling different from their peers and becoming isolated (Barlow & Ellard, 2006). They often feel different. It can mean that parents can be experienced as nagging their children to comply with complicated medical regimes, going to clinic appointments, completing physiotherapy exercises, etc. This can cause lots of conflict between children and their parents.

Once the brain injury is seen as separate from the child, it is possible to think about how co-operation and collaboration are a possibility. Parents and children can join together to become a team and take action against the effects of the "brain injury".

Witnessing and "thickening" preferred stories

For stories to live and breathe, they need an audience. Young people who are part of the "Beads of Life" group provide an audience. At this point, the group has already been together for a couple of hours. We have spent time making sure that we have created "islands of safety" (Lee, 2013) by setting "ground rules" and making sure through various activities that the group participants have had opportunities to get to know each other. They listen to the stories that each group member tells about his or her lives and then each group member gives a bead to the person who has been telling his or her story. They give the bead as a representation for the things that have touched them or resonated with their own lives. Many young people with a chronic medical condition have a sense of having very little influence on their own lives, let alone the ability to influence the lives of others. Hearing the impact of their story on others and the contribution their story makes to others' lives can be a validating experience. We literally see young people blossom as they hear others offer them beads for "your amazing attitude", "your persistence in making sure you received the right treatment", "your bravery in overcoming your fear of injections".

Therapeutic documents

Each young person takes home a string of beads, which represents their "preferred identity" stories and a pack which is a written and pictorial document of the many stories that are part of each young person's life. It could be seen as a therapeutic document. David Epston and Michael White conducted informal clinical research, where they found that a therapeutic letter was worth 4.5 individual sessions (Fox, 2003). We hope that the strings of beads and the packs will create curiosity in family members and friends who will ask about them and so news of the "preferred identity" will spread and have another audience. In this way, these alternative stories will be thickened.

A day in the life of a "Beads of Life" workshop

This full-day workshop is available to anyone who has a diagnosis of cancer and has been seen at UCLH and is between the ages of 12–24 years old. Before we run a workshop, we spend time telephoning the referred young people to explain to them what happens during the day. We may recruit the help of parents/carers or other medical professionals to speak to the young person if they are unable to speak on the telephone themselves. Interested young people are sent a leaflet about the day. We also get details of each person's abilities and disabilities, often young people may require extra help to take part – e.g. due to their poor sight, limited verbal abilities, poor motor control. For the younger children we run a series of shorter groups (roughly 1.5 hours).

The day begins with warm up exercises and setting ground rules, and we make sure we provide lots of food. We also ask that if people want to leave the workshop, they should let a member of staff know and explain that they can always come and speak to one of us if they are struggling at any point during the day.

Part 1 – choosing life beads

We provide plates of colourful beads of different shapes and sizes. When Emma attended a workshop, we made sure that there were plenty of large beads with different shapes and finishes (round, square, spikey, hard and metallic, soft and rubbery) so that she was able to see them and feel them. We give each person a colourful sheet to document their stories in five sections:

- Daily lives – how they spend their days, their interests, what keeps them going

- Skills and abilities – the things they are good at, what others appreciate about them
- Important people and their gifts – these people may be alive or dead, in their present lives or people they remember who have had an influence on their lives and the values or gifts (e.g. kindness) they learnt from these important people
- Where I am from – this is about their family's roots and their customs (e.g. if they have a special way of celebrating birthdays)
- Their hopes and dreams for the future for themselves or others that are close to them.

With the help of workshop facilitators, Emma used her Braille machine to document what each bead represented. Instead of drawing a picture of what the bead looked like, Emma wrote a description of what the bead felt like to her so that she could identify each bead on her string through touch.

Part 2 – thickening these stories

Once the young people have selected their life beads, we invite them, one at a time, to take a piece of twine and thread each bead onto the twine. As they thread, we use the beads as a prompt to extend their descriptions into a story line with questions like "Can you tell me more about that?", "How did you do that?", "How long have you had that hope?", "Who else shares that interest with you?", "Who would be least surprised to hear about that skill?" As they put the beads onto the twine, the facilitator draws the beads on the colourful sheet so that they have a record of what each bead represents.

Part 3 – witnessing

We invite all in the group, young people and staff, to identify something the young person said that was particularly meaningful to them. They choose beads as "gifts" for each young person to represent what they have learnt or valued from listening to their stories. They give these beads to the young person, and they are recorded on a separate sheet.

Part 4 – personifying the "injury"

Once we have created a safe place to stand for the young people, we invite them to externalise and personify the "problem" that has been dominating their life. We give them modelling clay and pieces of paper and coloured pens and ask them questions such as, "If the problem was sitting on an empty chair in this room, what would it be doing? Does an image or character come to mind that helps you describe the problem? Does the problem have a shape, colour or a voice? What name do you prefer to call it? Would it be saying anything?" (Morgan, 2000).

Externalising involves a process of separating the person from the problem. Our intention is to help young people see themselves as separate from the health problem, instead of having the illness (e.g. she has a brain tumour) or being the problem (he is the patient).

Part 5 – beading the journey since the incident

We give each young person a different pot of beads and a new thread with which to tell the medical story as well as a new chart with three sections on it labelled "Beginning", "Where am I now?", "What is next?" We usually begin with questions like "Where does the medical story start for you?" or "Where do you want to begin this part of the story?" and go on to ask, "What happened next?" Young people talk about the significant moments for them, such as when they first realised something was wrong, who they told and their first stay in hospital.

During this part, we both acknowledge the effects of the health problem as well as ask young people about their responses to some of the difficulties that they mention. For example, we asked Emma, "What did you do when you felt sicker than you had ever felt before?" And we learnt about how she distracted herself by listening to some favourite stories again and again. We asked Emma about the skills that she mentioned previously and if any of these skills helped her during this difficult time, and so we started to weave between the different stories in her life. It is another way of increasing the young person's feeling of personal agency.

Part 6 – sharing testimonies

When they have beaded their medical journey, we ask them to form a large group and move from their individual responses to hear about collective ideas. We ask them, "What changes happen as a result of "Brain injury" waltzing into your lives uninvited?" "What does it do to your body, your friendships, your family, your school, your jobs and your hopes and dreams for the future?" Then we ask about some of the non-medical things they have done to try and shrink and soothe "the problem". We then hear about how they have used humour and learnt to appreciate the small things in life.

Part 7 – certificates

The day ends with each participant receiving a certificate acknowledging that they have taken part. We ask family and friends to join for the certificate ceremony. Sometimes we ask members of the medical team to join. We are hoping that this may be the beginning of conversations with other people who have not been part of the day, and so the stories that the young people have started to tell will have an even wider audience.

Part 8 – peer trainers

After each "Beads of Life" day, we ask the participants if they would be interested in becoming a "peer trainer". We explain that the role of a "peer trainer" is to join us on subsequent workshops. Their role will be different; instead of taking part, we will be asking them to help the young people who are attending the day for the first time to feel comfortable and to facilitate the new attendees ability to participate.

Most of the participants want to remain connected with the project and become a peer trainer. Each year, we hold a day just for the peer trainers. We spend the morning thinking about how their role is different when they are a peer trainer. As one peer trainer said, *"We are like a buffer between the psychologists running the day and the young people coming for the first time, our job is to help the people coming for the first time feel more comfortable"*.

If during the day a young person asks for further psychological help, then they are usually referred to the psych-oncology team at UCLH.

Spreading the news

Emma decided to take her beads into school, and she told her classmates about all her beads. They were able to understand that she still had many skills, and she shared her hopes and dreams with them. She also told them about her journey since being diagnosed with a brain tumour (Lunn 2008).

Emma said, *"Talking about my beads at school helped me to see that I am so much more than my 'tumour'"*. She said that since talking about her beads she had noticed that the other children were asking her about hospital appointments when they had noticed she had missed some school, and they were including her more in their games. The beads can be a communication aid and allow young people to share the many stories of their lives, not just the "difficult" or "trau-matic" story.

What young people have said about being part of the project

"Beads of Life" helped me gain a different perspective about my tumour. An important part of the day was when I went home to my sister, my nephew asked me to tell him about the day instead of having a bedtime story. He learnt about me in a new way. He heard about me and not just about the tumour.

(McParland, Girling, & Portnoy, 2016)

Another young man said, "'Beads of Life' helped me come out of my shell and has increased my confidence. I used to be really shy. I was the person who went into a room and could not speak to anyone and now thanks to "Beads of Life" I have more confidence and I have even spoken at conferences in front of 200 people".

"For a long point in my life all that mattered was the fact that I had had Cancer and to one day go to the "Beads of Life" day and talk about what makes you special and what made you special before. It really does open up your world and gives you the motivation to want to be that person again or be better".

"I was an avid guitar player but as a result of the brain tumour I couldn't play my guitar anymore and from the first "Beads of Life" day, I got the motivation that I needed to play again and I play in a completely different style today and a lot of that is down to 'Beads of Life'".

(Portnoy, 2017, video Dulwich Centre website)

There are common themes that emerge from groups of children who have experienced a brain tumour. Children often talk about the impact of the tumour on their identities and question the impact that living through the rigorous treatment has had on them. They are often able to highlight how strong and resilient they have become. They talk about how they have learnt to appreciate those around them who have supported them. Young people have even commented on the "gift" that the brain tumour has given them, such as a new appreciation for life and a new determination to achieve as much as they can in life despite being left with physical health problems from the tumour or its associated treatment.

Using the 'Beads of Life' approach with an individual

Sometimes individuals are not able to get to groups, whether for practical reasons or personal. The "Beads of Life" can be adapted to be used during individual 1:1 therapy or as part of a family therapy session. The principles discussed at the beginning of this chapter remain the same, but the witnessing is done by the therapist and parents/family or another multidisciplinary team (MDT) member (if the young person is an inpatient). The advantages of using the approach with an individual include being able to take time to work through each section of the beads – e.g. spending a whole therapy session on "important people" or "interests and hobbies". This enables the young person to fully explain this aspect of themselves or their lives, which increase the strength of the therapeutic relationship as the young person feels listened to and understood in-depth and is more likely to engage in subsequent therapy sessions. Another advantage is that, as the therapist, you can flexibly adapt and scaffold to the young person's needs and level of ability, so that the individual is able to complete each section. Here is another example of how we adapted the "Beads of Life" approach for Adam:

Adam was 14 years old when he suffered a stroke resulting in difficulties with movement, memory and executive function. His parents said that Adam was "disinhibited" at times and would often get into a "rage". We hypothesised that the "rage" connected to frustration about what had happened to him, and the difficulties he was now experiencing. We also noticed that "rage" was connected with struggling to remember things important to him and that he was not always able to communicate this to others.

As Adam had difficulties with both fine and gross motor skills, he would not have been able to pick up or string beads. We decided to use different materials to represent the stories that he wished to tell. Adam chose from a selection of materials with different textures, such as satin, sandpaper, velvet, cotton and Velcro, and these were placed in a booklet which we called 'Adam's Book'. Prior to the stroke, Adam had been a keen musician and rugby player. He was able to use the materials to tell us about these stories of himself and to identify that these were still activities that he wished to pursue in life, even if he needed extra help or support. It was agreed that these would be communicated to his team to inform his rehabilitation. Due to Adam's cognitive changes since the stroke, he relied on his parents to identify some of the important events, such as "*who was that doctor I didn't really like?*". As Adam's attention span was limited, keeping a record of the "materials" in his book meant that when we met at each session, we could recap what we were talking about and together keep thickening each story. Over time, the 'rage' was mentioned less by his parents, and Adam became more motivated to engage in the sessions.

By completing the '*Materials* of Life', Adam could form a more complete narrative of what had happened to him. 'Adam's Book' became a resource prompting him of his preferred identity story and how his "medical story" did not need to be the dominant story. Having been "knocked off track" by the stroke, being reminded of his hopes for the future allowed him to identify rehabilitation goals and treatment options to realise his dreams.

Critiques of "Beads of Life"

One of the main critiques of the approach is that we chose the metaphor of the beads rather than finding a meaningful metaphor from the young people.

It has also been criticised for using a non-gender-neutral metaphor. Beads are seen as being more attractive to girls than boys. However, during one of our original pilot studies, we asked all the participants what they thought about using beads and whether they would prefer to use wristbands (seen to be more gender neutral). The boys were clear that it made no difference to them which one we used; the method would not influence their decision to take part in the project.

Another criticism of the "Beads of Life" workshop is that it takes a lot of time recruiting young people to attend. For most workshops, we usually phone at least 50–60 young people, and we usually have 8–10 young people attend on the day. When we run a workshop, we usually have one to two clinically trained members of staff present, and we invite two to three peer trainers. We always have a couple of trainees or assistant psychologists who are keen to learn about the project and join us for the day. Further criticism could be that running a workshop is not time efficient. However, within six months of the "Beads of Life" running consistently on our unit, the number of individual referrals to the cancer ward psychologist halved (Portnoy, Girling, & Fredman, 2016).

There are different ideas about whether a physical health issue should be "externalised". In our experience at UCLH, when the physical health issue is dominating a young person's life, "externalised" allows the young person to take a different position in relation to it, and from our clinical experience, the vast majority of young people find this re-positioning very helpful.

Summary

The "Beads of Life" is a therapeutic tool developed within paediatric hospital settings to enable young people to reconnect with and tell preferred identity stories of themselves. In these settings and situations, these preferred stories might have been overshadowed by stories of illness, disability or other health problems. The "Beads of Life" approach recognises that the child or young person is separate from the illness or injury and that by telling these preferred stories, the young person and those within the system are able to re-position themselves and the relationship they might have to the injury to allow new goals or achievements to be seen or recognised. In this chapter, we have set out guidelines for using the "Beads of Life" approach with groups and with individuals. We have also discussed ways to adapt the approach to best meet the needs of young people with ABI.

We have noticed that no matter what the level of illness or injury, it has been brilliant to see how engaged and connected young people have been in using this therapeutic tool to share their preferred identities. It is wonderful that some have connected to the approach so much that they have wanted to return as "peer trainers" to help and support other young people to do the same. We have also been humbled by the stories we have been able to hear from the young people who have taken part in the groups and individual sessions using this approach and feel privileged in what they have shared with us.

Ethics and patient consent

The young people mentioned throughout the article have had their names and identifying details altered to protect their anonymity. They have all given consent for their words to be quoted.

References

Anderson, H., & Goolishian, H. (1992). The client is the expert: A not-knowing approach to therapy. In S. McNamee & K. Gergen (Eds.), *Therapy as social construction* (pp. 25–39). Newbury Park, CA: Sage.

Barlow, J. H., & Ellard, D. R. (2006). The psychosocial well-being of children with chronic disease, their parents and siblings: An overview of the research evidence base. *Child Care, Health & Development, 32*, 19–31.

Baruch, J. M. (2010). *The beads of courage program for children coping with cancer* (unpublished doctoral dissertation), The University of Arizona. Retrieved October 28, 2011, from www.nursing.arizona.edu/Library/Baruch_Jean_Dissertation.pdf

Fox, H. (2003). Using Therapeutic Documents – A Review. *International Journal of Narrative Therapy & Community Work, 2003*(4), 26.

Freeman, J. C., Epston, D., & Lobovits, D. (1997). *Playful approaches to serious problems: Narrative therapy with children and their families.* New York: W.W. Norton & Company.

Lee, P. L. (2013). Making now precious: Working with survivors of torture and asylum seekers. *The International Journal of Narrative Therapy and Community Work, 1*, 1.

Lunn, S. (2008). Spreading the news: Coping tricks from the sickle cell clinic! *International Journal of Narrative Therapy & Community Work, 3*, 41.

McParland, J., Girling, I., & Portnoy, S. (2016). Supporting young people living with cancer to tell their stories in ways that make them stronger: The "beads of life" approach, a thematic analysis of young peoples' experiences. *Pscyho-oncology, 25*, 4–5.

Morgan, A. (2000). *What is narrative therapy? An easy-to-read introduction.* Adelaide: Dulwich Centre Publications.

Ncube, N. (2006). The tree of life project. *International Journal of Narrative Therapy & Community Work, 1*, 3–16.

Portnoy, S. (2017). Retrieved from http://dulwichcentre.com.au/beads-of-life-a-narrative-therapy-group-for-children-who-have-been-diagnosed-with-a-medical-condition-by-sara-portnoy/

Portnoy, S., Girling, I., & Fredman, G. (2016). Supporting young people living with cancer to tell their stories in ways that make them stronger: The beads of life approach. *Clinical Child Psychology and Psychiatry, 21*(2), 255–267.

Redshaw, S., Wilson, V., Scarfe, G., & Dengler, L. (2011). Narratives of the heart: Telling the story of children with a cardiac condition through a bead program. *Journal of Clinical Nursing, 20*(19–20), 2802–2811.

Reed, J., Byard, K., & Fine, H. (Eds.). (2015). *Neuropsychological rehabilitation of childhood brain injury: A practical guide.* Springer. London: Palgrave Macmillan.

Stutzer, C. A., & Gove, S. (2000). Creating meaning: A bead program for children with cancer. *Journal of Pediatric Oncology Nursing, 17*(2), 100–100.

White, M. (1984). Pseudo-encopresis: From avalanche to victory, from vicious to virtuous cycles. *Family Systems Medicine, 2*(2), 150.

White, M., & Morgan, A. (2006). *Narrative therapy with children and their families.* Adelaide: Dulwich Centre Publications.

Chapter 11

Systemic storytelling following childhood acquired brain injury

A family business

Sarah Helps

Introduction

Children and young people exist within family and caregiving systems. Each person in the family and caregiving system influences the actions and intra-actions between everyone else. This is no different for families and caregiving systems that include a child who has sustained a brain injury. As social, meaning-making beings, we tell ourselves and other people stories to understand and make sense of our experiences. Using a case example of the Bell family,[1] I show how exploring stories lived and told in different ways can start to guide storytelling between people living with and affected by brain injury to help the child, the family and the wider system find ways to go on together.

Systemic, relational ways of working with families

There are many ways in which parents can be coached, taught, trained and supported to help their brain injured child. Contemporary systemic practice focusses on working collaboratively with families, who are seen as experts in their own difficulties to help them find their own solutions (Dallos & Draper, 2005; Klonoff, 2010; Anderson & Goolishian, 1992)

Systemic practice privileges working with relationships and views difficulties as existing *between* rather than *within* people. This is not to deny the individual contribution that each member of a system brings to the issue of concern, but instead of trying to "fix" any individual person or part of the system, the aim of the work is to engage with the family and caregiving system to explore how to help them find ways to conduct their interactions in ways that work "better" whatever that means for each family (Rober, 2005, 2017).

A particular feature of contemporary systemic practice involves self and relational reflexivity – i.e. paying attention to what it is that *we* bring to the work and how this influences or is influenced by our practice (Burnham, 2005). This involves reflecting on our beliefs, assumptions and prejudices in relation to the work and paying attention to how they influence and are influenced by the work.

So, as a clinical psychologist, child neuropsychologist and systemic psychothera-pist, as a middle-aged, middle-class white mother whose children have not expe-rienced an ABI (there are many other ways in which I might position myself, but these are a selection that spring to mind). I will take a different position to you on the basis of your particular positioning. These positionalities are dynamic, evolv-ing and connected to local, global and societal patterns of behaviour, beliefs and pressures.

Working relationally with families of children who have sustained a brain injury

Palmer and Glass (2003) describe the primary goal of work with families of adults who have sustained a brain injury as to help the family system accommodate to functional and social changes of the affected adult, while also meeting the needs of all family members so as to ensure continuity of meaningful family relation-ships. The aim of work with children, young people and their families is similar, but a developmental perspective is emphasised, helping the family develop their ability to support an unexpected developmental trajectory. The overarching goal of the work involves helping the family to develop ways of living and relating that feel manageable, hopeful and hopefully more enjoyable.

Frameworks for storytelling – the coordinated management of meaning

The coordinated management of meaning (CMM) is a practical theory that explores how people make and manage meaning *together* (Pearce & Cronen, 1980; Barge, 2004). The theory falls within a broadly social constructionist epis-temology – i.e. taking a view that social reality is created by the stories that we tell about it. This is not to deny the reality of the material world, or indeed the reality of an acquired brain injury, but to emphasise that how we understand the world, and how we may story it, affects how we respond to it.

As meaning-making beings, we try to achieve *coherence* between our experi-ences and the ways in which we talk to ourselves and others about our experiences, but the theory suggests that this is never straightforward and often involves what Pearce and Cronen (1980) describe as *mystery* – i.e. processes that are ambigu-ous – that we cannot ever quite make sense of. Communication always involves other people, who themselves are trying to make meaning of their experiences. Generally, we try to *coordinate* our words and actions to fit with those around us. For example, a family might develop a particular script or story of how to deal with stressful events. The fit of the story will be more or less helpful for each fam-ily member and so tension can arise when the fit of the story is poor. All commu-nication exists within a cultural and societal frame. These bigger influences can influence and can be influenced by each episode of communication.

Stories lived, unknown stories, untold stories, unheard stories, stories told and storytelling: using LUUUTT to guide conversations

The LUUUTT model is an acronym for one of a suite of tools that were developed to explore aspects of the CMM. It provides one way of thinking about how communication works through constructing different kinds of stories of our experiences. The LUUTTT model provides an orientation to the tension between *stories lived* (how we act out our everyday experiences in our conversations and embodied exchanges with each other) and *stories told* (the way we put our experiences into words and actions in relationship with each other) (Pearce, 2004; Barge, 2004). As well as these two kinds of stories, stories *untold*, *unheard* and *unknown* can influence our ways of being and acting.

The LUUUTT model has been described in published work with families dealing with childhood asthma and bereavement (Wilson, 2012) but has not so far been described in relation to work where there is childhood ABI. It is a model that has influenced my work with families in the arena of fostering and adoption (Helps, 2018) as well as in the field of ABI.

Stories that help us go on

A useful story is one that helps us go on in ways that we find helpful and one that makes some sense to everyone in a communication network (White & Epston, 1989; Sluzki, 1992). The role of the therapist, therefore, is to create a conversational space in which people find ways of telling stories, unpacking those stories and weaving those stories within the experiences of others to open up new possibilities of understanding and action.

When working in the domain of explanation (Lang, Little, & Cronen, 1990), storytelling influences my practice, whether the task is the completion of a neuropsychological assessment, a piece of therapeutic work or reviewing progress with a family after a lengthy therapeutic engagement. The starting point for any therapeutic engagement is the exploration of the current story held by each person (including me the therapist) about the concern that brings them to the service. I see the exploration and negotiation of stories as an overarching approach that can be combined with a range of methods and techniques of practice.

The Bell family

The Bell family, depicted in Figure 11.1, were referred to me for a family intervention by their general practitioner (GP) 18 months after Patrick's moderately severe brain injury. Patrick, aged 11.5 at the time of the injury, and 13 at the time of the referral, had been knocked off his bike by an adult who was distracted by talking on his mobile phone while cycling through a local park.

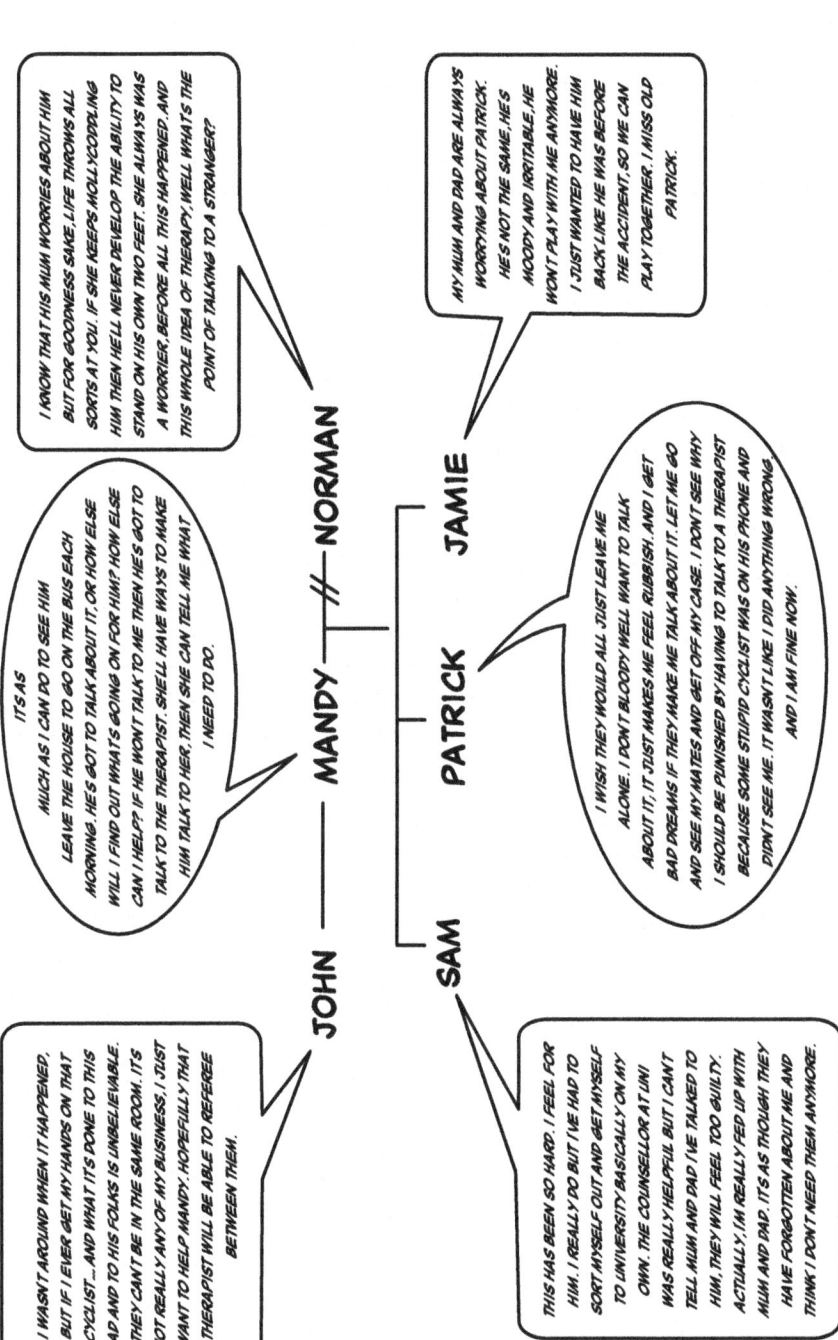

Figure 11.1 Stories told by the Bell family

Referrals to clinicians usually arrive with a problem-saturated description about a child's difficulties. Patrick's GP referral described how he was having frequent aggressive outbursts, seemed "all over the place" emotionally and seemed "different" to before the injury, and how they found him harder to manage. The first step in the intervention process was to clarify the concerns of the referrer in a brief telephone conversation. The GP expressed concern that the four members of the family that she knew (Patrick, mum Mandy and Patrick's siblings) had all been traumatised by the accident.

In line with the notion that the family members are the expert on their own lives, I asked the family to decide who should attend each of the five sessions we had. I first saw Patrick with his mum, Mandy, and his stepfather, John. Next, I met Mandy and John, and then I saw Mandy and Patrick's older brother, Sam. Later, I met with Jamie and Mandy and, finally, with Patrick's mum and dad, Norman.

Stories lived – Stories lived refers to our experiences. Stories are the explanatory narratives we use to make sense of our experiences (Pearce, 2004). As meaning-making beings, we are never passive recipients of our experiences. Every experience is unique to a person. Whether the experiences the person has are happy, mildly traumatic or life threatening, each person will start with a different perspective and so will construct a different story about an event (Ellis et al., 2016). There is, therefore, *always* a tension between stories lived and stories told. It is often the fallout from this tension that brings people into therapy. Patrick had one experience – his family, even when they were with him, had another.

Stories told – These stories reflect how we try to make sense, to ourselves and others, of our experiences. Stories evolve according to the context in which they are told and according to the meaning of the relationship they are given voice in. Whilst stories are dynamic, they can also become unhelpfully singular and fixed, particularly in relation to emotive or traumatic events. In the early stages of the work, I ask each member of the family to tell their stories of the thing that brought them to see me – in this case how the ABI affected each person, their lives and their relationships.

Family members are often concerned about sharing their thoughts and feelings with each other. Such concerns can lead to silencing, stuckness and poor communication. Therefore, early conversations often focus on talking about talking – i.e. exploring the benefits and risks of talking together, the worries about sharing thoughts and feelings (Rober, 2017).

When I met Patrick, I initially wanted to hear about him as a person separate to the ABI. I heard about how he loved playing on his PlayStation, and was great at making chocolate brownies. I heard about how he and his mum enjoyed 'hanging out' by walking on the Heath together. I heard how his mother appreciated his sense of humour and how she loved the hugs that he still occasionally gave her. In gathering a developmental history, Mandy described Patrick's determination right from birth. She told a story of how he was born prematurely, needing special care for a few days. With tears in her eyes, she told of how she remembered that Patrick had tried to pull out his feeding tube, just like he had tried to do so when he started to regain consciousness after his operation following the ABI. Patrick had not heard this story before. As he heard this story, Patrick smiled and leant into his mother for one of those infrequent hugs that she so loved. In sharing these stories together, Patrick and his mother started to hear 'news of a difference' (Bateson, 1972), which affected the way they understood each other's perspectives.

From hearing this and other stories, I talked to Patrick and his mum about my emerging sense of Patrick as a determined boy who would fight to survive, on his terms.

Patrick was ambivalent about talking therapy and so we explored his ideas about the risks and worries about talking to a therapist. He had an idea that talking made things worse, not better, and thought he was more of a doing kind of boy. At the end of our only conversation, we talked about the things that he could do to show his mum that he was OK.

John, Patrick's stepfather, shared some of Patrick's ambivalence about talking, believing that the past was best left unspoken about. Mandy felt that talking was a good way to deal with upsetting things. Talking together about talking led the family to the story that it was OK to do what felt right for each individual.

Talking with family members without Patrick enabled a focus on family relationships rather than the 'problems' seen as attached to Patrick. In session two, Mandy and John talked of how complex family life had become since the accident, describing how everyone at home walked around on eggshells, feeling so anxious to manage Patrick in the 'right' way that there were frequent arguments between everyone. They described how family life just wasn't fun anymore. In exploring this, I used the technique of interviewing the internalised other (Burnham, 2006) where I interviewed Mandy 'as' Patrick to get a richer sense of what life was like for Patrick. It was hard for them to imagine what life might be like, with a body that didn't work quite so well and a brain that sometimes got things a bit muddled. Mandy found talking as Patrick an emotive experience, but started to think about his strong desire to carry on being an 'ordinary teenager' as a positive survival strategy.

After witnessing Mandy talk as Patrick, with tears in his eyes, John told a story from his childhood of not being able to play sports as well as his brothers could, and how this had led him to push very hard for things that he found difficult to do.

Stories unheard – These are stories that have been told but have not been heard/noticed/responded to in hoped for ways. My task is to notice these stories and to shine a light on them.

In the third session, Sam described how he had felt excluded by his parents immediately after Patrick's accident. He described how they had complimented him for being such a resilient and competent older brother, when he had felt anything but resilient and had really wanted them to comfort him and reassure him that his little brother would be OK. When he told Mandy how he had felt, he was surprised and pleased that she could bear witness to his earlier experiences.

Stories unknown – These are stories that are somewhat out of the tellers' awareness or that other people have not been made aware of.

In the session with Jamie and his mum, Jamie talked of both the horror and the proudness that he had felt when left on his own to sit beside Patrick's hospital bed. He described the a clear image of this moment that he still held, the weight of the responsibility he had felt should anything happen to Patrick under his watch and the pride in knowing that his parents thought he was responsible enough to be able to do whatever was necessary to ensure that Patrick got the care he needed from the medical team.

In this session, we sculpted family relationships using toy animals. Jamie chose for himself a tall giraffe, looking carefully around, and for Patrick a lion with a slightly bent leg, which made him a bit wobbly. Jamie then described how he knew that Patrick's brain was a bit damaged but said how hard it was to remember this, as there was no clear external sign of damage. He said that, when the lion was still, it looked fine and strong but when it started to run, its bent leg got in the way. This led Mandy to talk to Jamie more openly about brains and brain injuries, in order that he could understand more about the hidden/invisible challenges that Patrick faced.

Stories untold – These stories relate to stories we have chosen not to tell or cannot tell, often for fear of how others will react. Working with the family involves developing an understanding of the perspective, beliefs, assumptions and prejudices of each family member. This might happen with everyone talking together but may require individual conversations with people. In these individual conversations, it is not at all unusual for people to talk about, or to give voice to, things that seem unthinkable. These unthinkable thoughts can range from wishing that a severely brain damaged child had not survived the accident, to feeling strong feelings of blame to the person – perhaps a family member – who was driving the car or the medics who were thought not to have responded quickly enough. It can be helpful to give voice to previously untold stories by exploring them in detail, by going closer to them rather than stepping in too quickly to close them down in order to loosen their grip.

The final session was with Patrick's mother and father, Mandy and Norman. The couple had separated when Patrick was nine. Their separation had not been amicable, and they had communicated mostly via the children, in the past few years. Meeting them together, they politely but robustly shared stories of blame, upset, loss and abandonment that still coloured their communication. They also described their shared but unspoken fear that Patrick might have died as a result of his injuries. They described how these worries had woven themselves into every single conversation that they had subsequently had with each other. They started to wonder whether everyone in the family had experienced the same fears. Mandy subsequently talked to James and Sam about their memories of the immediate aftermath of the accident. She later told me that she had felt saddened but also very connected to them when they told her that they had also been terrified that Patrick might die, but did not dare to say this.

Storytelling – As we tell stories and edit them, we can start to think and feel differently about ourselves and our experiences. As we start to understand things in a different way, we respond to things in a different way.

As Mandy started to tell herself that some of Patrick's irritability was due to being a teenager and to entering puberty, she started to offer him a little more independence, but with strict ground rules. He readily took this and, surprisingly to Mandy, kept in close contact with her whenever he went out.

Where we got to

Over five sessions, the Bell family, in different combinations, shared stories with each other of their experiences in relation to Patrick's accident. In doing so, they each came to a different and more shared understanding of each other's perspectives. The goals they had set at the start of the work – to find ways for Patrick to be less angry and to develop strategies to manage his behaviour – started to dissolve as they started to think differently about him and about relationships within the family unit. I wrote a therapeutic letter to the family members at the end of the work summarising their progress and sharing how I had been impressed by the risks taken by every family member in talking about feelings from the past and in the present.

The conversations we had together afforded Patrick an experience of having his strengths recognised, which the adults felt boosted his self-esteem, making him slightly happier and less irritable. The sessions opened space for family members to reflect on their interactions with all members of the family. The positive ripples of these different understandings of each other led to glimmers of different ways of being together when we said goodbye.

The task of the therapist in working with stories is to unpack, stretch and enrich those stories, to let light into them such that different ways of living and relating are possible (Cronen, Chen, & Pearce, 1988; Wilson, 2012). By the end of the work, not only were new stories being shared within our sessions but, more importantly, new stories and understandings were being shared and lived outside of the therapy room.

Therapist's stories of the self: self and relational reflexivity

Gone are the days of believing that therapists are neutral, unbiased or unprejudiced. Exploring our pre-session hypotheses, using supervision and working with a team can help us to understand and reflect on what we bring to the conversation and how we might use this in the service of the family. Sharing stories about and from within practice, therefore, enriches both our own and others' practice (Mattingly, 1991). I link this to the notion of intra-action, a new-materialist notion which suggests that we are permeable beings that in any moment affect and influence each other's next step and bodied response (Barad, 2007). If our every action and reaction is influenced by and influences every next step of our conversational partners, we have to carefully consider our own positions.

Working with children with ABIs, whichever way the injury was acquired, can be deeply moving (Klonoff, 2010) and may resonate with the therapists' own experiences. These resonances can be predictable but can also catch us off guard, leading us to lose our curiosity, compassion and openness (Bownas & Fredman, 2016).

In working with the family, some of their descriptions of Patrick in hospital reminded me of an experience I had when my own son was in hospital as an infant. I used supervision to explore the resonances I had experienced. These supervisory conversations made it possible for me to reflect on how my own experiences might draw me closer to nudge me away from exploring particularly resonant issues with the family. Using aspects of my own experiences, in conversation with Mandy, I asked more about her sensory memories from Patrick's time in hospital. She described how the smell of the hospital cleaning fluid had been an ongoing trigger for her since the accident, but one that she had never discussed for fear of sounding 'silly'. Talking further about her sensory memories opened space for conversations with other family members about the smells, sounds and sensations that they recalled from Patrick's inpatient stay.

Some concluding thoughts

There is growing evidence demonstrating the efficacy and effectiveness of a range of schools of systemic psychotherapy, including social constructionist, narrative and storying approaches, for a broad range of presenting problems (Denborough, 2014; Stratton, 2016; Gan & Ballantyne, 2016; Carr, 2018). A wealth of practice-based evidence demonstrates how systemic approaches can be helpful to families of both adults and children who have experienced ABI (Bowen et al., 2010; Klonoff, 2010). Contemporary systemic practitioners work from within attuned, embodied, collaborative relationships, acknowledging the ways in which we influence – and are influenced by – our conversational partners (Shotter & Katz, 1999; Barad, 2003; Gergen, 2009; Rober, 2017)

Within these relationships, close, compassionate and curious listening to the stories that families tell us, with a gentle focus to questioning about stories that are as yet unheard and untold, can transform understandings and can help families find their own ways of going on in situations where lives have unexpectedly changed.

As systemic practitioners, our task is not to tell people what to do, but to ask curious, dialogical questions and to tentatively offer our knowledge and expertise to scaffold the family's abilities. Telling stories about skills and abilities, sharing stories that have not previously been shared, is one way in which this can happen. Invitations to tell stories away from the problem, of strengths and resources, invites families into conversations about aspects of their experiences that have become hidden, buried, forgotten or not yet languaged.

In this chapter, I have shown how the LUUUTT model can serve as a useful starting point to guide conversations with families where a child has experienced an ABI. Whilst the model certainly provides only some exemplars of the kinds of stories that can be created, it is a useful model to orient the therapist to some kinds of stories that might be helpfully told in opening up space for thinking and acting in more helpful, hopeful ways together.

Note

1 Names and details have been changed to ensure confidentiality.

References

Anderson, H., & Goolishian, H. (1992). *The client is the expert: A not-knowing approach to therapy*. In S. McNamee & K. J. Gergen (Eds.), Inquiries in social construction. Therapy as social construction (pp. 25–39). Thousand Oaks, CA, US: Sage Publications, Inc.

Barad, K. (2003). Posthumanist performativity: Toward an understanding of how matter comes to matter. *Signs: Journal of Women in Culture and Society, 28*(3), 801–831.

Barad, K. (2007). *Meeting the universe halfway: Quantum physics and the entanglement of matter and meaning*. Durham: Duke University Press.

Barge, J. K. (2004). Articulating CMM as a practical theory. *Human Systems: The Journal of Systemic Consultation & Management, 15*(3), 13–32.

Bateson, G. (1972). *Steps to an ecology of mind: Collected essays in anthropology, psychiatry, evolution, and epistemology*. Chicago: University of Chicago Press.

Bowen, C., Yeates, G., & Palmer, S. (2010). *A relational approach to rehabilitation: Thinking about relationships after brain injury*. London: Karnac Books.

Bownas, J., & Fredman, G. (Eds.). (2016). *Working with embodiment in supervision: A systemic approach*. New York: Routledge.

Burnham, J. (2005). Relational reflexivity: A tool for socially constructing therapeutic relationships. In *The space between: Experience, context and process in the therapeutic relationship* (pp. 1–17). London: Karnac.

Burnham, J. (2006). Internalised other interviewing of emotions: From blame to strength. *Context, 85*, 32–35.

Carr, A. (2018). Family therapy and systemic interventions for child-focused problems: The current evidence base. *Journal of Family Therapy, 41*(2), 153–213.

Cronen, V. E., Chen, V., & Pearce, W. B. (1988). *Coordinated management of meaning: A critical theory*. In Y. Y. Kim & W. B. Gundykunst (Eds.), Theories in intercultural communication (pp. 66–98). Newbury Park, CA: Sage.

Dallos, R. & Draper, R. (2005). *An Introduction to Family Therapy*. Maidenhead: Open University Press/McGraw Hill.

Denborough, D. (2014). *Retelling the stories of our lives: Everyday narrative therapy to draw inspiration and transform experience*. New York, NY: W.W. Norton & Company.

Ellis, C., Bochner, A. P., Rambo, C., Berry, K., Shakespeare, H., Gingrich-Philbrook, C., Adams, T. E., Rinehart, R. E., & Bolen, D. M. (2016). Coming unhinged: A twice-told multivoiced autoethnography. *Qualitative Inquiry*, 1–15.

Gan, C., & Ballantyne, M. (2016). Brain injury family intervention for adolescents: A solution-focused approach. *NeuroRehabilitation*, *38*(3), 231–241. doi:10.3233/NRE-161315

Gergen, K.J., (2009). *Relational being: Beyond self and community*. Oxford, Oxford University Press.

Helps, S. (2018). Telling and not telling: Sharing stories in therapeutic spaces from the other side of the room. In L. Turner, N. P. Short, A. Grant, & T. E. Adams (Eds.), *International perspectives on autoethnographic research and practice* (pp. 55–63). New York: Routledge.

Klonoff, P. S. (2010). *Psychotherapy after brain injury: Principles and techniques*. New York: Guilford Press.

Lang, P., Little, M., & Cronen, V. (1990). The systemic professional: Domains of action and the question of neutrality. *Human Systems*, *1*(1), 34–49.

Mattingly, C. (1991). The narrative nature of clinical reasoning. *American Journal of Occupational Therapy*, *45*(11), 998–1005.

Palmer, S., & Glass, T. A. (2003). Family function and stroke recovery: A review. *Rehabilitation Psychology*, *48*(4), 255.

Pearce, W. B. (2004). *The coordinated management of meaning (CMM)*. Thousand Oaks, CA: Sage.

Pearce, W. B., & Cronen, V. E. (1980). *Communication, action, and meaning. The creation of social realities*. New York: Praeger.

Rober, P. (2005). Family therapy as a dialogue of living persons: A perspective inspired by Bakhtin, Voloshinov, and Shotter. *Journal of Marital and Family Therapy*, *31*(4), 385–397.

Rober, P. (2017). *In therapy together: Family therapy as a dialogue*. London, UK: Palgrave Macmillan.

Shotter, J. (2016). *Speaking, actually: Towards a new "fluid" common-sense understanding of relational becomings*. Farnhill, UK: Everything Is Connected Press.

Shotter, J., & Katz, A. (1999). Living moments in dialogical exchanges. *Human Systems*, *9*, 81–93.

Sluzki, C. E. (1992). Transformations: A blueprint for narrative changes in therapy. *Family Process*, *31*(3), 217–230.

Stratton, P (2016) *The Evidence Base of Family Therapy and Systemic Practice*. Association for Family Therapy, UK.

White, M. and Epston, D., (1989). *Literate means to therapeutic ends*. Adelaide, Australia: Dulwich Centre Publications.

Wilson, A. (2012). *Taking the private into the public*. Retrieved June 10, 2018, from http://uobrep.openrepository.com/uobrep/bitstream/10547/576433/1/REPOSITORY+WILSON+A.pdf

Chapter 12

Psychotherapy for children and young people with brain injury in conflict with the law

Huw Williams, James Tonks and Simone Fox

Introduction

Globally, traumatic brain injury (TBI) is the leading cause of mortality in young people (Maas, In Press). It is also a leading cause of disability in children and young people (CYP) (Graham, 2001; Luerssen, Klauber, & Marshall, 1988). Studies of child "head injury" presentation rates in hospital emergency departments demonstrate that both male and female children are at greater risk of brain injury (across all levels of severity) than adult populations. Forty percent of all patients attended to for TBI in the USA are under the age of 14 years (Guerrero, Thurman, & Sniezek, 2000). In the UK, as is often found worldwide, brain injury rates are higher in children than in adults (Yates, Williams, Harris, Round, & Jenkins, 2006). These rates remain relatively high up until 20 years of age.

The key points of risk are pre-school – with moderate to severe brain injuries in urban males and females under 5 years and mid-teenage to young adulthood, typically for males. Such incidence rates indicate that child brain injury is a "silent epidemic" (Perna, 2002). Symptoms of TBI are wide-ranging, but can include cognitive difficulties (including attention difficulties, poor memory or reduced processing speed), behavioural or mood-related changes. These important functions are essential for learning, emotion regulation, self-control and social behaviour.

The effects of TBI can be very subtle but can have wide and far-reaching consequences in both the short and longer-term. For example, TBI increases the risk of social isolation, behavioural disorder and psychiatric morbidity (Tonks et al., 2011).

Meanwhile, crime, a topic of major social concern – which has significant human and economic costs – is also an issue relevant to young minds. It peaks in late teenage years and early adulthood (Shulman, Steinberg, & Piquero, 2013). Indeed, prolific offenders tend to be early starters and go on to commit 77% of crime (Farrington et al., 2006).

Within a year of release from prison 73% of those under 18 years are reconvicted (Government, 2013). Although multiple factors play a role in crime, TBI has now been shown to be a risk factor for earlier, more violent, and persistent offending (Williams, Cordan, Mewse, Tonks, & Burgess, 2010). Therefore, a clear social problem can, to some extent, be explained by a "later emerging, or silent" disorder.

Theories of antisocial behaviour suggest "difficult" temperaments and neuropsychological problems are linked to crime (Hirschi & Gottfredson, 2000; Jolliffe & Farrington, 2004; Moffitt, Caspi, Harrington, & Milne, 2002). Social adversity might also increase the risk of crime and TBI – with TBI making a complex set of problems worse (Williams et al., 2015). This may particularly be so in the absence of protective factors, such as number of years of education and family support. We propose that improvement in the management of early TBI might improve outcomes and reduce costs associated with crime.

Traumatic brain injury

TBIs involve an insult to the brain, usually from an external mechanical force – a blow to the head in an assault, or car crash (Hutchinson & Kirkpatrick, 2002). Internal bleeding and hypoxia (oxygen starvation) often occur. These injuries lead to lacerations and bruising of the brain structures – often around bony protrusions on the base of the skull (Bigler, 2007). Frontal and temporal areas are often affected. High-speed or velocity-related injuries commonly exert excessive accelerating-decelerating and rotational forces upon the brain with devastating, shearing effects upon the white matter tracts that serve to "link" brain areas up (Caeyenberghs et al., 2014).

Injury is usually graded for severity at the time of the incident with Glasgow Coma Scale (GCS) – scores of 13 or above (out of a maximum of 15) denote mild injury, a score of 9–12 is moderate and 8 or below is severe. Loss of Consciousness (LOC) can also be used to indicate severity. Mild TBI is when the LOC is 0-to-30 minutes, with more than 30 minutes of LOC being called moderate to severe. With increased severity, there is a higher risk of chronic problems.

Neuropsychological functions and socio-behavioural problems

After medical recovery, survivors of TBI may often suffer neuropsychological problems, including poor memory, attention, concentration and planning. They may also have difficulty in managing feelings and communication with others, being impulsive and having poor social judgement. Milder TBIs can also affect attention and impulse control – albeit to lesser degree (Wall et al., 2006).

The "social brain system" is complex and distributed (Ryan et al., 2013). It comprises systems for deducing emotions from facial expressions and tone of voice, for "reading" others' minds for intentions and to feel and act empathically (Tonks, Williams, Frampton, Yates, & Slater, 2012). These key abilities for socialisation develop at different rates (Anderson & Catroppa, 2005). The parts of the brain that process reward (mesolimbic systems) become mature in mid-teens with increased sensation-seeking behaviour. Meanwhile the areas for control of impulses and making judgements – dorso-lateral prefrontal cortex – only reach maturity in the late teenage years (Lenroot & Giedd, 2006). This means that adolescents are particularly poor at stopping themselves to consider the long-term effects of acting on an impulse. This occurs particularly in the company of peers; hence, there is greater propensity for risk-taking behaviour (Steinberg, 2008; Tonks et al., 2012; Anderson, Damasio, Tranel, & Damasio, 2000; Best & Miller, 2010; Shulman, Steinberg, & Piquero, 2013).

Brain injury can disrupt these vital systems for social interaction as they develop and lead to poorer social decision making and impulsive aggression. A number of studies have shown how CYP after TBI can develop impulsive, irritable characteristics. Max and colleagues followed up 94 children with TBI aged between 5 and 14 years (Max, Robertson, & Lansing, 2001). Personality change occurred in 59% of those with severe injury and 5% of those with mild/moderate injury.

In a related and similar study, the same authors found lesions of the dorsolateral prefrontal cortex were associated with personality change. In a study with CYP with mild TBI, the same authors discovered novel psychiatric disorders (NPD) in 36%, with ADHD, "personality change" and oppositional defiance being most common (Max et al., 2013).

One of the effects of such injuries, in the medium period, is school related problems, however in the longer term a range of significantly more severe mental health disorders can be linked to brain injuries. Such difficulties include depression, anxiety disorders, phobias, obsessive compulsive disorder, bipolar affective disorder and schizophrenia. The authors indicate a biological rationale for causation, based upon increased impulsivity and disinhibition, which is linked to increased risk-taking behaviour (van Reekum, Cohen, & Wong, 2000).

In an eight year longitudinal study on children (N = 850) at risk from drop out from high school, head injury before young adulthood was linked to greater violence (Stoddard & Zimmerman, 2011). In two cohort studies adults who had TBI as children were poor at emotion perception, had externalising behaviour, poor pragmatic communication ability and, in one study, greater "trouble with the law"(Ryan, Anderson, Godfrey, Beauchamp, et al., 2013; Ryan, Anderson, Godfrey, Eren, et al., 2013).

TBI and risk of crime

There have been a range of studies showing how TBI in childhood may be linked to crime. In a birth cohort study (of around 12,000 subjects in Finland), there was a fourfold increased risk of mental disorder with coexisting offending in adult males who had had a TBI during childhood or adolescence (Timonen et al., 2002).) In a birth cohort study, in South-West England, however, although the TBI group was at increased risk of criminal behaviour (by age 17) compared to the non-TBI group, they were not when compared to an orthopaedic group (Kennedy, Heron, & Munafo, 2017). The TBI group was, though, more likely to have increased risk of hazardous alcohol use and having conduct problems, and ADHD. A data linkage study in Northern Finland – with adolescents admitted to psychiatric care – found that TBI history had increased risk of "any criminality" conduct disorder and criminality (Luukkainen, Riala, Laukkanen, Hakko, & Rasanen, 2012).

In a meta-analysis of studies of TBI in juvenile offenders (Farrer, Frost, & Hedges, 2013) the rate of TBI was approximately 30%. When compared to normative groups (in five of the studies) the odds of TBI being present in those who offend versus. those who did not was 3.37. Williams and colleagues assessed 197 young incarcerated male offenders (average age 16–38). They found that 60% reported a "head injury" – with a TBI with a LOC in 46% of the sample, and 16% had moderate or severe TBI (LOC for ten minutes to six hours or six hours or more) (Williams, Cordan, Mewse, Tonks, & Burgess, 2010), with violence being the main cause of injury. Those with three or more TBIs were more violent.

Adversity factors are very common in young offenders. Chitsabesan and colleagues showed that young people with TBI who offend often have comorbid issues with even higher levels – compared to non-TBI – being at risk of deliberate self-harm (57% vs. 43%) and suicidality (50% vs. 24%), and to have had a background of having been in care (64% vs 34%) (Chitsabesan, Lennox, Williams, Tariq, & Shaw, 2015). Similarly, Vaughn and colleagues in the USA with "adjudicated adolescents" found that those with TBI had higher levels of bullying, peer delinquency, significantly greater violent victimisation and to have witnessed violence (Vaughn, Salas-Wright, DeLisi, & Perron, 2014).

The following case study highlights some of these themes.

Client 1 – A missed opportunity – the typical experience of young people after TBI

Rachel did not display any mental health difficulties under the age of ten years. Rachel sustained a brain injury aged ten years after a fall of approximately 2 metres from a roof. This injury included right frontal contusions. By 12 years, Rachel was referred to Child and Adolescent Mental Health Services, and for a few months after this referral, Rachel received some support, but by 15 years Rachel was reportedly displaying problems with memory, she displayed difficulties controlling her temper and interactions with her siblings were problematic. Her progress in school was reportedly slowing and she was displaying concrete thinking. Family therapy was offered, and a psychiatric assessment was undertaken. By 21 years, Rachel was identified as having depression and anxiety. At around this time, Rachel received a diagnosis of probable bipolar affective disorder, type II, with obsessive thoughts and compulsive behaviour also noted. She was by this time in the criminal justice system based upon multiple incidents of assault.

Rachel's early positive educational psychology test results on verbal and non-verbal tasks probably reflected her learning and abilities that developed normally up until the point of injury. This masked the depth and severity of her injury so that no link between her injury and behaviour was made. She frequently experienced socioemotional behavioural difficulties in her teens, when the proficient application of these skills in social situations becomes more challenging. Hence, deficits involving executive synthesis in Rachel's case did remain hidden until later adolescence, when problems emerged to disadvantage her in social interactions and relationships.

The potential for the effects of earlier brain injury to emerge at a later stage of adolescent development has important clinical implications in terms of monitoring and tracking from the point of injury. Children like Rachel, with earlier TBI, typically make a good recovery, receive swift discharge from paediatric follow-up and, in most cases, are returned to mainstream schools. The future need for psychological support can remain unmet, and in most cases, it may be misattributed to other causes.

In Rachel's case, early intervention would have taken the form of considerable liaison with school staff well ahead of her return. Part of this would have meant having a clear and well-defined plan in place for managing difficulties as and when they arose. This may have involved a single person working with her on managing behaviour to avoid multiple negative mixed messages from other staff. It may have been appropriate to have sourced extra provision which might have included a single teaching assistant trained in the effects of her injury based upon regular repeat neuropsychological assessments.

Support could have included monitoring of peer-groups and actively seeking to manipulate peer-group support to ensure her integration. Time-out areas may have been helpful to give spaces to promote emotional regulation. Individual work with Rachel from a cognitive behavioural approach could encourage her to notice the building signs of stress, and to withdraw independently before situations escalate. Part of her therapy could have utilised a 'Wellness Recovery Action Plan', which alongside listing strategies Rachel could do to help herself, it would also list how others could help Rachel, and how she would like to be treated when she was no longer in control. A multidisciplinary approach to her recovery could be involved linking health professionals such as occupational therapy and education colleagues. This would set clear learning and behaviour goals for Rachel to achieve (based upon awareness of her limitations – as identified by neuropsychology), and these would be reviewed every six months.

Summary of traditional interventions for young offenders

There are a variety of risk factors in the onset and development of antisocial behaviour that range from the individual (for example, poor self-regulation, problems solving and skills deficits), to family (such as harsh and inconsistent parenting practices, low supervision and monitoring) and other contextual factors (such as antisocial peers) (Farrington & Welsh, 2003; Loeber, Burke, Lahey, Winters, & Zera, 2000). Bronfenbrenner's (1979) theory of social ecology suggests that human behaviour is multi-determined, and the young person is influenced by the multiple systems and contexts in which they exist. For interventions to be effective they need to target the multiple factors across the various domains, be individualised to the strengths and needs of each young person and their family and be delivered in the naturally occurring systems in which the behaviours occur and implemented in "ecologically valid" ways.

Traditionally interventions for young people within the criminal justice system (CJS) have typically meant services to individuals in a group setting either in custody or in the community (Ashmore & Fox, 2011). Wilson (2013) conducted a study to fill the gap in the youth justice evidence base by assessing the range of interventions delivered by Youth Offending Service (YOTs) (Wilson, 2013). This study used data from the Juvenile Cohort Study (JCS) which comprised a broadly representative sample of 13,975 young people in contact with YOTs between February 2008 and January 2009. The intervention plans consisted of face-to-face meetings, group work, programmes or packages or a combination of these. YOT resources were found to be aimed at young people who were most likely to re-offend. Interventions were more likely to address lifestyle, perception of self/others, thinking and behaviour, attitudes to offending and motivation to change. Therapy is considered to target the individual risk factors with the young person (such as those around emotion regulation and poor problem-solving abilities), and there is no, or limited, consideration of the systems around the young person, including the neighbourhood, living arrangements and family and personal relationships. Several child-focussed interventions are offered to target conduct problems and NICE guidelines recommend group social and cognitive problem solving programmes (2013). It should be noted that there is limited research in the area of psychological treatments for adolescents with TBI in the CJS.

Limitations of these traditional interventions

These traditional interventions have a number of limitations. A significant concern is that the wider systemic variables are not targeted as the interventions focus on the young person and the onus is on them to engage. Many of these interventions are offered in a group context, which means that young people are brought into contact with other peers who are engaging in similar behaviours. We know that this is a significant risk factor for future offending behaviour (Lahey, 2003). Many of the programmes offered within the CJS have been manualised on a particular population and have not been individualised to the needs of the young person, such as those with additional developmental needs or those with a TBI.

Furthermore, offenders with specific needs such as a TBI may not be suited to many of the traditional interventions. These generic interventions may assume a level of verbal and cognitive ability. Furthermore, many of the researched interventions have a number of treatment components (Staniforth, 2015); young people with TBI are likely to have information processing difficulties which affect how they can retain information and generalise to other settings. The individual may not have the insight that he or she has learnt a new skill (Staniforth, 2015). Specific needs and learning styles can affect ability to engage in interventions intended to support rehabilitation. As a consequence, adolescents with TBI may be more likely to drop out of treatment and may not achieve positive outcomes (Fox & Jones, 2017). It is, therefore, felt that a multidisciplinary and/or a multi-systems approach would be better able to meet the needs of this group.

Systemic approaches to antisocial behaviour

A number of family-based systemic interventions have been shown to be effective for a proportion of childhood behaviour problems (Carr, 2009). NICE (2013) recommend multimodal interventions for the treatment of conduct disorder (CD) for 11–17-year olds. Multimodal interventions should have the following characteristics: involve the young person and their parents/carers, have an explicit and supportive family focus, be based on a social learning model with interventions provided across the different systems around the young person, be provided by specially trained case managers; typically consist of three to four meetings per week over a three to five month period and adhere to a developer's manual and employ all of the necessary materials to ensure consistent implementation of the programme.

A meta-analysis of eight family treatment studies of adolescent CD found better outcomes for three family-based interventions: multisystemic therapy (MST), functional family therapy (FFT) and treatment and foster care Oregon (TFCO) (formerly multidimensional treatment and foster care [MTFC]) (Woolfenden, Williams, & Peat, 2002). In their review of 47 RCTs of therapies for children and adolescent externalising disorders, Sydow and colleagues found that systemic (family) therapy was equally as or more efficacious than other evidence-based interventions (e.g. individual and group CBT, family psychoeducation) (von Sydow, Retzlaff, Beher, Haun, & Schweitzer, 2013). Their "systematic review" considered the "big four" therapies; brief strategic family therapy (BSFT), FFT, multidimensional family therapy (MDFT) and MST.

Brief overview of MST, FFT and TFCO

MST is an intensive, brief (three to five month) intervention for 11- to 17-year-olds that works primarily with the parent/caregiver (Henggeler et al, 2009). The main aim is to provide them with the skills to tackle future difficulties and to reduce further antisocial behaviour in order to prevent the risk of out-of-home placements, either in care or custody. The MST therapist works with the family to overcome barriers that prevent effective parenting and management of child behaviour (for example, systematic monitoring, reward and discipline systems, prompting parents to communicate effectively and problem solve day-to-day conflicts).

The theory is that as the parents' effectiveness increases, so will their impact on the other systems around the young person, thus reducing the risk of antisocial behaviour. One MST team consists of a supervisor and three to four therapists who come from a range of disciplines. Supervision is provided weekly onsite by the supervisor and an off-site expert consultant. There is a strong emphasis on drawing upon evidence-based psychological approaches to intervention development such as behavioural, cognitive and structural/strategic family therapy models. The therapist has a small caseload of four to six families and delivers all of the intervention with the family and the systems around the young person.

FFT is a manualised systemic, cognitive behavioural model of therapy that targets 11- to 18-year-olds with antisocial and violent behaviour. It is predominantly home based, but can also be carried out in clinics, schools and other community settings (Alexander, 2013). There are distinct stages of engagement, motivation, relational assessment, behaviour change and generalisation. The intervention uses a strength-based relational focus, with behavioural components, and is for three to six months in duration. Those with moderate need have eight to 12 sessions compared to 26–30 sessions for those with high needs. All practitioners are trained family therapists and there is a comprehensive system of training and supervision built into the model which ensures fidelity.

Treatment Foster Care Oregon (TFCO-UK) is an evidence-based treatment programme for children and young people aged 3–17 years. It is a community-based programme that lasts between 9 and 12 months and involves a team of clinicians working intensively with children placed with specially trained foster carers. Foster carers are recruited, trained and receive 24-hour professional support in providing single treatment placements. They are at the centre of treatment implementation and are seen as part of the TFCO-UK treatment team, attending weekly meetings and contributing to the development plans.

Common themes of these approaches

There are a number of commonalities of these systems interventions that were highlighted in a report to the Department of Health and the Prime Minister's Strategy Unit in 2007 by Utting and his colleagues (Utting, 2007). These principles can be grouped into three overall themes: flexibility and collaboration, model of delivery and evaluation and outcome, which will be discussed in turn (Fox & Jones, 2017).

Flexibility and collaboration with families and key stakeholders has a big impact on increasing engagement and reducing drop out. As such, they do not rely on the individual to engage. Engagement and retention rates of systemic (family) therapy have been found to be superior to other therapy approaches for externalising disorder (Hamilton, Moore, Crane, & Payne, 2011; Ozechowski & Liddle, 2000). Externalising disorders refer to a broad topic that includes several clinically recognised disorders such as attention deficit/hyperactivity disorder (ADHD), CD and oppositional defiant disorder (ODD). In terms of flexibility, the majority of the programmes are delivered within the family home, school or the community.

One of the advantages of providing a service out of the office is that the family does not have to travel to a clinic. These practical barriers are frequently reported by parents as a reason for treatment drop out (Garvey, Julion, Fogg, Kratovil, & Gross, 2006). Furthermore, the therapist is better able to understand the environment within which the problems are occurring (and often witness the issues live during sessions such as how arguments might escalate), thus the interventions are more ecologically valid. Some of the interventions operate outside of office hours (for example, MST and TFCO), enabling parents who work to attend sessions with minimal disruption. These are factors which families have reported to increase engagement (Tighe, Pistrang, Casdagli, Baruch, & Butler, 2012).

The second theme is around model of delivery. The interventions target both the individual and the contextual risk factors that have been shown to contribute to the development of antisocial behaviour. This socio-ecological approach supports the systems to address the strengths and needs around the young person, thus increasing generalisation and sustainability post treatment. For young people with TBI, the emphasis would be on working with the systems to identify, assess and support the needs related to the problem behaviours. All the models have a strong, coherent and clearly articulated theoretical basis. They are multimodal and multidimensional. They are delivered by professional, qualified and trained staff who provide a high level of face-to-face contact for a sustained, but time-limited, treatment period.

The final theme is around evaluation and outcome. Each intervention is monitored to ensure high levels of "programme fidelity" (core elements of the intervention are consistently delivered). There are clearly defined, operationalised goals and a strong emphasis on outcome measurement (with clear definitions of outcome such as reduction in offending and substance misuse, and improvements in education). There is a strong evidence base for the interventions, especially from the US but increasingly from other countries too, with a large number of Randomised Control Trials (Borduin, 1999; Henggeler et al., 2009; Hansson et al., 2004; Westermark et al., 2010). However, it should be noted that there is a dearth of research and thus evidence base for specific populations, including TBI. Further research is required to look at whether these interventions might be as effective for this specific population.

Opportunities for change

There has been growing recognition of the need for action on neurodisability in vulnerable groups who offend. The British Psychological Society (BPS) recommended a range of actions that would be important to act on to address the issues of young people vulnerable to offending who have neurodisabilities (Society, 2015). Very recently the Justice Committee of the Parliament of United Kingdom and Northern Ireland recently reported,

> We received compelling evidence that another important consideration for young adults in the criminal justice system is the potential presence of atypical brain development . . . those who persist in criminal behaviour into adulthood are more likely to have neuro-psychological deficits, including cognitive difficulties with thinking, acting, and solving problems, emotional literacy and regulation, learning difficulties and language problems associated [often due to] traumatic brain injury.
>
> (Justice Committee of the Hosue of Commons, 2016)

They add, how "neurological impairments impact on [the] . . . capacity [of affected individuals] to desist from crime".

They recommended a range of initiatives for prisons, including, screening, awareness training for staff, appropriate specialist support, data gathering for service deign and commissioning, etc. There have also been, at the same time, in the UK, new standards for improved care for vulnerable young people in custody that emphasises such issues as assessing and managing neurodisabilities and there are plans to develop a new set of services for trauma focussed care for young people who offend (RCoPaCH, 2013). Such a groundswell of understanding of such matters offers hope that there would be more action in future to address neurodisabilities in the context of crime – and the criminalisation of those who are affected.

In this context we argue that the following are vitally important. Recognition that any form of rehabilitation early on could offset the risk of violent crime (LeÓn-CarriÓn & Ramos, 2003). A study in Spain showed that, in adult offenders with TBI, those who had had any kind of neurorehabilitation were less likely to be violent (LeÓn-CarriÓn & Ramos, 2003). Improved linkage between emergency departments, community mental health services (CAMHS), GPs and school systems might lead to early identification management of TBI in children and young people, particularly in lower socioeconomic areas. This may reduce chances of school exclusion and social isolation.

On entry into the justice system (police, courts or admission to probation or secure care) there should be routine screening for TBI and providing treatment options. We note that for young people in courts in UK there is now recognition (as of June 2017) that TBI should be taken into account in sentencing council guidelines (Council) (2017) Furthermore, there has been screening for neurodisability in entrants into youth secure estate in England and Wales (Chitsabesan et al., 2015). Provision of brain injury link workers within prisons should be nationally available to enable improved screening and support for those with TBI, and training and support for staff (Chitsabesan et al., 2015). Such link workers (see report for case examples) provide a vital role in helping prison staff identify TBI, provide advocacy, and one-to-one neurorehabilitative support to affected individuals (Williams & Chitsabesan, 2016).

Client 2 – Timely recognition and support: an early intervention approach

Callum, aged 15 years, was referred to MST by his YOT worker. He was involved in a road traffic accident when he was 13 years old. Following this incident, his mother reported noticing a deterioration in his concentration, memory and attention. He was also more reactive at home and there were weekly incidents of verbal aggression towards her. Callum's attendance at school had been deteriorating, and he was at risk of permanent exclusion due to his aggressive behaviour. He had also started to hang around with other young people who were truanting. He had come to the attention of the YOT due to several arrests for possession of cannabis, shoplifting and antisocial behaviour in the local community.

The MST therapist met with Callum, his mother, the YOT worker and the school to gather their desired outcomes. A primary concern was the risk of exclusion (being out of school was also a driver to much of his offending behaviour). The therapist met with mum initially around three times a week, as well as Callum and staff at the school. The therapist gathered sequences of incidents of aggression in order to understand the 'fit' of the aggressive behaviour at school. 'Fit circles' are ways that MST conceptualises a referral behaviour – the behaviour is placed in the centre of the circle and drivers are factors that are assessed as contributing to the behaviour. A number of individual drivers were identified which included poor emotional regulation, difficulty following instructions and poor concentration/attention. These linked with school drivers around staff not knowing how to support him and his learning needs not being adequately addressed.

The therapist worked with mum, Callum and school to develop strategies to support Callum to manage his emotions better (including practising relaxation techniques, having time-out and seeking support from an identified staff member). The therapist empowered mum to link more closely with the school and develop a clear school-home communication plan so that she could build in a behaviour management plan to support both positive and negative behaviours at the school more consistently. Regular meetings between mum and the school were arranged to review progress and whether the drivers on the fit were being addressed.

Some further work was done with staff around psychoeducation and the potential impact of the RTA. Developing awareness in the staff meant that they were more understanding towards Callum, less blaming and increased their support in helping him within the classroom environment.

The therapist worked with the family for four months, which included developing 'fits' on the other referral behaviours and developing interventions to address the drivers on these. At the end of this time, Callum's attendance at school had increased and school reported a significant improvement in his behaviour. He had started to develop some more pro-social peers and was no longer coming to the attention of the police.

Conclusions

TBI is linked to earlier age of incarceration, greater violence and more convictions. Life histories of abuse, neglect and trauma appear elevated in those with TBI. TBI could amplify any neuro-cognitive problems due to adverse life events. Incarceration is costly and potentially counter-productive – as may offer "schooling" in crime. It is imperative that more is done to provide support in least restrictive environments for enabling such young people to develop the skills to thrive in society.

References

Alexander, J., Waldron, H. B., Robbins, M. S., & Neeb, A. A. (2013). *Functional family therapy for adolescent behaviour problems* (ist ed.). American Psychological Association.

Anderson, S. W., Damasio, H., Tranel, D., & Damasio, A. R. (2000). Long-term sequelae of prefrontal cortex damage acquired in early childhood. *Developmental Neuropsychology*, *18*(3), 281–296. doi:10.1207/S1532694202Anderson

Anderson, V., & Catroppa, C. (2005). Recovery of executive skills following paediatric traumatic brain injury (TBI): A 2 year follow-up. *Brain Injury*, *19*(6), 459–470. doi:10.1080/02699050400004823

Ashmore, Z., & Fox, S. (2011). How does the delivery of Multisystemic therapy to adolescents and their families challenge practice in traditional services in the Criminal Justice System. *The British Journal of Forensic Practice*, *13*(1), 25–31.

Best, J. R., & Miller, P. H. (2010). A developmental perspective on executive function. *Child Development*, *81*(6), 1641–1660. doi:10.1111/j.1467-8624.2010.01499.x

Bigler, E. D. (2007). Anterior and middle cranial fossa in traumatic brain injury: Relevant neuroanatomy and neuropathology in the study of neuropsychological outcome. *Neuropsychology*, *21*(5), 515–531. doi:10.1037/0894-4105.21.5.515

Borduin, C. M. (1999). Multisystemic treatment of criminality and violence in adolescents. *Journal of the American Academy of Child & Adolescent Psychiatry, 38*(3), 242–249. doi:10.1097/00004583-199903000-00009

British Psychological Society. (2015). *Children and young people with neuro-disabilities in the criminal justice system.* https://www.bps.org.uk/news-and-policy/children-and-young-people-neuro-disabilities-criminal-justice-system-2015

Bronfenbrenner, U. (1979). *The ecology of human development.* Experiments by Nature and Design Cambridge, MA: Harvard University Press.

Caeyenberghs, K., Leemans, A., Leunissen, I., Gooijers, J., Michiels, K., Sunaert, S., & Swinnen, S. P. (2014). Altered structural networks and executive deficits in traumatic brain injury patients. *Brain Structure and Function, 219*(1), 193–209. doi:10.1007/s00429-012-0494-2

Carr, A. (2009). The effectiveness of family therapy and systemic interventions for child-focused problems. *Journal of Family Therapy, 31*(1), 3–45. doi:10.1111/j.1467-6427.2008.00451.x

Chitsabesan, P., Lennox, C., Williams, H., Tariq, O., & Shaw, J. (2015). Traumatic brain injury in juvenile offenders: Findings from the comprehensive health assessment tool study and the development of a specialist linkworker service. *The Journal of Head Trauma Rehabilitation, 30*(2), 106–115.

Farrer, T. J., Frost, R. B., & Hedges, D. W. (2013). Prevalence of traumatic brain injury in juvenile offenders: A meta-analysis. *Child Neuropsychology, 19*(3), 225–234.

Farrington, D. P., & Welsh, B. C. (2003). Family-based prevention of offending: A meta-analysis. *Australian & New Zealand Journal of Criminology, 36*(2), 127–151. doi:10.1375/acri.36.2.127

Farrington, D. P., Cloid, J. W., Harnett, L., Soteriou, N., Turner, R., & West, D. (2006). *Criminal careers and life success: New findings from the Cambridge study in delinquent development.* Retrieved from www.homeoffice.gov.uk/rds/pubintro1.html: Crown/HMGovernmnet

Fox, S., & Jones, H. (2017). Systemic treatment approaches in young people with risky behaviours. In P. C. S. Bailey & P. Tarbuck (Ed.), *Forensic child and adolescent mental health: Meeting the needs of young offenders.* Cambridge: Cambridge University Press.

Garvey, C., Julion, W., Fogg, L., Kratovil, A., & Gross, D. (2006). Measuring participation in a prevention trial with parents of young children. *Research in Nursing & Health, 29*(3), 212–222. doi:10.1002/nur.20127

Graham, D. I. (2001). Paediatric head injury. *Brain, 124*(7), 1261–1262. doi:10.1093/brain/124.7.1261

Guerrero, J. L., Thurman, D. J., & Sniezek, J. E. (2000). Emergency department visits associated with traumatic brain injury: United States, 1995–1996. *Brain Injury, 14*(2), 181–186.

H. Government. (2013). *Proven re-offending statistcs – July 2010 – June 2011.* London: H. Government.

Hamilton, S., Moore, A. M., Crane, D. R., & Payne, S. H. (2011). Psychotherapy dropouts: Differences by modality, license, and DSM-IV diagnosis. *Journal of Marital and Family Therapy, 37*(3), 333–343. doi:10.1111/j.1752-0606.2010.00204.x

Hansson, K., Johansson, P., Drott-Emnglen, G., & Benderix, Y. (2004). Funktionell familjeterapi I barnpsykiatrisk praxis: Om behandling av ungdomskriminaliet utanfor universitesforskningen. *Nordisk Psykologi, 56*(4), 304–320.

Henggeler, S. W., Schoenwald, S. K., Borduin, C. M., Rowland, M. D., & Cunningham, P. B. (2009). *Multisystemic Therapy for Children and Adolescents*. 2nd Edition. The Guildford Press. New York. London.

Hirschi, T., & Gottfredson, M. R. (2000). In defense of self-control. *Theoretical Criminology*, *4*(1), 55–69. doi:10.1177/1362480600004001003

Hutchinson, P., & Kirkpatrick, P. (2002). Acute head injury for the neurologist. *Journal of Neurology, Neurosurgery, and Psychiatry*, *73*(Suppl 1), i3–i7. doi:10.1136/jnnp.73.suppl_1.i3

Jolliffe, D., & Farrington, D. P. (2004). Empathy and offending: A systematic review and meta-analysis. *Aggression and Violent Behavior*, *9*, 441–476. doi:10.1016/j.avb.2003.03.001

Justice Committee of the Hosue of Commons, U. P. (2016). *Young adults in criminal justice system: Change in policy needed.*

Kennedy, E., Heron, J., & Munafo, M. (2017). Substance use, criminal behaviour and psychiatric symptoms following childhood traumatic brain injury: Findings from the alspac cohort. *European Child & Adolescent Psychiatry*, No-Specified.

Lahey, B. B., Moffitt, T. E., & Caspi, A. (2003). *Causes of conduct disorder and juvenile delinquency*. New York: The Guildford Press.

Lenroot, R. K., & Giedd, J. N. (2006). Brain development in children and adolescents: Insights from anatomical magnetic resonance imaging. *Neuroscience Biobehavioral Review*, *30*(6), 718–729. doi:10.1016/j.neubiorev.2006.06.001

LeÓn-CarriÓn, J., & Ramos, F. J. C. (2003). Blows to the head during development can predispose to violent criminal behaviour: Rehabilitation of consequences of head injury is a measure for crime prevention. *Brain Injury*, *17*(3), 207–216. doi:10.1080/0269905021000010249

Loeber, R., Burke, J. D., Lahey, B. B., Winters, A., & Zera, M. (2000). Oppositional defiant and conduct disorder: A review of the past 10 years, part I. *Journal of the American Academy of Child & Adolescent Psychiatry*, *39*(12), 1468–1484. doi:10.1097/00004583-200012000-00007

Luerssen, T. G., Klauber, M. R., & Marshall, L. F. (1988). Outcome from head injury related to patient's age. A longitudinal prospective study of adult and pediatric head injury. *Journal of Neurosurgery*, *68*(3), 409–416. doi:10.3171/jns.1988.68.3.0409

Luukkainen, S., Riala, K., Laukkanen, M., Hakko, H., & Rasanen, P. (2012). Association of traumatic brain injury with criminality in adolescent psychiatric inpatients from Northern Finland. *Psychiatry Research*, *200*(2–3), 767–772.

Maas, A. I. R., Menon, D. K., et al. (In Press). Traumatic brain injury – integrated approaches to improving clinical care and research. *Lancet Neurology*.

Max, J. E., Robertson, B. A. M., & Lansing, A. E. (2001). The phenomenology of personality change due to traumatic brain injury in children and adolescents. *Journal of Neuropsychiatry Clinical Neuroscience*, *13*(2), 161–170. doi:10.1176/jnp.13.2.161

Max, J. E., Schachar, R. J., Landis, J., Bigler, E. D., Wilde, E. A., Saunders, A. E., . . . Levin, H. S. (2013). Psychiatric disorders in children and adolescents in the first six months after mild traumatic brain injury. *Journal of Neuropsychiatry Clinical Neurosciene*, *25*(3), 187–197. doi:10.1176/appi.neuropsych.12010011

Moffitt, T. E., Caspi, A., Harrington, H., & Milne, B. J. (2002). Males on the life-course-persistent and adolescence-limited antisocial pathways: Follow-up at age 26 years. *Developmental Psychopathology*, *14*(1), 179–207.

N. I. f. H. a. C. E. N. (2013). *Antisocial behaviour and conduct disorders in children and young people: Recognition, intervention and management.*

Ozechowski, T. J., & Liddle H. A. (2000). *Clin Child Fam Psychol Rev.* Dec; *3*(4): 269–98.

Perna, R. B. (2002). "Brain injury: Does age really matter." *Brain Injury Source 6*(2): 32–34.

RCoPaCH. (2013). *Healthcare standards for children and young people in secure settings.*

Ryan, N. P., Anderson, V., Godfrey, C., Beauchamp, M. H., Coleman, L., Eren, S., . . . Catroppa, C. (2013). Predictors of very-long-term sociocognitive function after pediatric traumatic brain injury: Evidence for the vulnerability of the immature "Social Brain". *Journal of Neurotrauma, 31*(7), 649–657. doi:10.1089/neu.2013.3153

Ryan, N. P., Anderson, V., Godfrey, C., Eren, S., Rosema, S., Taylor, K., & Catroppa, C. (2013). Social communication mediates the relationship between emotion perception and externalizing behaviors in young adult survivors of pediatric traumatic brain injury (TBI). *International Journal of Developmental Neuroscience, 31*(8), 811–819. doi:https://doi.org/10.1016/j.ijdevneu.2013.10.002

Ryan, N. P., Catroppa, C., Godfrey, C., Noble-Haeusslein, L. J., Shultz, S. R., O'Brien, T. J., . . . Semple, B. D. (2016). Social dysfunction after pediatric traumatic brain injury: A translational perspective. *Neuroscience and Biobehavioral Reviews, 64,* 196–214.

Sentencing Council. *Sentencing children and young people overarching principles and offence specific guidelines for sexual offences and robbery definitive guideline.* Retrieved from www.sentencingcouncil.org.uk/wp-content/uploads/Sentencing-Children-and-young-people-Definitive-Guide_FINAL_WEB.pdf

Shulman, E. P., Steinberg, L. D., & Piquero, A. R. (2013). The age – crime curve in adolescence and early adulthood is not due to age differences in economic status. *Journal of Youth and Adolescence, 42*(6), 848–860. doi:10.1007/s10964-013-9950-4

Staniforth, C., & Griffin, Y. (2015). Intellectual disabilities. In A. Rogers & H. Law (Eds.), *Young people in forensic mental health settings; Psychological thinking and practice.* London: Palgrave Macmillan.

Steinberg, L. (2008). A social neuroscience perspective on adolescent risk-taking. *Developmental Review: DR, 28*(1), 78–106. doi:10.1016/j.dr.2007.08.002

Stoddard, S. A., & Zimmerman, M. A. (2011). Association of interpersonal violence with self-reported history of head injury. *Pediatrics, 127*(6), 1074.

Tighe, A., Pistrang, N., Casdagli, L., Baruch, G., & Butler, S. (2012). Multisystemic therapy for young offenders: Families' experiences of therapeutic processes and outcomes. *Journal of Family Psychology, 26*(2), 187–197. doi:10.1037/a0027120

Timonen, M., Miettunen, J., Hakko, H., Zitting, P., Veijola, J., von Wendt, L., & Rasanen, P. (2002). The association of preceding traumatic brain injury with mental disorders, alcoholism and criminality: The Northern Finland 1966 birth cohort study. *Psychiatry Research, 113*(3), 217–226.

Tonks, J., Williams, W. H., Frampton, I., Yates, P., & Slater, A. (2012). The neurological bases of emotional dys-regulation arising from brain injury in childhood: A "When and Where" Heuristic. *Brain Impairment, 8*(2), 143–153. doi:10.1375/brim.8.2.143

Tonks, J., Yates, P., Frampton, I., Williams, W. H., Harris, D., & Slater, A. (2011). Resilience and the mediating effects of executive dysfunction after childhood brain injury: A comparison between children aged 9–15 years with brain injury and non-injured controls. *Brain Injury, 25*(9), 870–881. doi:10.3109/02699052.2011.581641

Utting, D., Monteiro, H., & Ghate, D. (2007). *Interventions for children at risk of developing antisocial personality disorder.* http://www.prb.org.uk/research%20projects/project%20summaries/P182.htm

van Reekum, R., Cohen, T., & Wong, J. (2000). Can traumatic brain injury cause psychiatric disorders? *Journal of Neuropsychiatry & Clinical Neuroscience, 12*(3), 316–327. doi:10.1176/jnp.12.3.316

Vaughn, M. G., Salas-Wright, C. P., DeLisi, M., & Perron, B. (2014). Correlates of traumatic brain injury among juvenile offenders: A multi-site study. *Criminal Behaviour and Mental Health, 24*(3), 188–203.

von Sydow, K., Retzlaff, R., Beher, S., Haun, M. W., & Schweitzer, J. (2013). The efficacy of systemic therapy for childhood and adolescent externalizing disorders: A systematic review of 47 RCT. *Family Process, 52*(4), 576–618. doi:10.1111/famp.12047

Wall, S. E., Williams, W. H., Cartwright-Hatton, S., Kelly, T. P., Murray, J., Murray, M., . . . Turner, M. (2006). Neuropsychological dysfunction following repeat concussions in jockeys. *Journal of Neurology, Neurosurgery & Psychiatry, 77*(4), 518.

Westermark, P.K., Hansson, K., & Olsson, M. (2010). Randomised control trial of MTFC in Sweden with 35 anti-social youths receiving either MTFC or treatment as usual. *Journal of family therapy*, 1–23.

Williams, W. H., & Chitsabesan, P. (2016). *Young people with traumatic brain injury in custody: An evaluation of a linkworker service for barrow cadbury trust and the disabilities trust*. Retrieved from www.barrowcadbury.org.uk/wp-content/uploads/2016/07/Disability_Trust_linkworker_2016Lores.pdf

Williams, W. H., Cordan, G., Mewse, A. J., Tonks, J., & Burgess, C. N. W. (2010). Self-reported traumatic brain injury in male young offenders: A risk factor for re-offending, poor mental health and violence? *Neuropsychological Rehabilitation, 20*(6), 801–812.

Williams, W. H., McAuliffe, K. A., Cohen, M. H., Parsonage, M., Ramsbotham, J., & David, G. T. L. (2015). Traumatic brain injury and juvenile offending: Complex causal links offer multiple targets to reduce crime. *The Journal of Head Trauma Rehabilitation, 30*(2), 69–74. doi:10.1097/htr.0000000000000134

Wilson, E. (2013). *Youth justice interventions – findings from the Juvenile Cohort Study (JCS)*. https://core.ac.uk/download/pdf/19438493.pdf

Woolfenden, S., Williams, K., & Peat, J. (2002). Family and parenting interventions for conduct disorder and delinquency: A meta-analysis of randomised controlled trials. *Archives of Disease in Childhood, 86*(4), 251–256. doi:10.1136/adc.86.4.251

Yates, P. J., Williams, W. H., Harris, A., Round, A., & Jenkins, R. (2006). An epidemiological study of head injuries in a UK population attending an emergency department. *Journal of Neurology, Neurosurgery & Psychiatry, 77*(5), 699.

Zoë, A., & Simone, F. (2011). How does the delivery of multisystemic therapy to adolescents and their families challenge practice in traditional services in the criminal justice system? *The British Journal of Forensic Practice, 13*(1), 25–31. doi:10.5042/bjfp.2011.0047

Chapter 13

The road to transition

A SHARED model

*Laura Carroll, Elizabeth Roberts
and Gemma Costello*

I've always had this feeling that it's been more fighting against the system than the system being there for us.

(Parent)

Transition: bridge or gap?

Transition post-ABI for children or young people (CYP) refers to the process by which their needs transfer from being met primarily within the health system to more long-term support within the community. Most frequently this involves transferring directly from hospital to school with or without specialist outreach support. In some cases, CYP may access residential rehabilitation prior to returning to school.

Rehabilitation following paediatric ABI is a long-term process. It is not possible to know the full impact of the ABI until the brain has reached maturity, which is thought to occur around age 25. As such, schools inevitably become a primary service provider for children following an ABI. Despite this, the health to education transition following ABI is an under-developed aspect of the rehabilitation process.

There are only a few studies in the UK that comment on how the transition back to school for CYP with ABI is being managed. For example, in one particular study, it is reported that only 32 of the 82 CYP had an educational planning meeting prior to hospital discharge (Tomlin, Clark, Robinson, & Roach, 2002). A planned return to school was only achieved in half of their study's population. Other research suggests that only one-third of teachers knew about the CYP's ABI and only 24% had special educational needs (SEN) identified with 9% receiving specialist support (Hawley, Ward, Magnay, & Mychalkiw, 2004). In a recent systematic review of hospital to school interventions (Lindsay et al., 2015), it was noted that studies seemed to focus on community integration rather than school integration and that very few studies coordinated services between health and education.

The guidance at both a national and local level is patchy. A review of available guidance uncovered the following:

- Recent guidelines from the International Paediatric Brain Injury Society emphasise a multidisciplinary approach as well as sharing of information. Amongst 14 recommendations, they call for greater collaboration between health and education services, a family-centred approach to assessment and intervention, and a focus on long-term outcomes (McKinlay et al., 2016).
- In the US, the recent Report to Congress on the Management of Traumatic Brain Injury (TBI) by the Centers for Disease Control and Prevention (CDC, 2018) highlights key policy strategies to address both short- and long-term strategies for TBI, including, amongst many calls for action, systematic examination of health to education transition programmes and practice, the need for hospital systems and healthcare providers to work together with community services (including education services) and families to ensure optimal long-term care and for enhanced training for education staff.
- In Britain, the only explicit government document "Best Practice Guidance" relating to ABI transition was written by both the Department for Education and Skills and the Department of Health (2004). It outlines the exemplar journey of a child called Jack who transitions from health to education services. Emphasis is placed upon collaboration between health and education professionals with clear reference to the role of psychologists within the transition process.
- In Northern Ireland, more recent government guidance is available. The "Acquired Brain Injury Pathway for Children and Young People" (2014) is a five-phase pathway, one of which focusses on effective transitional practices. It promotes the inclusion of education services as a critical component of optimal provision.
- There are pockets of examples of regional pathways around the UK which outline mutual liaison between health and educational professionals. Some of which involve hospitals directly referring to educational services and/or special-ist outreach support which is sometimes delivered by charitable organisations.

A solid transition has been linked to increasing the likelihood of young people staying in education (Todis & Glang, 2008), which, in turn, is likely to positively influence future outcomes and quality of life. It is, therefore, of utmost importance for supportive systems to be established during the time of transition to ensure positive reintegration back into the education system. This should set the foundation for a continuum of integrative support which considers psychosocial, physical, and cognitive aspects of ABI.

The SHARED model

To guide and support an optimal transition from a rehabilitation setting, the authors have developed and put into practice the SHARED model. We propose that our model (Figs. 13.1 and 13.2) could inform future guidelines and practice during transitions from health to education settings.

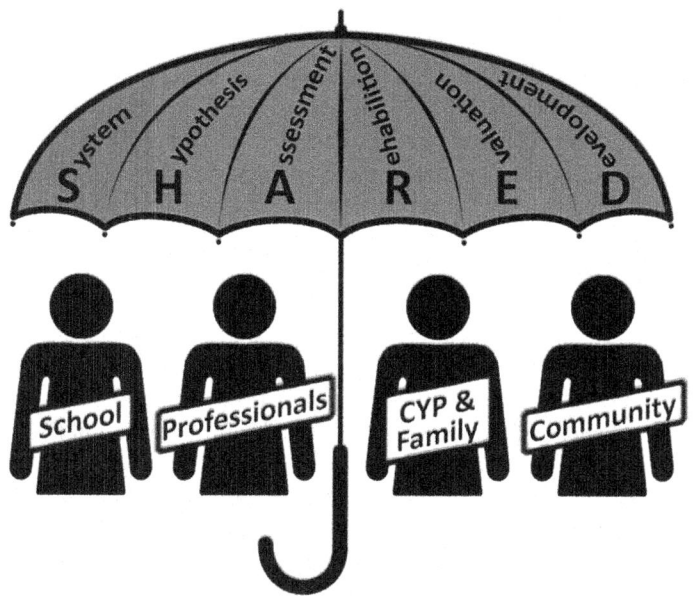

Figure 13.1 The SHARED Model

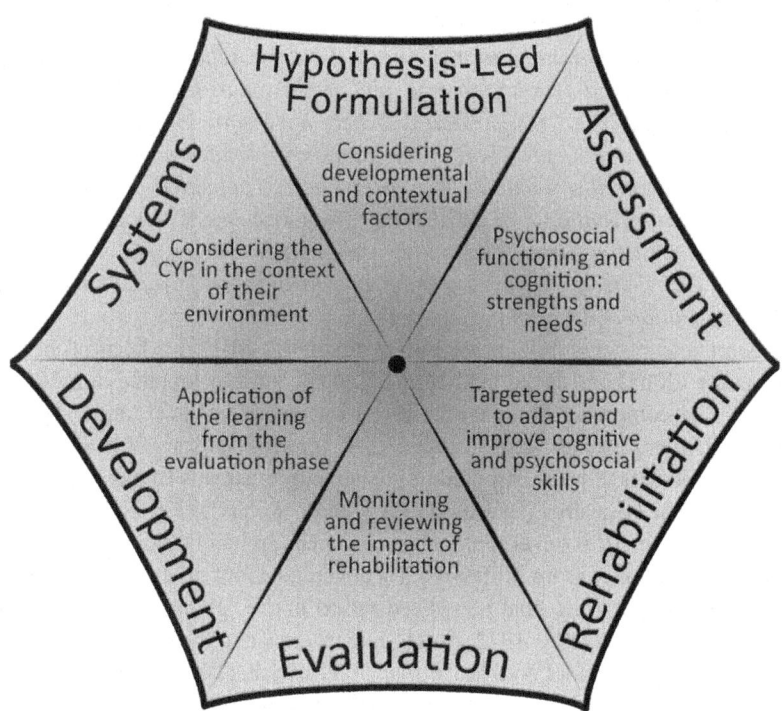

Figure 13.2 The SHARED model in focus

The model can be applied in an interactive way to support the needs of CYP and their families both during the initial transition from health setting to education and throughout their educational years. The overall concept of the model is underpinned by SHARED understanding and sharing information between professionals (both health, social and educational, as well as with CYP and families).

Systems

CYP and their families live within multiple systems which can impact on development and long-term functioning and outcomes – for example, the family system, the school and health systems, their peer group, their culture and society. Bronfenbrenner's ecological systems theory describes this in greater detail (Bronfenbrenner, 1979).

Teamed with the knowledge that children with ABI rarely meet clinical thresholds for support services but present with complex needs across domains, a systems model allows for contextual understanding of needs while opening up the opportunities for intervention through a collaborative system. If children are unlikely to meet local service thresholds for learning needs and/or psychosocial support, it adds to the argument that specialist ABI services need to upskill the adults in the CYP's family lives well as being available to be called upon or accessed when issues arise.

When planning the transition from a health setting to an education setting for John, a discharge planning meeting was held at his school prior to discharge. Attendance consisted of John, parents, and professionals from across education, health and social care. This ensured that there were representatives from organisations that could influence change and plan a coordinated action plan that was holistic and ensured streamlined support services. The action plan included the initiation of an educational health and care plan assessment, home visits from the community nurse, community activities with a youth worker, drawing on John's teacher's experience of supporting complex transitions and brain injury information to education and health professionals.

Theoretical systems models relating to paediatric ABI have been proposed by McCusker (2005) and Bozic and Morris (2005), and, in practice, a randomised control trial comparing clinician-delivered intervention versus family-supported intervention groups has demonstrated that working intensively within CYP's everyday routines at home resulted in greater improvements to physical and cognitive outcome measures (Braga, Da Paz Junior, & Ylvisaker, 2005). Braga has acknowledged that this novel approach to support and rehabilitation was initially met with some resistance from professionals concerned about giving away expertise – this echoes the concerns that have been raised in the "giving away psychology" debate (Miller, 1969; Kay, 1972; for specific reference to the educational psychology profession, see MacLeod, Macmillan, & Norwich, 2007). However, given the evidence for a systems-level approach, coupled with the cost-effectiveness of this way of working (i.e. Braga reported that the family-supported intervention was four times less expensive to operate), this is the approach we advocate.

Hypothesis-led formulation

Best practice is to develop a formulation that reflects the skills and resources of CYP in the context of their family and school. This approach allows for a shared understanding of the interacting factors that may be strengthening or impacting upon capacity within the system and, thus, builds resilience towards long-term rehabilitation (e.g. King et al., 2017). In our experience, optimal transition planning benefits from such a holistic approach as it promotes structured-thinking and transparency.

Throughout Jakob's residential neurorehabilitation placement, information was gathered to inform a systems formulation (see Chapter 4 *for further description of formulation models used within our service). Jakob's formulation was a working document, reviewed with both the family and the education setting at key points throughout Jakob's placement. At the point of transition, the formulation was handed over to the education setting to continue to inform long-term rehabilitation outcomes. This helped Jakob and his parents to feel that rehabilitation occurred along a continuum rather than something that ended upon discharge from the health setting. It also supported the education setting to feel more empowered and secure in their role in meeting Jakob's long-term rehabilitation needs.*

In planning for transition for CYP with ABI, it is important to include in the formulation the potential unique challenges that ABI poses in comparison with other medical conditions. For example, children with traumatic brain injury (a subgroup of ABI), miss a similar number of days of school in comparison to orthopaedically injured children but have more complex transitions and longer-term needs (Yeates, 2011). A range of factors are important to consider when developing a hypothesis-led formulation (see Table 13.1).

We must consider that although there are common challenges raised within the literature, CYP with ABI are not a homogenous group in terms of need. Formulation allows for these differences through the systematic testing of hypotheses on an individual level and prevents misunderstandings and assumptions at transition.

This can often be a challenging time for CYP and their families as their current profile of strengths and needs may be different to their pre-injury sense of identity and future aspirations. As such, there is frequently a role for clinicians to support the process of getting to know themselves post-injury, to develop a sense of identity that will support them to advocate for themselves during transition and beyond.

Max is a young person whose pre-injury sense of identity was a sporty, sociable individual who liked to "go with the flow". This led to challenges for him post-injury due to his changed physical skills and the impact of his injury on his communication skills which in turn affected his confidence. Psychology sessions helped him to develop a narrative of his experiences, reflecting upon his interests, strengths and skills pre- and post-injury. This helped to give him a voice, and to understand what matters to him. He was able to share his perspective through videos, photographs and a PowerPoint presentation, which he first showed to his parents. This gave him the confidence to later share his experiences and views with his teachers and peers in preparation for his transition back to school and to inform his future education planning.

Table 13.1 ABI: Challenges for transition.

ABI: Challenges for Transition	Associated Research
More than missed schooling	Difficulties with a sense of belongingness (Sharp, Bye, Llewellyn & Cusick, 2006) and changes in sense of identity (Ylvisaker, Turkstra, & Coelho, 2005).
Hidden and emerging needs	Hidden cognitive and psychological needs that may not be seen and are not in keeping with physical recovery (Hawley et al., 2004).
Challenges in assessment	Sensitivity of different attention measures (Cooper et al., 2014). Assessment tools may assess pre-injury skills and not the ability to learn new and novel concepts following ABI (Ewing-Cobbs et al., 2004).
Communication	Poor transfer of information from health to educational professionals (Carroll, 2011). Absence of direct communication between hospital and schools (Hawley et al., 2004).
Medicalisation of needs and professional's confidence	Persistent misconceptions and knowledge gaps amongst educators regarding ABI (Ettel, Glang, Todis, & Davies, 2016).

Assessment

For the purpose of this chapter, we will discuss assessment in relation to transition from health to education settings. Thorough neuropsychological assessment is important to test hypotheses and to inform evidence-based formulation. Neuropsychological assessments are typically not carried out until CYP are six-months post-injury. This first assessment post-injury provides a baseline of ability against which future development can be compared as well as informing educational planning.

Due to the time-frames, the transition from health to education setting may occur prior to the assessment. As such, it is important that the assessment remains a priority and is followed up post-discharge from health settings. Carrying out an observation in the education setting alongside gathering qualitative feedback about the settling in period provides rich information that can support quantitative assessment interpretation.

It is key that assessment is not seen as a one-off measure of intelligence, but a means to document the CYP's strengths and needs over time, being wary of any deterioration or lack of progress. This is particularly pertinent given that some difficulties may only become apparent as developmental and academic expectations of the CYP increase – e.g. some academic skills such as literacy and numeracy may only become noticeable over the five years post-injury (Ewing-Cobbs et al., 2004). Furthermore, CYP often experience more transitions than the initial transition back to school. Sometimes a good transition can be implemented but information is lost in the next transition. Or, sometimes, the CYP's needs evolve over time resulting in a need for more up-to-date information. Ongoing assessment is typically needed to ensure monitoring of the rehabilitation trajectory over time.

Wing was referred for specialist outreach support following concerns about her academic progress and behaviour. It had been five years since her ABI. Although she had been assessed within a year of her injury, and her scores had ranged from low average to average, there had not been any initial concerns about her cognitive functioning. However, following her transition to secondary school, Wing's teachers expressed concerns about her organisational skills and her social integration. Follow-up assessment from a specialist outreach team included classroom observation, neuropsychological assessment, and consultations with her parents and key teachers. This provided new information about difficulties Wing was having with executive functioning, novel learning and initiation. The teachers had not known about her ABI. Together, it was possible to formulate a changed narrative of Wing's needs. Wing's behaviours were reframed and agreed to be better understood in light of her executive functioning and initiation difficulties. This altered the education plan for Wing and led to a more positive relationship between her and her teachers.

Wing's practice example highlights that, whilst teaching staff are often aware of the CYP's ABI immediately post-injury, future teachers and/or schools are not always informed as the CYP transition into new classes or even to new schools (e.g. Hawley, Ward, Magnay, & Long, 2004). CYP are particularly vulnerable if there are no physical symptoms of the injury which can lead to the child's needs not being considered in the context of their ABI.

Rehabilitation

Rehabilitation post-ABI should be considered as a continuum, which starts in the health setting and continues in the education and home setting following transition. In practice, rehabilitation is often viewed as a discrete package typically delivered by health professionals with a focus on medical and physical needs. Whilst there is growing understanding of the need for more long-term community-based rehabilitation, this is still not the norm for CYP and, as such, there is a role for psychologists, and other clinicians, to promote ongoing systems-based rehabilitation with a wider focus on cognition, learning and emotional well-being.

The remit of rehabilitation can be varied. For example, a recent systematic review of hospital to school interventions classified the interventions into arts-based activities, problem-solving activities, clinician-led information sessions, behavioural and cognitive interventions, family or social support interventions, online interventions and multi-component interventions (Lindsay et al., 2015). It was noted that studies seemed to focus on community integration rather than school integration and that few emphasise educating teachers or peers. This highlights the need for greater collaboration between health and education settings in relation to rehabilitation.

Muhammad's formulation highlighted significant needs in relation to attention. As such, he was offered individual and group cognitive rehabilitation sessions whilst in the health setting. This provided an opportunity to test out strategies and established that Muhammad was able to sustain attention longer when tasks were broken into step-by-step sequences and visual distractors minimised. Despite the limited ABI knowledge of Muhammad's school staff, they were able to bring their expertise and experience in classroom pedagogy and make suggestions regarding what may help Muhammad in their school context. The teachers also found it helpful to visit Muhammad at the health setting and observe his cognitive rehabilitation sessions as this helped to demystify the strategies being used and supported them in making links between Muhammad's rehabilitation and their own teaching methods. On the basis of this, an individual education plan was devised, and the teachers felt more confident about being responsible for Muhammad's learning going forward.

Whilst teachers have good knowledge of pedagogical theory and practice, and are typically able to apply this to support CYP with ABI, there is also an evidence base for using teaching strategies that would not typically be implemented in the classroom and might contrast with usual teaching styles. One example of this is the errorless learning approach which is specifically aimed at those with memory impairments who are learning by implicit rather than explicit memory processes. For CYP with ABI of this type, the education methods need to adapt from the more commonly used trial-and-error approach. In our experience, teaching this way is typically new to teachers and can feel overwhelming without training, time to prepare lessons and appropriate supervision. As such, there is a role for clinicians in helping education staff to understand the ABI-specific terminology and strategies and the reasoning and evidence base behind recommendations.

Evaluation and development

The SHARED model is a continual process which requires constant evaluation to ensure further development. Whilst good practice exists, the reality is that this is not happening consistently. For example, in the aforementioned systematic review of hospital to school interventions, very few studies coordinated services between health and education, and of the studies that did, these lacked evaluated outcomes (Lindsay et al., 2015).

The importance of contextual follow-up evaluation became apparent with Salma, a young girl who presented with significant orientation and memory difficulties in the health setting. It was, therefore, hypothesised that Salma may have difficulties navigating her way around school and was likely to need constant adult supervision. Neuropsychological assessment helped to explore the issues further by highlighting challenges with novel learning. This led to a revised hypothesis that Salma may be able to orientate herself when in familiar settings. During a visit to the school prior to discharge, it was confirmed that Salma was able to navigate around her previous school. This led to a revised plan that amended her support from constant adult supervision to support only if in unfamiliar environments. Without this continual evaluation and development, the level of support provided to Salma would have been unnecessarily high and likely to have impeded on her independence.

The SHARED model in practice

In practice, using the SHARED model can look different depending on the CYP's needs, priorities of them and their family and the local resources available upon discharge. No two transitions are the same. However, here is an example of a recent transition from health to education setting which highlights key aspects of the transition pathway.

Lucas is an 11-year-old who sustained a brain injury following a road traffic accident. It occurred during the summer holidays between primary to secondary school. Lucas was an inpatient at a hospital before commencing a three-month residential neurorehabilitation placement. Brain scans indicated significant diffuse axonal injury, a common sequelae of traumatic brain injury which disrupts the connections throughout the brain.

Meeting with family members and the CYP to establish their views and priorities

Parents reported no cognitive or learning difficulties prior to his brain injury. According to his end of year school report, Lucas was working at age-expected levels although he sometimes had difficulties with attention.

The psychologist met with Lucas and his parents to consider their goals relating to school and learning. Parents felt strongly that Lucas should still attend the local mainstream secondary school at which he was enrolled. Using visual resources to facilitate communication, Lucas expressed that his main goal was to be able to play football with his friends. He emphasised that he did not want to start at the secondary school until he could do this.

Establishing direct communication between health and education settings

Contact was made with the local special educational needs (SEN) service to ensure that they were aware of Lucas. They highlighted that Lucas's school had an allocated educational psychologist (EP) and that there was a local special school that could provide outreach support to mainstream schools.

Contact was made with Lucas's school and the school special educational needs coordinator (SENCo) was identified as the link person. The transition pathway was explained. The school staff arranged for a card to be sent from his form class and teachers and for regular communication. This helped to support Lucas's feelings of belonging to his new school.

Support family or school staff to access educational funding

Parents were provided with a template letter to request an Educational, Health and Care Plan (EHCP) assessment from their local SEN Service. Although it was a sensitive topic to broach while Lucas was making his recovery, parents appreciated being informed about local services, funding and supported to get this process underway promptly due to the lengthy timescales involved. The EHCP process helped parents to feel that Lucas's needs were officially recognised at the local level with an answerable system in place if Lucas's needs were not supported.

Identify the CYP's cognitive and learning strengths and needs

A neuropsychological case summary was written and shared with the multidisciplinary team. This outlined the background information, the details of the accident, the brain injury and hypotheses about Lucas's strengths and ongoing needs.

To have a clear understanding of Lucas's cognitive and learning strengths and needs, a variety of assessment methods were used. For example, standardised neuropsychological assessments were administered to determine a current profile of Lucas's needs which acted as a baseline for future assessment and monitoring of progress. Dynamic assessment was used to understand how Lucas responded to mediation and varying levels of adult support. In addition, Lucas was observed in his school sessions. The evidence from the assessments suggested that Lucas was having significant difficulty in relation to executive functioning and attention.

Provide cognitive rehabilitation in line with the CYP's cognitive and learning strengths and needs within the health setting and/or education setting

The information from Lucas's assessments was then used to inform a cognitive rehabilitation plan. To address his executive functioning difficulties, efforts were made to use visual and organisational tools to help him to plan and organise his day as independently as possible. A laminated checklist was put on his bedroom door to help him to know what to bring in the morning. To address his attentional needs, Lucas had attended group sessions which had a focus on sustained attention through the use of games and music. Advice was given to parents and staff around the use of metacognitive questioning and descriptive praise.

Meet with the CYP and family members to support their understanding of CYP's brain injury

Lucas's parents were keen to learn more about Lucas's brain injury and its implications for his education. Lucas was not so interested but was open to thinking about what might help him. Two sessions were held with the parents, the first to discuss the basic information about the brain, what the different parts do and how they connect with each other. The second session focussed on Lucas's brain injury, the cognitive and learning implications from the neuropsychological assessment and what support he may require at school. Colourful books with large diagrams of the brain and foam brain models were used.

Regular sessions were held with Lucas to help him to explore what his brain injury means for his understanding of himself and to think about what he may find helpful at school. Books about ABI written for CYP were introduced to guide initial discussions. These triggered Lucas's interest and he began to ask questions about his own brain injury. Digital resources about the brain were used to expand Lucas's knowledge and to provide interactive forums which he could access both with parents and at school.

Ensure there is a discharge planning meeting prior to discharge and that the relevant local professionals are identified

The psychologist and another member of the multidisciplinary team attended the discharge planning meeting. To support the local team in taking ownership of the transition, a decision was made to hold this at the new secondary school. This also helped to ensure maximum attendance of local professionals.

At this meeting, firstly, Lucas's views and goals were represented using photographs. The health professionals shared information with the local team about Lucas's ABI, and initial hypotheses and formulations. As well as planning for health and social needs, facilitators and barriers to the transition were identified and action plans were drawn up as a team. For example, it was decided that Lucas would visit the school twice in preparation for his return and that he would have a staggered return to school, prioritising core subjects and time with peers.

Prepare the CYP for returning to school

Having learnt more about his brain injury and his strengths and needs, Lucas was supported to create a PowerPoint presentation about his life so far including information he had learnt about his brain injury. Lucas chose aspects of his PowerPoint story to include in a short presentation to be shared with his classmates. He focussed on things he likes to do, what he wants others to know and how they can help. Lucas was supported to develop scripts and strategies around responding to difficult questions that his peers may have.

Two visits to the school were set up, as previously agreed. The first visit took place at the end of the school day and provided an opportunity to familiarise himself with the school premises and key members of staff. For the second visit, Lucas was met by an identified 'buddy' before meeting his form class to present his pre-prepared presentation about himself. In addition, the visits helped to develop the educational professionals' confidence in working with Lucas and allowed the health professionals to observe Lucas in a real-world environment meaning that they could better advise on what his needs would be in an educational setting.

Follow-up post-transition

One month after Lucas's return to school, a training session was provided for all school staff and any local professionals who wanted to attend. This focussed on facts about the brain injury, rehabilitation and knowledge gathered from assessment. At the end of the training, a consultation was held with a smaller group of staff to review the transition plan, share what was working well and to explore any challenges that had arisen. Following this, a handover was completed to the local team for long-term monitoring and advice.

Conclusion

Drawing on practice guidelines, research examples and our own practice and application of the SHARED model, there is growing evidence that applying a systems model to transition for CYP with ABI promotes optimal rehabilitation. As discussed, intervention should not be restricted to the CYP with ABI, rather a key aspect of transition support is skilling up and empowering the education professionals who will most likely become the primary service providers for the CYP in the long-term. This also has the additional benefit of maximising the support on offer to the CYP in comparison to what can be achieved through intervention solely directed at the CYP. Communication and transfer of information between health and education professionals alongside parental involvement is essential. The CYP's perspective should also be paramount. Providing consultation and training to schools allows for the development of a shared understanding of the CYP and the sharing of expertise between professionals. A professional shift in focus is needed. This will support a move away from viewing assessment and rehabilitation as a discrete intervention, primarily delivered in the health setting, towards the view that rehabilitation is a long-term process that should be seen as a continuum, moving from health to education services.

References

Bozic, N., & Morris, S. (2005). Traumatic brain injury in childhood and adolescence: The role of educational psychology services in promoting effective recovery. *Educational and Child Psychology*, *22*, 108–120.

Braga, L. W., Da Paz Junior, A. C., & Ylvisaker, M. (2005). Direct clinician delivered versus indirect family-supported rehabilitation of children with traumatic brain injury: A randomized controlled trial. *Brain Injury*, *19*, 819–831.

Bronfenbrenner, U. (1979). *The ecology of human development*. Cambridge, MA: Harvard University Press.

Carroll, L. (2011) *Childhood Acquired Brain Injury: The experiences of children, their parents, their teachers and educational psychologists* (unpublished doctoral dissertation), The Institute of Education, University of London. Retrieved June 19, 2019, from http://discovery.ucl.ac.uk/10019982/

Centers for Disease Control and Prevention. (2018). *Management of traumatic brain injury in children*. Retrieved July 26, 2018, from www.cdc.gov/traumaticbraininjury/pdf/reportstocongress/managementoftbiinchildren/TBI-ReporttoCongress-508.pdf

Children and Families Act. (2014). *Office of public sector information*. Retrieved January 11, 2015, from www.legislation.gov.uk/ukpga/2014/6/contents/enacted

Cooper, J. M., Catroppa, C., Beauchamp, M. H., Eren, S., Godfrey, C., Ditchfield, M., & Anderson, V. A. (2014). Attentional control ten years post-childhood traumatic brain injury: The impact of lesion presence, location and severity in adolescence and early adulthood. *Journal of Neurotrauma*, *32*(8), 713–721.

Ettel, D., Glang, A. E., Todis, B., & Davies, S. C. (2016). Traumatic brain injury: Persistent misconceptions and knowledge gaps among educators. *Exceptionality Education International*, *26*, 1–18.

Ewing-Cobbs, L., Barnes, M., Fletcher, J. M., Levin, H. S., Swank, P. R., & Song, J. (2004). Modelling of longitudinal academic scores after pediatric traumatic brain injury.

Hawley, C. A., Ward, A. B., Magnay, A. R., & Long, J. (2004) Outcomes following childhood head injury: A population study. *Journal of Neurology, Neurosurgery, and Psychiatry*, *75*(5), 737–742.

Hawley, C. A., Ward, A. B., Magnay, A. R., & Mychalkiw, W. (2004). Return to school after brain injury. *Archives of Disease in Childhood*, *89*, 136–142.

Kay, H. (1972). Psychology today and tomorrow: Bulletin of the births. *Psychological Society*, *25*(88), 177–188.

King, G., Imms, C., Stewart, D., Freeman, M., & Nguyen, T. (2017). A transactional framework for pediatric rehabilitation: Shifting the focus to situated contexts, transactional processes, and adaptive developmental outcomes. *Disability and Rehabilitation*, 1–13.

Lindsay, S., Hartman, L. R., Reed, N., Gan, C., Thomson, N., & Solomon, B. (2015). A systematic review of hospital-to-school reintegration interventions for children and youth with acquired brain injury. *PLoS One*, *10*(4), 1–19.

MacLeod, F., Macmillan, P., & Norwich, B. (2007). Giving psychology away: Helping pupils at risk of reading failure by means of a self-voice feedback programme. *School Psychology International*, *28*, 555.

McCusker, C. (2005). An interacting subsystems approach to understanding and meeting the needs of children with acquired brain injury. *Educational and Child Psychology, 22*(2), 18–28.

McKinlay, A., Linden, M., DePompei, C., Jonsson, A., Anderson, V., Braga, L., Castelli, E., de Koning, P., Hawley, C., Hermans, E., Kristiansen, I., Madden, A., Rumney, P., & Wicks, B. (2016). Service provision for children and young people with acquired brain injury: Practice recommendations, *Brain Injury, 30*, 1656–1664.

Miller, G. A. (1969). Psychology as a means of promoting human welfare. *American Psychologist, 24*(12), 1063–1075.

Sharp, N. L., Bye, R. A., Llewellyn, G. M. & Cusick, A. (2006) Fitting back in: Adolescents returning to school after severe acquired brain injury. *Disability Rehabilitation, 28*, 767–778.

Todis, B., & Glang, A. (2008). Redefining success: Results of a qualitative study of postsecondary transition outcomes for youth with traumatic brain injury. *Journal of Head Trauma Rehabilitation, 23*, 252–263.

Tomlin, P., Clark, M., Robinson, G., & Roach, J. (2002). Rehabilitation in severe head injury in children: Outcome and provision of care. *Developmental Medicine and Child Neurology, 44*, 828–837.

Yeates, K. (2011). Educational outcomes and intervention in children with traumatic brain injury. In P. Rankin (Chair), *2nd paediatric neuropsychology symposium.* Symposium conducted at the UCL Institute of Child Health & Great Ormond Street Hospital, London.

Ylvisaker, M., Turkstra, L. & Coelho, C. (2005) Behavioral and social interventions for individuals with traumatic brain injury: a summary of the research with clinical implications. *Seminars in Speech and Language, 26*(4), 256–267.

Part III

What differences can we make?

Chapter 14

Reflections on outcome measurement in child neuropsychological rehabilitation

A child-centred approach

Katie Byard and Sophie Gosling

Introduction

Aims of the chapter

In writing this chapter, we are choosing to take a practical approach to outcome measurement, and we focus on a discussion of the contextual and process issues of outcome measurement, in childhood acquired brain injury (ABI). We want to share our ideas and signpost to the models, theories and ways of working with outcome measurement in ABI. Specifically, we will be focussing on outcome measurement of interventions contributed to by the clinical (neuro-) psychologist covering a range of neuropsychological domains of functioning, usually delivered within an interdisciplinary setting. We aim to demonstrate the contribution of the social constructionist and narrative position in outcome measurement. Further, we hope to explain how measuring outcome can be helpful in childhood rehabilitation and that it is possible to pay attention to systemic complexity and measure change within a goal and outcomes framework.

Reflections on our positioning

We are clinical psychologists working in a community setting with children with ABI. We work mostly in the family home or in schools supporting the development and maintenance of rehabilitation programmes, often for 12 months or more.

As clinical psychologists we are trained within a scientist-practitioner model which values scientific methodology and quantitative and qualitative research. We value the clinical application of child developmental and neuropsychological knowledge to rehabilitation. We draw on this knowledge and our clinical experience from working in other settings, in the delivery of child neuropsychological rehabilitation. Further, as scientist-practitioners, we believe that a key component of rehabilitation is measurement of its success across time. We view outcomes as central to the planning, direction, delivery and measurement of rehabilitation for a child and their family across time. We place value on demonstrating outcome at an individual level and contributing to the development of an evidence base at a population level in order to build a narrative of evidence and outcome in this clinical field.

Alongside these values, we acknowledge our positioning as systemic practitioners and hold a perspective on systemic thinking and practice in rehabilitation as not simply a recommendation and intervention at one point in time, but an ongoing process and perspective on the planning and delivery of rehabilitation. We consider that the clinician must be continually mindful of the multisystemic context for the child with brain injury and intervene at a level that is most likely to ameliorate the effects of brain injury at an individual, family and wider systems level (Byard, 2015).

We value a post-modern and social constructionist perspective, conceptualising the complexity of the human condition within the different narrative perspectives that we hold and the social systems within which we reside. As we reflect on the practice of outcome measurement within different settings and within the wider socio-political systems within which rehabilitation takes place, we recognise that supporting patient choice, service user-involvement and the rights of the child, and the measurement and reporting of outcomes and use of evidence to inform practice, are values widely held within national educational and health policies and guidelines (National Service Framework for Long-term Conditions, Department of Health, 2005; Children and Families Act, 2014; United Nations, 1989).

Why measure outcome?

An "outcome" can be defined in a number of ways. Within the medical model where an intervention is "done to" a patient (e.g. surgery) there can be an assumption of a clear and definable outcome (e.g. was the surgery successful in ameliorating the medical complaint?). However, even within the medical model there is growing recognition of the fluidity and personalised nature of outcomes, particularly with respect to chronic conditions. In psychological therapy, an outcome can be a client's own goal for change and can be measured subjectively and arguably objectively (i.e. are symptoms of distress reduced in frequency and intensity? Does the client feel better? Is the client able to "function" better?). Even these terminologies can be perceived as patronising or patriarchal; what might be "better functioning" is likely to differ between people and for some the expression of distress is understandable and necessary (e.g. grieving).

The social model of disability

There is also a growing "anti-(dis)ableism" movement which seeks to reject normative definitions of a "positive outcome", which are only defined from an able-bodied perspective instead arguing for the "social model". This model says that it is society's perspective that is at fault, and that the environment and social system is set up only for able-bodied people therefore the cultural, societal, attitudinal and environmental contexts/barriers should be the focus of change, not the person themselves (for example, see www.scope.org.uk/about-us/our-brand/social-model-of-disability; www.scope.org.uk/support/families/books/kids/social-model-disability). This leaves the practitioner in a potential bind about measuring outcomes and can result in a paralysing position where no one is sure what to measure and so nothing is measured at all.

A child-centred focus

We would argue that there is a way through these dilemmas, through the use of a collaborative and child-centred framework, close attention to and reflection about our assumptions about what is "right" for a child or family and through using a range of different ways to examine outcomes. In this way, the use of multiple outcome lenses helps us to build a rich, meaningful and measurable narrative about changes, progress and development of a child.

An understanding of child development and child neuropsychology also helps to move the argument away from that of static, "end-point" outcomes to a more fluid, ongoing and responsive standpoint. Systemic models of the family life cycle (Carter & McGoldrick, 1988; Rolland, 1988a, 1988b, 1994) and consideration of culture, gender, class and religion are explicitly held as part of the process (Burnham, 1992). Holding the social model in mind also helps the practitioner to consider this important perspective about where the focus of change could be.

Measuring complexity

Outcomes help us to monitor and track the progress of an intervention. Simply asking a person if he or she feels better or if things have improved for them does not capture the complexity, particularly in a rehabilitation context where multiple interventions may be underway concurrently. Psychologists have a tradition of trying to measure the esoteric using rating scales, subjective units of distress and symptoms checklists. Whilst one can argue that these will always be subjective and difficult to validate, the use of triangulation (using several viewpoints or different measures that examine a similar domain) can strengthen validity.

"Putting a number" on a measure of change also helps the child and family to narrate their story of change in another way and children often find scaling a very useful tool in expressing how they feel. Measurement of psychological and systemic outcomes can be challenging; we argue that using both individualised and standardised measures of outcomes enriches the story being told about the child's journey, and gives more information about their progress and what could be the next steps or goals for that child. Lastly, outcome measurement is a tool to help practitioners demonstrate the effectiveness of their work to others; commissioners, families and other stakeholders.

Measurement at a population level

In addition to the value of measuring outcomes at an individual level, we would suggest that using standardised measures allows us to begin to understand what helps a group of people with similar conditions. This population level of measurement is the domain of most medical and psychological research interventions where participants' outcomes are grouped together and subjected to statistical analysis thereby ascertaining whether a clinical change has occurred.

It is outside of the scope of this chapter to detail research methodology and an assumption is made that most readers will be familiar with methods used. More sophisticated analysis can now help us to draw out the sub-groups that are more likely to benefit from an intervention and those who are not; within the heterogeneous population of children with a brain injury this is of great value as we still know very little about which interventions are most effective.

What models of outcome are out there?

We will focus on the models most commonly applied within the health and rehabilitation field, other models may be relevant and not mentioned here. In considering outcomes, the type of intervention chosen and implemented, and the evidence base for its effectiveness should underpin the rehabilitation process.

In the child brain injury field, the evidence base for neuropsychological and systemic interventions is weak (see the Canadian project, Evidence-Based Review of Moderate and Severe Acquired Brain Injury projects, or EBRABI, Teasell et al., 2017). Longer-term follow-up outcome studies are emerging (e.g. Taylor et al., 2001; Anderson, Brown, Newitt, & Hoile, 2011) and there are some specific intervention studies (Shari Wade's work on problem solving in teens and parenting; Felicity Brown's work on group parenting interventions; also see Cole, Paulos, Cole, & Tankard, 2009). To our knowledge there are no studies that have examined long-term rehabilitation with all its complexities, nor have studies of long-term outcome teased out the "active ingredients" of a complex rehabilitation intervention to show which result in the best outcomes, recognising the challenge of untangling the relationship between what is spontaneous recovery from the elements of rehabilitation associated with positive outcome (Forsyth, Salorio & Christensen, 2009).

However, it is known that there is a bidirectional relationship between family functioning, severity of the brain injury and outcome and that intervening at a family level does seem to be associated with better outcomes for both the child and their family (see Tal & Tiosh, 2013; Byard, 2015, for a summary of relevant studies). We often "borrow" and adapt our interventions creatively from other closely related fields such as work with trauma, paediatric chronic conditions and learning disability (Novak, 2014; Gosling, 2016; Hastings, 2014).

In the UK, the National Institute for Health and Care Excellence (NICE) considers the best evidence for interventions to produce guidelines and recommendations for practitioners. Evidence can be at a number of levels from the medical model "gold standard" of the RCT to case study series and single case studies (www.nice. org.uk/article/pmg20). We would argue that there is value in the latter approaches when a heterogeneous and highly individualised approach is taken to intervention. Tate et al. (2015) outline the "best practice" for conducting a single case study based on the single case experimental design (SCED) protocol.

Evidence cited for current rehabilitation guidelines focusses mainly on the cost-benefit analysis of specialist inpatient rehabilitation and not specific interventions per se. The key measurable outcomes for all ages are reported through the UK Rehabilitation Outcomes Collaborative or UKRoC database (see Turner-Stokes, Vanderstay, Eager, Dredge, & Siegert, 2015) and includes: functional gain measurement (FIM+FAM, Turner-Stokes, Nyein, Turner-Stokes, & Gatehouse, 1999; Turner-Stokes & Siegert, 2013); and attainment of individual goals for rehabilitation measured using GAS (Goal Attainment Scaling; NHS England, 2013). Whilst useful for inpatient, acute post-injury rehabilitation, we would argue that purely focussing on functional gain misses the longer-term processes of psychological and family adjustment, does not account for the development of a child and needs a broader focus when considering longer-term community rehabilitation. We do agree that the use of a goals/GAS framework allows for individualised progress to be captured in a measurable and comparable way and we will discuss this further later in the chapter.

Measuring functional change

International classification of diseases framework (ICF)

Developed by the World Health Organisation (2001), the ICF framework is the most ambitious and comprehensive framework that incorporates both the social and medical models of disability and seeks to measure outcomes at the level of function rather than a focus on the impairment itself. It directly uses the UN Convention of Human and Children's Rights as underpinning the framework. Therefore, philosophically, ICF encompasses objective elements (nutrition, sanitation, access to education) and subjective elements (the right to a full and decent life, self-reliance and dignity).

Considering the effects a health condition has on body function and structure, activities and participation, the ICF coding is the best way of profiling how an impairment or disability affects a person's everyday life. Additionally, it allows for cross-cultural adaptations in defining specific domain sets (Prodinger et al., 2016) and, therefore, is both flexible and sensitive to the needs of the population (see Figure 14.1).

Of great interest to therapists and psychologists is that although the ICF acknowledges personal and contextual factors as important moderators of outcome, it does not attempt to classify or measure these directly, arguing that these are too complex and individualised to do so. However, it is often these very factors

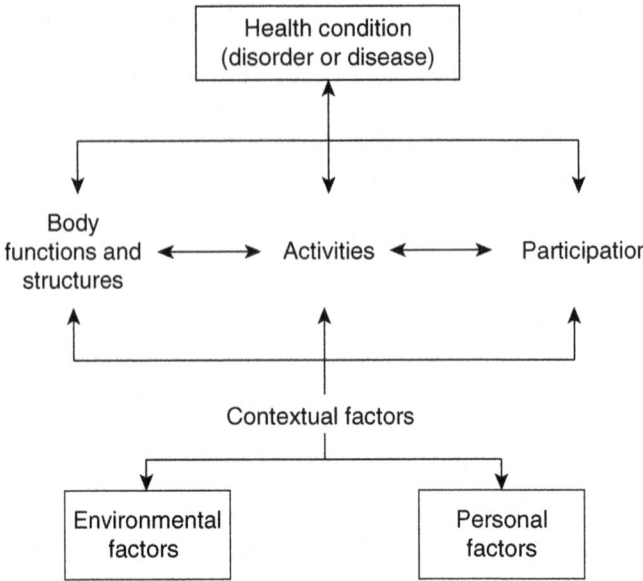

Figure 14.1 The ICF model depicting interaction between the components of functioning and disability and contextual factors. Adapted from the *International Classification of Functioning, Disability and Health* by World Health Organisation. Geneva: World Health Organisation.

Source: Copyright 2001 by the World Health Organisation.

that are our focus when supporting a family and their child and so although the ICF model is useful at the level of function and activity; it loses its measurement power when emotional, psychological and relationships are the focus of an intervention.

Goal setting and scaling

One possible solution to this dilemma is the use of a goal-based approach. Tucker (2015) eloquently outlines why this approach to brain injury rehabilitation is psychologically powerful. In essence, rehabilitation is a process of adjustment and working towards functional restoration; the resulting progress or deterioration and the affective (emotional) response to this process. He argues that goal setting helps to gradually rebuild a sense of integrated self, post-injury in a more graded bearable way.

Goal setting is therefore both a tool that measures progress and a philosophical, psychological approach to rehabilitation which is sensitive to the pace, focus and motivations of the child and the system around them. By using a collaborative approach, as well as being aware of developmental tasks and cognitive/

neuropsychological functioning, skilful goal setting helps to regulate the system, take account of readiness to change and also be clear about what are realistic and achievable goals for that particular child.

Goals should be "SMART" – that is, specific, measurable, achievable, realistic and timed. Goal Attainment Scaling (GAS) (Turner-Stokes, 2009) can also be applied to the goals setting and review framework. GAS enables goals to be scaled (in relation to expected performance of the client in achieving the goal) and weighted (in relation to ratings of difficulty and importance to the client). At the point of review, calculations can then be made that provides a numerical value in how far the goal has been achieved thereby providing a measure of change alongside standardised measures (see Tucker, 2015, for a more detailed explanation of GAS).

Cooper and Law (2018) widen this lens further in their discussion of the rationale for, and development and application of goal-oriented practices in psychotherapy and counselling. The book provides a forum for debate about the value and efficacy of the goals process as a method to promote therapeutic alliance and as a measure of change and progress across diverse therapeutic practices.

Using standardised measures

Common data elements collaboration (CDE)

Measuring outcome using standardised tools allows population-level analysis and some comparison against norms within a population for an individual. The international collaboration of the common data elements group (McCauley et al., 2012) brings together recommendations for both domains of measurement and best tools available for the paediatric ABI population. The strength of this work is its scope, measuring cognitive impairment, quality of life, participation, behaviour, emotional and psychological adjustment, as well as family functioning to guide and inform research and clinical practice towards a consistent use of a suite of applicable standardised measurement tools in order to build a richer and more nuanced picture of outcome in neurorehabilitation.

Measuring outcomes across a service: a practical combined approach

CAMHS outcomes project: 'COOP' (Law & Wolpert, 2014)

CAMH services have developed a suite of outcome measures and discuss the processes involved in giving, interpreting and discussing measures with their clients. They use a trio of measurement domains: standardised questionnaires and scales (mainly mental health-focussed but includes behaviour, social and family functioning), collaborative goal setting and measures of process (i.e. therapeutic alliance, ratings of the usefulness of each therapy session). They helpfully suggest that therapists should always be considering the "4M" principles when using out-come measures with their clients, which we would agree are laudable aims:

- Minimal burden (for the client and practitioner)
- Multiple perspectives (consider collecting different views)
- Meaningful use (do the measures make sense for the presenting problems?)
- Missing something? (using the form to fill gaps/areas not considered)

A detailed document, it has strengths in incorporating service user views, tak-ing a reflective stance to measurement and in attempting to capture the differ-ent processes and aims of an intervention. Reflecting on how other services and therapeutic orientations have approached measuring outcomes, and learning from those with lived experience of accessing services (see Feltham, Martin, Walker, & Harris, 2018) will help us to improve and develop.

Measuring the active ingredients of rehabilitation

PRISM (paediatric rehabilitation ingredient model, Forsyth et al., 2018)

Forsyth et al.'s (2018) recent paper addresses the challenging issue of teasing out the active ingredients or content of rehabilitation. In response to this dilemma, the authors introduce the PRISM model, an online ingredient-mediator matrix tool that lists 11 possible content-mediator rehabilitation combinations ("ingredients" associated with practice, management, family and advocacy) for selection by the therapy team involved in delivering rehabilitation. The PRISM model is signifi-cant in its scope, and in the questions, it is attempting to address in the context of outcome measurement in rehabilitation.

In addition, other methodologies are being developed in different settings – e.g. in CAMHS (Law & Wolpert, 2014) and in adult rehabilitation (Turner-Stokes et al., 2015). To date, as far as we are aware it remains an elusive challenge to develop methodology which identifies exactly which of the ingredients are the active components of a given intervention.

How outcome is measured across settings

In our community rehabilitation setting, we have developed a core process of outcome measurement (Gosling, 2015) that integrates a functionally based goal framework and collection of outcome measures that map onto the CDE work-group's suite of measures (McCauley et al., 2012). Other settings were surveyed (ABI inpatient and outpatient and community NHS services). About half of these settings (and all inpatient settings) reported using a goals system, either setting SMART goals and/or using GAS (see Table 14.1).

Table 14.1 CDE recommended outcome measures for children with ABI, comparison with measures used in different settings (see McCauley et al., 2012)

Domain	CDE Core Measures	CDE Supplemental Measures	CDE 'Emerging' Measures	Recolo (Community) Core Measures (Supplemental)	Inpatient Settings (Acute Phase)	Inpatient Settings (Post-acute)	Outpatient Settings
Rehabilitation measures							
Academics/school functioning	CBCL-SC (School competencies)	WJ-III	CTOPP Key math-3 TOWRE ABAS-2 MPAI	School reports/levels of attainment (WIAT-II) observation (ABAS)		SFA (School function assessment) PASS (Pupil attitudes to self and school)	School attendance
Adaptive/ daily living skills	PEDI Wee FIM	Vineland-III			PEDI FIMFAM	PEDI FIMFAM MPOC (Measures of Processes of Care)	BASC-3
Family and environment	Family assessment device (FAD)	Family burden of injury interview format	Child and adolescent scale of environment	Family assessment device, PedsQL family impact module		Family needs survey (FNQ) currently being validated	
Global outcome	GOS-E Peds or King's outcome scale for childhood head injury	PedsQL	Paediatric test of brain injury	PedsQL core module: parent report (self-report where possible)	KOSCHI	RCS NPNTDA/NPDS (Northwick park dependency assessment/score)	
Health-related quality of life	PedsQL core module		NeuroQoL	PedsQL core module (PedsQL cerebral palsy module) WASI/WISC-IV	PedsQL-core	PedsQL	PedsQL GTS-QOL
Language and communication	WASI-II Vocabulary scale						LaTrobe, CCC
Social role	PedsQL social scale SDQ Peer and pro-social scales	CASP		PedsQL social scale SDQ CASP			CASP

(Continued)

Table 14.1 (Continued)

Domain	CDE Core Measures	CDE Supplemental Measures	CDE 'Emerging' Measures	Recolo (Community) Core Measures (Supplemental)	Inpatient Settings (Acute Phase)	Inpatient Settings (Post-acute)	Outpatient Settings
Psychological functioning	CBCL SDQ			SDQ (BYI) (CRIES)	RCADS	SDQ IES-R PROMS SCORE Birleson depressions scale Spence anxiety scale Self-esteem measure	SDQ CRIES SCAS BYI SPIN RCADS
Fatigue				PedsQL Multidimensional fatigue module			
Parental psychological functioning				PedsQL family impact: HRQL (BAI, BDI, IES)		BAI-II BDI-II	
Neuropsychological impairment measures							
Attention and processing speed	WISC-V Processing Speed Index	Connors CPT-2 TEA-Ch2		WISC-V, WPPSI-III (Connors parent/ teacher report)			
Executive functioning	Delis-Kaplan (D-KEFS)	BRIEF		BRIEF-II (D-KEFS)		BRIEF-II	BRIEF-II YGTSS CYBOCS
General Intellectual functioning	WASI-II			WASI/WISC-VI/ WPPSI-III			
Memory	RAVLT CVLT-C	WRAML-2 TOMAL-2		CMS			Children's memory questionnaire
Visuo-spatial	–	WISC-V Block design VMI		WISC-V/WPPSI-III, VMI			

Source: Our thanks to our colleagues who contributed to the development of the table of outcome measures used within different clinical settings

Functional goals framework

We incorporate a goal setting and scaling framework centred on functional gains based on the aims of the ICF framework that seeks to measure outcome at the level of function and activity rather than impairment. Further, we apply goal setting and scaling into our assessment, intervention and review protocols, and report templates. These ensure that as standard, goals are set clearly and collaboratively with routine reviews within rehabilitation.

In our view, the functional goal framework also provides a structure within which the child, their family and team/wider system can develop a shared language and understanding about the aims of rehabilitation, and more widely still it creates opportunities to hold conversations about change, progress and recovery and expectations of, and engagement with rehabilitation. We value this framework because it actively and creatively supports the collaborative development of functional goals that by their idiosyncratic nature can be child and systemically focussed.

We are building a database of goals and we are noticing that goals are being set at an individual child level, but do also include whole families and the wider system. As outlined by Todd (2013), goals can be set with a narrative focus. In our setting, we are working with recurring concepts and narratives associated with self-identity post-injury, and adjustment, loss and adaptation; and goals are being created within a narrative frame to, for example, promote the development of shared language and terminology or develop coherent and shared narratives that focus on meaningful stories post-injury related to themes such as recovery, the future and family life, strengths and resiliencies.

Core standardised outcome measures

Alongside the goals framework, we use a range of standardised measures that focus on a child's behaviour and social functioning and participation, child and parental psychological/emotional functioning, fatigue levels, child and parental quality of life, and family functioning. We have chosen to measure those areas of functioning that from a rehabilitative perspective are typically key areas identified for change. All measures we use are included in the CDE recommendations. These measures are completed at baseline and 12 months, (and at later data points if rehabilitation is ongoing). As shown in Table 14.1, other services report using some of these measures, in particular those measuring quality of life and psychological adjustment.

The child's neurocognitive profile and a measure of executive functioning are also included to contextualise the child's difficulties, particularly with respect to understanding specific cognitive deficits and how this may relate to what they experience and may struggle with day to day. This information may also highlight areas that may be subject to amelioration or compensation via rehabilitation. In addition (and as listed as being used by other services in Table 14.1), individualised measures can be included – usually attached to a specific goal – such as the following:

- Measurement of the frequency/intensity of a specific behaviour
- Measurement of a new skill
- Use of analogue scales: (e.g. measuring perceived changes in mood, confidence, quality of friendships or relationships with family members)

Contextualisation

We recognise the importance of contextualising the outcome data in order to enrich and give meaning to the changes in scores (Todd & Weatherhead, 2013). As an example of this, we have noticed occasions when a score deteriorates at review; for example, a parent or child reports increased levels of fatigue or greater executive function difficulties. Although it is important to assess whether there has been decline in functioning, it has been our experience that a worsening score may in fact reflect greater awareness about the issues associated with brain injury rather than a frank deterioration.

Other services report using verbatim feedback, interviews and also pay attention to the need for outcomes to be individualised. It is important to take into account the accessibility of measures to families, the timing of giving these and the applicability of different methods of measuring outcome at different stages of rehabilitation, as well as ensuring that data is meaningful at an individual as well as at a service level. For example, during the inpatient phase, our colleagues report that using a quality of life measure does not seem appropriate, as the child is in the acute stage of recovery and therefore it is not sensitive to their needs, whereas setting goals around functional gains and in relation to this stage of recovery is reported to be much more meaningful. We are continually monitoring and are sensitive to these dilemmas and suggest that choosing which measures are used and when, should be adapted according to the family and child's context and their stage of recovery.

Database

We hold a cumulative database capturing data and contextual narrative at baseline and review for each child that participates in rehabilitation. We use the database on a case by case basis to demonstrate change over time. The database is also showing us which standardised measures are most sensitive to change in our clinical setting, thereby automatising the process of outcome measurement at a group as well as individual level. In our service audit (Gosling et al., 2015), we found that our community rehabilitation interventions resulted in self-reported improvements in quality of life and family functioning after a year of intervention, but less change on measures of impairment such as the Behaviour Rating Inventory of Executive Function.

The challenge of outcome measurement

There is an implicit concern or question about whether outcome measurement can capture the nuances of the narrative journey of the child, their family and the wider team. Here again, we acknowledge the challenge for those of us working in rehabilitation to identify and measure the active components of rehabilitation and that the psychological elements almost always combine with other therapies and medical interventions that will also affect outcome. In our view, for the psychological input, the triangulation of (1) standardised measures, (2) goals, and (3) the narrative contextualisation of the data, goes some way in capturing and describing the distinct idiosyncrasies of a child's story through the journey of rehabilitation. Further, this data can be used to more widely evaluate process and outcome in rehabilitation.

However, the concept and practice of outcome measurement is a philosophical and practical challenge. At both levels, there are value-laden assumptions about what should be measured, what constitutes a good enough outcome, and how quality of life should be defined. Further, alongside our own values and assumptions, there are dominant narratives within public policy and held at a societal level regarding definitions of rehabilitation, disability, outcomes and evidence, and a child's rights and welfare (and in this context making decisions with and in the "best interests" of the child). It is important as clinicians to be aware of the dominant narratives and inherent assumptions and values that we bring to our work. More widely, this may influence service delivery, and our definition and measurement of an outcome and what may be considered a "good enough" outcome. In addition, these narratives can influence both within a service setting, and at a wider societal level (see Gosling, 2015, for a more detailed discussion of these issues).

Members within a rehabilitation team do not always hold the same views on the priorities and goals for clinical input, and how change should be measured. Collaboration is not always possible due to conflicting or competing perspectives held within the professional system and/or family; it may be difficult to determine the child's views because of their level of disability; and to ascertain the family member's and/or rehabilitation team's views due to issues of power and powerlessness, and beliefs and prejudices held within different levels of the system.

As an example, there is sometimes tension between goals that a clinician may want to set "for" the child, and in this regard how the clinician guides the child and the family to consider goals that they may at that point not be valuing. Although, as far as possible, goals are most effective when they are collaboratively set, there are times when the work is to help a family move to a greater understanding of their child's needs, in order to set a goal that is in an area hitherto not considered a priority by them. Acknowledging that the clinician is holding knowledge about what can aide a positive outcome and so needs to use this in guiding goal setting, a goal is often to develop a *shared understanding* of the child's needs in order to guide the process and, thereafter, a new phase of intervention.

In these situations, questions can arise about who owns the goal, and whose goal is being worked on and how aligned the outcome of that goal is with the overall guiding principles of rehabilitation held by individuals and at a wider systems level. Although a goal and outcomes framework promote collaboration and the development of a shared understanding and language, these processes and ideas should not be considered a panacea with respect to dilemmas of power, prejudice and competing narratives.

There are parallels with the CAMH service outcome measurement framework and our approach. Both use a combination of standardised measurement tools and collaborative goals. One difference is that currently we do not use measures to evaluate process, engagement or the therapeutic alliance as seen in the CAMH services. Although it can and does form part of conversations as we work with families, especially within the goals process, we do not *systematically* seek feedback about how our clients are experiencing the service we are providing. We are often working with different parts of the system and may not be engaging in one focussed piece of "therapy"; work with the child and/or their family may be indirect and so capturing process meaningfully is more complex than simply asking for a rating after a therapy session. This could be a useful addition to gain a richer picture of the process of experiencing rehabilitation, whilst bearing in mind who to ask, the additional burden of more measures and adapting questions to be relevant to this context. Our practice example reflects this, with the child's parent being an active participant in the writing.

Practice example (all names and personal details have been anonymised)

A story

There was a little girl who was 7 years old. We will call her Lizzie. She was *terrified* of hospitals, dentists and seeing anyone with a bandage, plaster or illness. This little girl had had a traumatic start to her life. She was in hospital for weeks after being born. Her mum and dad didn't know if she would make it. Now she is fine, but she had a brain injury at birth resulting in cerebral palsy that affects her body movements and her speech production. Her neuropsychological profile showed that she also has memory difficulties, in areas of episodic memory, recall and memory for faces. She still needs to go to hospital for lots of check-ups.

Using outcome measures and goals

What did our measures tell us about Lizzie? At assessment, the PedsQL (parent and self-report) picked up her emotional difficulties – more so Lizzie's own report – feeling angry, worried and sad. The PedsQL (cerebral palsy module) measures also showed the impact of her physical disability on her everyday self-care, mobility and communication. Family functioning was not problematic, although understandably, stresses and strains were evident. Her memory difficulties emerged as she developed; her family and school noticed her weak memory for events and that she was not recognising people she had met; formal assessment was able to specify her areas of strengths and weaknesses.

Goals were collaboratively set and initially the work focussed on assessing Lizzie's cognitive functioning, helping her mum and Lizzie to manage her physical frustrations, changes in routine and learning to wait. As the work continued, it emerged that she also found hospital visits terrifying and also became uncontrollably upset when she saw someone with a plaster or a bandage. A new goal was set to address this, as it became a priority with upcoming hospital appointments and the unpredictability of when she might see someone with a bandage. It was hypothesised that this emotional response stemmed from her early experiences (precognitive) of being in hospital and the understandable worry around her as a vulnerable baby.

Using a therapeutic storytelling approach

Lizzie and her mum were seen for five sessions at home. We used a therapeutic storytelling approach based on the Lovett adaptations to working with trauma in younger children (Lovett, 2008). Lizzie's mum wrote a story in the third person, based on Lizzie's start in life. The story includes the present day where the young girl is no longer unwell or in danger, and introduces some coping strategies to build on in the sessions jointly. Lizzie's mum was present at all the sessions and her mum and dad worked between sessions, re-reading the story with her, elaborating and strengthening the narrative of a young girl who had had a scary and unpleasant time in hospital as a baby, but who was fine now and was strong enough to be brave when she went back for appointments. Lizzie strongly identified with the story and so it was personalised, driven by Lizzie.

As she was just 6 years old, this included a strong element of emotional support from her parents in helping her be brave, preparing her for the visits and being with her throughout.

Outcomes

Using the SMART goals approach meant that we could measure the outcome of this intervention by comparing her behaviour at the start of the intervention and at the end: after one false start, Lizzie was calm when visiting a hospital and no longer became upset in any way when she saw someone with a bandage or plaster. She was able to visit her grandparent in hospital and had her ears pierced. The standardised measures also showed an improvement in her emotional well-being on the PedsQL scales, giving another indication of a positive outcome.

There are a number of other elements to the psychological intervention that focus on the educational, neuropsychological and multidisciplinary aspects of her rehabilitation. Her memory difficulties are being supported using compensatory strategies and her neuropsychological functioning continues to be monitored. Further work continues using the narrative approach, focussing on Lizzie's identity as a girl with CP, her frustrations and triumphs with her physical limitations, and how she views herself, not with a "disability" but with "diff-ability". As Lizzie grows up her needs, priorities and goals will also develop alongside those of her family and work continues with Lizzie and her family.

Lizzie's mother's perspective

To say Lizzie was petrified was an understatement; hospital visits loomed over me for days before with me trying to think of ways I could goad her into even just getting into the car. If we got that far without an utter meltdown, it was then the dreaded period waiting to be seen! With my talking endlessly with nerves just hoping, I could distract her long enough to not go into sheer panic & fright! It never worked!

That seems now like another lifetime ago. The story we put together, the method in which I told it to her, the teddy I always made sure she had while I was telling her the story all contributed to her overcoming this gut-wrenching fear she had of hospitals/doctors or come to think of it anything that you would associate with being medical.

I was sceptical, however trusted [the psychologist] and was willing to try anything. It's funny because it actually became a lovely five minutes I shared with Lizzie every day, as not only was I reading to her I was helping her in so many ways that she had no idea about.

Lizzie is not 'cured' of this fear; however, it seems to have built a way of dealing with this inner terror that she had. I have recalled the story to Lizzie only last week when due to an illness I thought we may have to go to hospital, even though weak, poorly and not best pleased she still understood and accepted we may need to go. To me that is a massive achievement for her. She has come such a long way.

Future directions

There is work to be done regarding the concept and application of outcome measurement and the advancement of consistent protocols across settings and disciplines that allows for the capture and measurement of change in rehabilitation. This will inform us and those who commission our services about what interventions produce meaningful change both at an individual and population level. Cultivating networks of clinicians willing to share ideas and work collaboratively will support the development of outcome protocols, and potentially data-pooling. Ultimately, this will inform what interventions work best for whom which can then be implemented across services more systematically. In our view, the addition of single case study methodology (as outlined by Tate, Perdices, McDonald, & Rosenkoetter, 2014) would also be a valuable asset to this process.

We have much to learn from our colleagues that work within systemic and mental health settings with respect to the measures and processes they use to define and measure change/outcome, acknowledging that there are other ways to capture change than those described in this chapter. Further, it is important to create space to listen to the voice of people with lived experience who access rehabilitation services and integrate their perspective into service development plans including outcome protocols.

The process of writing this chapter has helped us to think carefully about our current practice, where we could develop and improve our protocols, including the development of ways to listen to the perspectives of those with lived experience routinely and the importance of not just "measuring for measuring" sake. There needs to be meaning: a contextual, collaborative interpretation of the measures being completed. We want to know what has enabled a good outcome for a child and conversely when an intervention was not good enough and why. This is a rich question and is in itself an area for further discussion, exploration and research by the community of professionals working in child rehabilitation. After all, this is why we measure outcome; we want to know what works so we can deliver the best possible rehabilitation to children and their families, as they are always at the heart and centre of what we do.

References

Anderson, V. A., Brown, S., Newitt, H., & Hoile, H. (2011). Long term outcome from childhood traumatic brain injury: Intellectual ability, personality and quality of life. *Neuropsychology, 25*, 176–184.

Brown, F. L., & Whittingham, K. (2015). A structural behavioural family intervention with parents of children with brain injury. In J. Reed, K. Byard, & H. Fine (Eds.), *Neuropsychological rehabilitation of childhood brain injury* (pp. 60–81). Palgrave Macmillan.

Burnham, J. (1992). Approach – method – technique: Making distinctions and creating connections. *Human Systems, 3*(1), 3–27.

Byard, K. (2015). A contextual, systemic perspective in child neuropsychological rehabilitation. In J. Reed, K. Byard, & H. Fine (Eds.), *Neuropsychological rehabilitation of childhood brain injury* (pp. 173–190). Palgrave Macmillan.

Carter, B., & McGoldrick, M. (1988). *The changing family life cycle: A framework for family therapy*. New York: Gardner Press.

Cole, W. R., Paulos, S. K., Cole, C. A. S., & Tankard, C. (2009). A review of family intervention guidelines for paediatric acquired brain injuries. *Developmental Disabilities Review, 15*, 159–166.

Cooper, M., & Law, D. (Eds.). (2018). *Working with goals in psychotherapy and counselling*. Oxford University Press.

Department for Education. (2014). *Children and families act*. London: Department of Education.

Department of Health. (2005). *National service framework for long-term conditions*. London: Department of Health.

Feltham, A., Martin, K., Walker, L., & Harris, L. (2018). Using goals in therapy: The perspective of people with lived experience. In M. Cooper & D. Law (Eds.), *Working with goals in psychotherapy and counselling*. Oxford: Oxford University Press.

Forsyth, R., Salorio, C. F., & Christensen, J. R. (2009). Modelling early recovery patterns after paediatric traumatic brain injury. *Archives of Disease in Childhood, 95*(4), 266–270.

Forsyth, R., Young, D., Kelly, G., Davis, K., Dunford, C., Golighty, A., Marshall, L., & Wales, L. (2018). Paediatric rehabilitation ingredients measure: A new tool for identifying paediatric neurorehabilitation content. *Developmental Medicine & Child Neurology, 60*, 299–305.

Gosling, A. S., Smart, C., Byard., K, Reed, J., Fine, H., & Tucker, P. (2015, September). *Measuring outcomes in a clinical service: An audit of Recolo UK Ltd neuropsychological rehabilitation.* Poster presented at the First International Paediatric Brain Injury Symposium, Liverpool.

Gosling, S. (2015). Measuring outcomes for children with brain injury: Challenges and solutions. In J. Reed, K. Byard, & H. Fine (Eds.), *Neuropsychological rehabilitation of childhood brain injury* (pp. 131–150). Palgrave Macmillan.

Gosling, S. (2016). Recent developments in the neuroimaging and neuropsychology of cerebral palsy. *Applied Neuropsychology: Child*, 1–9. Retrieved from www.tandfonline.com/doi/full/10.1080/21622965.2015.1074914

Hastings, R. (2016). *Handing the power to families and careers through positive behaviour resources.* Retrieved from http://pavingtheway.works/whats-new/handing-power-family-carers-positive-behavioural-support-pbs-resources/

Law, D., & Wolpert, M. (Eds.). (2014). *Guide to using outcome and feedback tools with children, young people and families.* CORC Ltd.

Lovett, J. (2008). *Small wonders: Healing childhood trauma with EMDR.* New York: The Free Press.

McCauley, S. R., Wilde, E. A., Anderson, V. A., Bedell, G., Beers, S. R., Campbell, T. F., et al. (2012). Recommendations for the use of common outcome measures in pediatric traumatic brain injury research. *Journal of Neurotrauma, 2*, 678–705.

NHS England. (2013). *Specialist rehabilitation for patients with highly complex needs (all ages).*

Novak, I. (2014). Evidence-based diagnosis, health care and rehabilitation for children with cerebral palsy. *Journal of Child Neurology, 29*(8), 1141–1156.

Prodinger, B., Reinhardt, J. D., Selb, M., Stucki, G., Yan, T., Zhang, X., & Li, J. (2016). Toward system-wide implementation of the international classification of functioning, disability and health (ICF) in routine practice: Developing simple, intuitive descriptions of ICF categories in the ICF generic and rehabilitation set. *Journal of Rehabilitation Medicine*, doi:10.2340/16501977-2066

Rolland, J. S. (1988a). A conceptual model of chronic and life threatening illness and its impact on the family. In C. Chilman, E. Nunnally, & F. Cox (Eds.), *Chronic illness and disability.* Newbury Park, CA: Sage.

Rolland, J. S. (1988b). Chronic illness and the family life cycle. In B. Carter & M. McGoldrick (Eds.), *The changing family life-cycle: A framework for family therapy.* New York: Gardner Press.

Rolland, J. S. (1994). *Families, illness & disability: An integrative treatment model.* New York: Basic Books.

Tate, R. L., Perdices, M., McDonald, L. T., & Rosenkoetter, U. (2014). The design, conduct and report of single-case study research: Resources to improve the quality of the neurorehabilitation literature. *Neuropsychological Rehabilitation, 24*, 315–331.

Todd, D. (2013). Narrative approaches to goal-setting. In S. Weatherhead & D. Todd (Eds.), *Narrative approaches to brain injury* (pp. 51–76). London: Karnac.

Todd, D., & Weatherhead, S. (2013). Outcome evidence. In S. Weatherhead & D. Todd (Eds.), *Narrative approaches to brain injury* (pp. 185–208). London: Karnac.

Tucker, P. (2015). Goal setting and goal attainment scaling in child neuropsychological rehabilitation. In J. Reed, K. Byard, & H. Fine (Eds.). *Neuropsychological rehabilitation of childhood brain injury* (pp. 151–170). Palgrave Macmillan.

Turner-Stokes, L. (2009). Goal attainment scaling (GAS) in rehabilitation: A practical guide. *Clinical Rehabilitation, 23*, 362–370.

Turner-Stokes, L., & Siegert, R. J. (2013). A comprehensive psychometric evaluation of the UK FIM+FAM. *Disability Rehabilitation, 35*(22), 1885–1895.

Turner-Stokes, L., Nyein, K., Turner-Stokes, T., & Gatehouse, C. (1999). The UK FIM+ FAM: Development and evaluation. Functional assessment measure. *Clinical Rehabilitation, 13*(4), 277–287.

Turner-Stokes, L., Vanderstay, R., Eager, K., Dredge, R., & Siegert, R. (2015). *Cost-efficient provision in neuro-rehabilitation: Defining needs, costs and outcomes for people with long term neurological conditions.* Draft report submitted to the National Institute for Health Research.

Wade, S. L., & Hung, A. (2015). Online family problem solving for adolescent traumatic brain injury. In J. Reed, K. Byard, & H. Fine (Eds.), *Neuropsychological rehabilitation of childhood brain injury* (pp. 43–59). Palgrave Macmillan.

World Health Organisation. (2001). *International classification of functioning, disability and health.* Geneva: World Health Organisation.

United Nations. (1989). *UN convention on the rights of the child.* London: UNICEF.

Chapter 15

Our children do deserve better

*Jenny Jim, Heather Liddiard
and Esther Cole*

Overview

This chapter aims to speak to the heart of the recommendations of the chief medical officer's annual report (2012), "Our Children Deserve Better" (Davies, 2013), by addressing the need for (1) early intervention (and prevention), (2) proactive innovation and (3) interventions with lasting impact to optimise our children's well-being into later life. "Our Children Deserve Better" recognises that we are failing to meet the needs of our children and young people with ABI. The writing of this chapter pre-dates the recent All Party Parliamentary Group debate for ABI held on 18 June 2018 (HC Deb, 2018) – we were very pleased to read that many of the dilemmas we outline reflect national concerns and are now being heard at the highest level. We will try to formulate these core issues and make suggestions for intervention including service development.

Children and young people with ABI live with varied primary and secondary impacts which fundamentally alter their life, making them more dependent on others and systems, and more vulnerable to negative influences. Throughout their natural development, our children must transition into and out of different services and pathways of care. This has its own inherent stressors, because comprehensive psychological formulation and information sharing within a multi-agency approach is vital. Currently, most services are not designed to work like this. Consequently, transition is often fraught with individuals falling between services with information not being shared. For families, this can be psychologically distressing and inefficient, which should be preventable.

Whilst improvements are definitely required, there is much to be optimistic about in current practice (and research). The innovations in this book outlined across the chapters reflect the knowledge that is growing internationally about psychosocial risk and protective factors in childhood brain injury. This is the compelling force for the need for integrative, systemic, narrative and multisystem approaches. Furthermore, we have the privilege of being able to intervene at a time when the brain is most sensitive, and we are most likely to have lasting developmental impact. CYP at this point are developing their identities, learning social, emotional and educational skills, to name a few. The psychological and rehabilitative work is paramount to the best recovery possible and to increasing their quality of life. The potential for poor outcomes (evidenced by research studies on trajectories for this group) underlines the importance of our work.

What could "better" look like?

To consider what "better" might look like for our children with ABI, we would like to share our thoughts about how the current mismatch between demand and available resources has occurred.

What do we think are the core issues?

We feel the core issues relate to both the complexity of brain injury as well as the ability of the systems around the CYP to respond. CYP with ABI can have multiple problems across all social, physical, emotional, cognitive and spiritual domains that go beyond the primary direct impact of the injury. These problems can be unmet and misunderstood by current services. Frontline staff often face barriers to providing tailored support within service structures.

How have we got here?

As mentioned in earlier chapters, medical advances have led to increased survival rates of children and adults with ABI. Therefore, we have an increased population of more severely injured individuals who require services. This is coupled with a contextual change in public services, whereby criteria for accessing services and receiving ongoing support are more tightly monitored. At one time, a person with ABI might receive support from a variety of services, such as those for people with intellectual disability or mental health diagnoses; this is now less likely to happen. Paradoxically, advances in services which were meant to result in more person-centred care have also led to unintended consequences, such as leaving many people underprovided – i.e. a person with a diagnosis of secondary autism as a result of an ABI who did not have an intellectual disability could not access a learning disability service. This is even though they may have needs more consonant with this population.

One geographical borough will have a unique service structure that does not correspond to other boroughs. In reality, this means that families and health professionals alike have to negotiate complex referral and discharge pathways that all have different criteria within them. Restricted funding can also lead to a culture of protectionism where services cannot be more flexible as they must justify and protect their resources.

What makes this a difficult problem?

Over medicalising our CYPs needs can be part of the difficulty because ABI represents an organic condition, this can lead to the assumption that it is treated solely within a medical model. This overshadows myriad other sequelae especially psychological and cognitive problems. Whilst it is obvious when a person experiences hemiparesis that they require physical rehabilitation, the need for psychological and cognitive effects of this injury are largely invisible and risk being under-recognised. A further complicating factor is that the person themselves may not be fully aware of their multiple challenges as lack of insight frequently co-occurs.

Brain injuries can cause or be linked to severe mental health difficulties, such as psychosis, depression, self-regulatory problems and existential issues. These presentations could be primary and/or secondary to the brain injury. For instance, a young person who has been in a car accident may shows signs of low mood and have difficulties regulating high emotion. This could be due to the brain injury itself or may be a reactive response to becoming aware of what they are going through. Services can have different perspectives on how to understand their needs – if a CAMHS views this as a direct result of brain injury, it is unlikely to accept a referral for support. Furthermore, even if the young person had been depressed previous to their brain injury, this still would not guarantee that they would receive help from CAMHS. Often, it feels to clinicians that the presence of a brain injury can be used by services to exclude.

If there is a latent belief that if the cause is organic then treatments should be medical and, as such, psychological interventions can be seen as being pointless. This may be related to a societal belief of a Cartesian split between mind and body. Thus, if the body (i.e. the brain) is injured then the discourse is that you do not necessarily require any intervention for the mind as it should be unaffected.

A further contributing factor is a widely accepted belief that children "bounce back". There is a misunderstanding of the long-lasting impact of ABI, where in fact the true effects of the injury may not be obvious until a later developmental stage. There is a high risk that the brain injury is forgotten by the time services are needed. This leads to misdiagnoses and inappropriate interventions. This can result in a young person being "blamed" for their behaviour without any sense of linking this to the impact of their earlier injury that fundamentally affects their self-regulation skills. At the recent parliamentary debate, Dr. Lisa Cameron, MP and clinical psychologist, expressed so well that ABI represents a "hidden disability". This echoed Chris Bryant, leader of the All Parliamentary Group for ABI and MP for Rhondda who stated that ABI is an "invisible epidemic" (HC Deb, 2018).

What keeps the problem going?

Often serious untoward incidents (SUIs) highlight, albeit all too late, myriad factors that have led to failures of care. It is vital we learn from root cause analysis of SUIs to identify the major contributory factors and to address them appropriately.

A key example of this is the Somerset Case Review (Flynn, 2016) that investigated why "Tom", a 43-year-old man with a history of multiple head injuries spanning back to very early childhood, took his life in 2014. At age 3, Tom was knocked down by a car; at age 8, he received a concussion; at age 14, he suffered a reported sports injury, with a minor head injury at age 17. When Tom was 22, he suffered a significant brain injury from another road traffic accident.

Tom was left with extensive medical (epilepsy, chronic pain), psychological (depression, aggression, insomnia and substance misuse) and cognitive (problem-solving, speed of processing and memory) in addition to communication (dysphasia) needs. Tom was accessing services for multiple and complex needs relating to these issues and had contact with the criminal justice system. Whilst he was linked into Headway – a national brain injury charity – it appears that ongoing intensive specialist support was missing. In addition, he was a full-time carer for his partner who also sustained a head injury. His role as a carer was rarely taken into account in his support plans.

Multiple failures include a lack of coordinated services especially in the management of the risk of harm, poor documentation, not following policy (which would have acknowledged him as a vulnerable adult) and not recognising severe cognitive impairments that impacted on his mental capacity and ability to engage in traditional interventions. In addition, services did not invite Tom's family to be part of his care planning, did not appear to take interest in his personhood and were not flexible enough to engage an individual who was clearly living in chaos. No organisation took a lead role in advocating and determining a coordinated, multi-agency response. This resulted in services minimising his distress, the family's distress and his actual extensive support needs.

Tom's story highlights to us key areas that require urgent change in order to protect others like Tom and to prevent this situation and devastating outcome to occur again. A key "learning lesson" from Somerset Safeguarding Adults Board was that brain injuries must be taken into account and their impact on cognitive impairment and capacity. This points to limitations in workforce readiness. Often, there is a lack of knowledge of working with paediatric ABI, the majority of children and adults affected by ABI will come across more non-specialists than specialists throughout their life. The illness or injury will continue to be "hidden", which creates problematic interactions with services who lack knowledge of how ABI can present.

A lack of knowledge and awareness of paediatric ABI and its impact is not only engrained in society but perpetuated by the training pathways for psychologists and other therapists in the UK. In clinical and educational psychology qualifications, neuropsychology has not always been firmly embedded. This leads to difficulties in psychologists formulating the heterogeneous and complex presentations of paediatric ABI that encompass many different levels of needs. The opportunities for specialist neuropsychology placements are rare, as there are so few trained paediatric neuropsychologists in the UK.

Furthermore, clinical and educational psychologists need to complete their doctorates first before being eligible to train as a clinical neuropsychologist. Adult and child clinical neuropsychology qualifications have historically focussed on cognitive assessment and cognitive neurorehabilitation. However, there is a need for courses to train therapists to adapt their existing skills to work with the whole child and family's need for emotional and psychological support, and mental well-being. Clinicians often report feeling overwhelmed and under skilled. Other allied health professionals and social services are likely to experience similar gaps in knowledge and confidence. Often, nurses are the first professionals that people come into contact with and contribute to the triaging of CYP with ABI. More training and support are required for all professionals.

What are the positive changes?

Shifts in policy and funding are beginning (HC Deb, 2018). In 2016, NHS England published further rehabilitation guidance on commissioning services for both adults and children (NHS England, 2016). This provides local service planners with a commissioning model, a range of case studies and crucially, an evidence base for the economic benefits of delivering high-quality rehabilitation services. There is now recognition that access to high-quality rehabilitation both improves outcomes for patients and can save money. Effective rehabilitation can pay for itself (HC Deb, 2018).

The government have also invested £29 million for education, health and care plans (EHCPs) for children at schools. This will enable different teams and services working with children and young people in education to have a coordinated plan for any additional needs, reasonable adjustments, therapies and services required to optimise their well-being and learning. There is also increasing awareness of trajectory research that refutes the "earlier the better" argument for ABI with more children growing up from ABI with evident multiple problems. Researchers are beginning to see links such as those in the criminal justice system and early head injuries (Hughes et al., 2015).

How do we intervene?

(i) Early intervention (and prevention)

There is a clear case for increasing public and professional awareness of the vulnerabilities that our children with ABI must live with. If we are to fully acknowledge and not minimise the potential need for help, we must also put into place mechanisms to increase confidence and skills in working with this group. This is likely to include specific training and supervision, increasing the interface between and within specialist services and community services. This requires fundamental changes to commissioning in both inpatient and community services. The ultimate goal would be that a lifespan model be used to provide a range of specialist brain injury services from low to high support with intensive and ongoing follow-up where necessary. We would like there to be established links between specialist and mainstream provisions such as schools and CAMHS.

Continuing professional development and research is also required to further identify risk and resiliency factors. This would promote our ability to bridge the gaps between theory/research and practice. Prevention would include increased involvement in public health campaigns to reduce frequency and severity of head injuries. Brain injury is a major cause of death and disability for children in England, the majority of which are unintentional, "predictable and preventable" (NIHCE, 2010). An example of this is the recent recognition and development of monitoring systems for safe return to play after a mild concussion sustained in contact sports (i.e. Return 2 Play, 2019).

There is also a financial argument for early intervention and prevention. The Child Accident Prevention Trust have demonstrated that the lifetime cost to care for a child with severe TBI in the UK can amount to £4.9 million, including medical costs, social care, educational costs, government benefits and missed employment opportunities. Given the prevalence this potentially amounts to a total societal cost of £640 million – £2.24 billion annually (Davies, 2013).

(ii) Proactive innovation

We hope the contributions within the book have showcased a diversity of ways in which clinicians are innovating practice. Embedded in all chapters is an ethos that we see children with ABI as children first rather than being defined by their injury. Seeing a child as a child rather than thinking about children with ABI as a specialist group is important. This is a key attitudinal change advocated by the chief medical officer to think of all children as children, with various socioeconomic, psychological, health and well-being needs, and not to think of children with ABI in a separate category. If we separate them, we risk thinking we cannot meet their needs because they are perceived to be too complex and require too much specialist expertise.

On the frontline there are many small developments that any service can consider, including ensuring that assessments routinely enquire about early ABI and the impact this has had. Every 30 minutes, a child sustains a brain injury through accident, illness, abuse or injury (CBIT, 2017). Practically, this means that up to five children in every classroom in the UK will have a brain injury (HC Deb, 2018). Therefore, always asking the question is vital. For example, routine screening of prisoners for brain injury is now in the early stages of being piloted by the Ministry of Justice (HC Deb, 2018).

Clinicians need to be supported in thinking around how to deliver more flexible interventions taking into account the CYP's ability levels. Other developments might include supervision networks, case management and other continuing professional development activities which have a focus on ABI. Some services already harness the energy of service users/ experts by experience to empower relevant change for our children with ABI.

Within the book, we have also presented examples where people have developed new approaches, have influenced service design and put forward and actioned arguments that bring new ways of service delivery. Policy development and strategic development must reflect the everyday experience of our children, young people and their families.

(iii) Interventions with lasting impact to optimise our children's well-being into later life

We need to avoid interventions that are unlikely to make meaningful sustainable change. These would typically be short-burst treatments requiring a high level of engagement and no ongoing support. They often are not tailored to the idiosyncratic neuropsychological profile of the person as well as their physical and other sensory impairments. Some approaches require a degree of self-directed work in between sessions which can be inordinately more difficult or impossible for our children and young people with ABI. Not engaging or completing set work should not be interpreted as a sign of poor motivation for change (as it was in Tom's case).

Rather, we need to prioritise and focus on key principles that will guide what support is provided, when, how and how long for. This has cost and time implications as truly person-centred working with this group often requires *translating concepts* of assessment and intervention into accessible resources taking into account the child's cognitive, physical and sensory needs. For instance, if a child has receptive or expressive aphasia (or both), this would invalidate most traditional neuropsychological tests and mean that talking therapies would need high levels of augmentation. Translating concepts in this example may involve heavy use of visual material, drawings and pictures, music and song to circumvent obvious cognitive and sensory barriers. Unfortunately, there is no easy way of creating new resources which conceptually match the original test/therapy/approach. Often, much trial and error are required, combined with qualitative interpretation by a skilled clinician. The next step is to use the results in improving their everyday functional rehabilitation.

On a more macro-level, we need to heed the lessons from research and serious case reviews for services to improve and align themselves more closely to the recommendations made. This would include greater understanding of trajectories and vulnerable periods of development, whilst also being able to make economic arguments to gain longer-term funding, more joined up service delivery which would encompass multiservice and global collaborations. This is also necessary to advance the empirical evidence base. Key to all of this is that our children, young people and families are listened to and their views and ideas are the foundation for innovation.

Effecting change

We have attempted to present both micro and macro-level ideas for making better services for our children and young people with ABI. As we write this, we are aware that our thoughts may come across as an unachievable wish list. As clinicians ourselves, it can evoke a sense of being overwhelmed and feeling under-equipped to make any change.

Change is possible and requires interagency/global and grassroots level development. This might include services, clinicians and service users developing practice guidelines; disseminating learning points from everyday work; collecting outcome data; and finding means to share information across services (perhaps using frameworks such as SPECS). We should not strive for perfection as this inevitably results in paralysing creativity and innovation. It is true to say that the voices of the child and family need to be listened to more closely so that there is a genuine partnership that leads innovations.

Summary and conclusions

We hope that we have been able to reflect on why our children and young people with ABI frequently do not receive the support they desperately require. We also present some ideas to address the shortfalls both at a clinician and service level. It is important to bear in mind that a perfect service does not exist but small changes in everyday practice are key to wider changes.

What our children do deserve are services that are attuned to their needs as they develop and change following their ABI. This may mean specialist input at some points and mainstream support at other times. We also anticipate that for long periods of time, the best support may not be professional in nature. However, we want an easy way for re-engaging services, as rehabilitation will continue across their lives.

References

Child Brain Injury Trust (CBIT). (2017). Retrieved October 29, 2018, from https://child braininjurytrust.org.uk/

Child Accident Prevention Trust. *The costs of head injuries*. Retrieved July 2013, from www.makingthelink.net/costs-head-injuries

Davies, S. C. (2013). *Annual report of the chief medical officer 2012, our children deserve better: Prevention pays*. London: Department of Health.

Flynn, M. (2016). *The death of "Tom": A serious case review*. HL, Somerset: Somerset Safeguarding Adults Board.

HC Deb. (2018, June 18). Vol. 643, col. 132. Retrieved July 24, 2018, from https://han sard.parliament.uk/commons/2018-06-18/debates/6619D69D-616C-4EEC-A2A5-5F3A5C082FA1/AcquiredBrainInjury

Hughes, N., Williams, H., Chitsabesan, P., Walesby, R.C., Mounce, L.T., Clasby, B. (2015). The prevalence of traumatic brain injury among young offenders in custody: A systematic review. *Journal of Head Trauma Rehabilitation, 30*(2), 94–105.

National Institute for Health and Clinical Excellence. (2010). *Strategies to prevent unintentional injuries among the under-15s – NICE public health guidance 29*. London: National Institute for Health and Clinical Excellence.

NHS England. (2016). *Commissioning guidance for rehabilitation*. Retrieved July 14, 2018, from www.england.nhs.uk/wp-content/uploads/2016/04/rehabilitation-comms-guid-16-17.pdf www.return2play.org.uk

Return2Play. (2019). Retrieved June 13, 2019, from https://www.return2play.org.uk

Experts by Experience Reflections on the Book – Jackie Solaiman

Jackie Solaiman, mother of Rafi kindly read through our book manuscript and gave us the following reflections:

"Some of the approaches in the book (Structured Narrative Therapy) may have been effective but we had no access to them at a time that was appropriate for Rafi at The Children's Trust as his insight was too poor and he was suffering from post-traumatic amnesia.

When we were at The Children's Trust the clinical psychologist helped us maintain the family relationships which is so difficult when going through the trauma of having a brain injured child. I feel that having a strong family around him was one of the most important factors that helped his recovery (there is a mention of better outcomes for parent-delivered rehabilitation). In the chapter that presented an imagined therapeutic interview with The Brain – the ideas of the 'Torch' versus 'the doom' resonated with me - after reading an autobiography about a woman who recovered from a similar injury to Rafi I used this as my 'torch' to keep me positive and hopefully pass positivity onto Rafi".

Theory-practice links in "Narrative-inspired interview with the brain"

Narrative process
Paraphrased by Nolte (2016) from Michael White's 'Maps of Narrative Practice' (2007; New York: W.W. Norton)
Two stages:
Deconstruction of the dominant story/identity
Reconstruction of alternative preferred story/identity

Narrative therapeutic focus	Areas focussed on in interview	Examples of questions used in interview
Deconstruction of the dominant story/identity	Describe the problem and ask What happened/happens? What were/are the circumstances? Who was/is involved?	Please tell me what is troubling you and what you hope I can help with? What happened? What troubles you the most? If you can, do tell me a bit more so I really understand where you are coming from.
Deconstruction of the problem story/identity Externalising conversations: The objectification or personification of the problem Four steps to externalising conversations Mutually acceptable name for the problem Name linguistically separates the person from the problem The person is not the problem, the problem is the problem Explore the relative influence of the problem Explore the impact of the problem on different areas of the person's life, relationships and views of themselves – e.g. home, university, friends, actions, emotions, physical, relationships with self and others.	Agree mutually acceptable name for the problem Explore relative influence of the problem Evaluation of the effects of the problem Justification of evaluation	I wonder if we can capture what you are saying distinctly perhaps by giving it a name? What could we call this feeling of 'never getting better … being damaged'? So, if I can ask more about 'The Doom' – when is the 'The Doom' most likely to be around? Before 'The Doom' was around what had you hoped for yourself – your ambitions? Tell me if you can, how has affected other parts of your life?

How has the problem been disrupting, dominating and discouraging regarding hopes, dreams, aspirations and values? Impact on identity and person's view of themselves?	I can see that you are saying that the damage has made emotions and behaviour hard to control, plus 'The Doom' then gets in on the act and brings thoughts of 'what's the point?' – I guess this connects to the idea that you will never get better. I am also hearing that because of this combination of the damage and 'The Doom' that your life is more limited in terms of hanging out with others.
Evaluation of the effects of the problem? Person to judge (justify) whether the impact of problem on life is preferred (or not)? Person to take a stand against the impact of the problem on the various areas of their life Is this okay with you? How do you feel about this?	I am hearing very strongly a very dominant idea from you that 'you will never get better' – is that right? How do you feel about the power of 'The Doom' on your life?
Justification of the evaluations Person gives an account/reasons <u>why</u> the influence/impact of the problem in their life, relationships and view of themselves are unacceptable Why is this not okay for you? Justification elicits the person's hopes, dreams and aspirations and preferred identities	It is OK with you that it has such a strong effect? It sounds like you have enough to cope with besides 'The Doom' making you feel worse? Why do you think it's not OK that 'The Doom' affects you like this?
Reconstruction of alternative preferred story/identity: Re-authoring conversations Identifying exceptions (unique outcomes) to dominant story and thicken the unique outcomes/alternative stories and their meanings	Can you think of anything new you have learnt or made progress with? But how? Tell me. It doesn't just happen! What did you have to do? But what I am hearing is that 'The Doom' could not have been that powerful all of the time; otherwise, how would you have go to where you are now?
Finding a mutually acceptable name for the unique outcome Map potential effects/influences of unique outcome Evaluation of the effect of the unique outcome Justification of evaluation	

(Continued)

Narrative therapeutic focus	Areas focussed on in interview	Examples of questions used in interview
Four steps for re-authoring conversations: Finding a mutually acceptable name for the unique outcome Map potential effects/influences of unique outcome Evaluation of the effect of the unique outcome Justification of evaluation	Explore the (potential) effects of the unique outcome/exception on the various domains of living and views of the self	I guess this is a sort of 'Anti-Doom' – what would you call it? When 'The Torch' is around, what does it allow you to do? So it sounds like you have hope when 'The Torch' is around? . . . Hope about achieving something and changing? The Torch certainly seems to change a lot about what you think about yourself, being social and putting things in perspective. Is it OK for you that 'The Torch' has this power?
Unique outcomes/exceptions: Moments in past or present when the person was able to escape the influence/resist the dominance of the problem in their life Deconstructs the notion that the problem is all-powerful Exceptions (or unique outcomes) provides the starting points for alternative story lines and re-authoring conversations		So you would prefer if 'The Torch' was on all of the time because . . .? Now that we realise 'The Torch' exists, when else have you experienced it as being on? I guess we both didn't know about 'The Torch' until today – I am wondering if there are others who *wouldn't* be surprised about the times the 'The Torch' exists?
Negotiate a mutually acceptable name for the unique outcome: What shall we call this development? Negotiate an experience-near definition for the unique outcome/counterplot Definition remains fluid and evolving		If you were to invest more in 'The Torch' and less in 'The Doom', where do you think that would get you?
Mapping of the influence/effect of the unique outcome: Explore the (potential) effects of the unique outcome/exception on the various domains of living and views of the self? Home, workplace, university, friendships, actions, emotions, physical, relationships with self and others What does the unique outcome tell you about yourself?		What could you do or think that would help you listen more to 'The Torch' and less to 'The Doom'? I agree it won't be easy as 'The Doom' has gotten so much power in the past. What seems to switch 'The Torch' on?

Regarding your hopes, dreams, aspirations and values?	So do you need to see if you can make more of those times happen? Also it might be good to think more about what flicks the on button for 'The Torch'.
Evaluation of the (potential) effects of the unique outcome:	I'm interested also in giving you some time to think about what our conversation about 'The Torch' now makes you feel about yourself.
Clients to judge (justify) whether the effects of the unique outcome/ exception/ problem-solving skills are preferred (or not):	
Is this okay with you?	
Is this a positive or negative development?	
Justifications of these evaluations:	If we think together about where the 'The Doom' and 'The Torch' come from … 'The Doom' connects to a very strong idea for you 'that Brains never recover' but 'The Torch' must resist connecting to this idea? Do you know what could be another idea that powers the 'The Torch'?
Person gives reasons why the influence/ implications of the unique outcome is preferred	
Justification elicits clients' hopes, dreams and aspirations and preferred views of themselves	How does that make you feel about "never getting better and being damaged"?
	When you think about what you just said, how does it make you feel!
History of the unique outcome:	
Drawing out a history of the unique outcome (i.e. behaviours/skills/events)	
Accepts a history already exist but has not been noticed or given credence	
Situates the unique outcome in sequence of events across time according to particular plots/themes:	

(Continued)

Narrative therapeutic focus	Areas focussed on in interview	Examples of questions used in interview
Remembering conversations, who from your past would be least surprised regarding this unique outcome? What did s/he know about you that would result in them not being surprised?		
Future implications of alternative story: Let person reflect on and determine the meaning of developments/unique outcomes Richly develop conclusions about identity if alternative story could hold ground in future		
Generate new proposals/steps for action Identify post-session tasks or rituals to anchor and reconfirm the new story Finding an audience and 'telling others' How might you put others in touch with these developments/discoveries about yourself?		So thinking about a new way of talking about what you are going through gives you a way to switch on 'The Torch'. What else could you do? Who can we tell about it, give it more airtime?
Finding an audience Definitional ceremonies Outsider-witness practices		

Name index

Subject index

Note: Page numbers in *italics* indicate figures and in **bold** indicate tables on the corresponding pages. Page numbers followed by an "n" refer to a note and the subsequent note number.